Managing Health
Care for the Elderly

Managing Health Care for the Elderly

Cynthia Polich
Marcie Parker
Deborah Chase
Margaret Hottinger

JOHN WILEY & SONS, INC.

New York • Chichester • Brisbane • Toronto • Singapore

RA
564.8
.M35
1993

This text is printed on acid-free paper.

Copyright © 1993 by John Wiley & Sons, Inc.

This publication is designed to provide accurate and authoritative information in regard to the subject matter covered. It is sold with the understanding that the publisher is not engaged in rendering legal, accounting, or other professional services. If legal advice or other expert assistance is required, the services of a competent professional person should be sought. *From a Declaration of Principles jointly adopted by a Committee of the American Bar Association and a Committee of Publishers.*

Library of Congress Cataloging in Publication Data

Managing health care for the elderly / Cynthia Polich . . . [et al.].
        p.   cm. — (Employee benefits human resources library)
    Includes index.
    ISBN 0-471-57277-2 (cloth)
    1. Aged—Medical care—United States.   I. Polich, Cynthia Longseth.   II. Series.

RA564.8.M35   1992
362.1'9897'00973—dc20   92-28511
                                                                CIP

Printed in the United States of America

10 9 8 7 6 5 4 3 2 1

Foreword

There is little question that our nation is facing a crisis in health care: Our population is increasing and aging. The development and use of new health care technologies continues to grow. Add to this the fact that many people are not receiving care appropriate to their needs in the most cost-effective way possible, and we have a formula for continued explosion of costs and utilization, as well as dissatisfaction with the "system" of providing health care.

This dilemma is even more pronounced for the elderly population. Of the nearly 35 million elderly in our country today, 1.5 million reside in nursing homes and nearly a quarter are over age 85. Health costs for these individuals exceed $160 billion, a substantial portion of which is spent for care that is both unnecessary and ineffective. Aging of the population alone will drive health care costs and utilization to ever-increasing levels. Today the elderly consume a third of all health care resources. By the year 2000, this is projected to increase to 50 percent.

Regardless of who pays for these services, this care must be managed. Ineffective management will either bankrupt the nation's economy or deny millions of elderly the care they truly need . . . and neither prospect is appealing or acceptable.

This is more than a societal problem, however. It is a personal problem for each of us. With any luck, I will be in my 80s in the 2030s, along with many of the large population group popularly known as the baby boomers. My parents will be there well before then. I want to ensure that when their time comes, and when my time comes, appropriate, necessary, cost-effective health care is available and affordable.

I want a system that is sensitive to the needs of the elderly. One that is, in the jargon of today's business, "customer-focused." I want health-care providers who understand how to care for the elderly and who do not consider *any* disability or functional impairment to be "normal aging." And if I ever have to enter a nursing home, I want to be as independent as possible in my decision making and life style. In other words, I do not want to be an elderly patient in today's health care system. I want something different, something better. And I don't believe I am the only one.

This is not unreasonably demanding, but it does require significant changes in the health and long-term care delivery system for the elderly. This book begins to lay out the direction that could be taken to meet this challenge. Unlike so many others, the authors of this book do not provide a doomsday prediction of high costs and deteriorating quality of care for the elderly. While the numbers are daunting, they should spur us on to innovation and reform rather than elicit despair and hopelessness. This book is about exploring new ideas and innovative programs to effectively manage care for the elderly. It also challenges prevailing wisdom about how to organize, finance and deliver care to the elderly and builds understanding that it is possible to create a system that manages costs while providing appropriate, quality care.

Good ideas and understanding are necessary, but not sufficient. It also takes the work and dedication of all those in the health care system to create change. United HealthCare Corporation is committed to meeting the challenge of effectively managing health and long-term care for the elderly and creating financing and delivery systems that facilitate that effort. We hope that the ideas and information presented in this book will spur others to join that effort.

WILLIAM W. MCGUIRE
Chairman and CEO
United HealthCare Corporation

September 1992

Preface

Americans are living longer than ever before. In fact, it is no longer uncommon to see active people who are in their 80s or 90s. The number of elderly (those 65 years and older) in the United States has grown over the past several decades both in size and in proportion to the general population, and will continue to grow at an even faster rate during the 21st century.

The growth of the elderly population will have a profound effect on the health care delivery system. Current resources—both in terms of workers and financing—will not be adequate to meet their needs. In addition, as the elderly live longer, the nature and complexity of their health status change, and they require different care than the current system is designed to provide.

This book examines the need for a health care management system that integrates acute and long-term care as well as social and medical services for the elderly. Such a system would alleviate much of the fragmented, inappropriate, and inefficient service delivery that occurs in the current health care system.

Chapter 1 outlines the demographics of the aging population, their health status, and their use of health and long-term care services. Chapter 2 examines the current financing system, its impact on service delivery, and the medical and institutional bias that often fails to meet the chronic care needs of the elderly. Chapter 3 defines and describes managed care and its application to an older population. Chapters 4 and 5 give an overview of managed care approaches for the elderly, for both acute and long-term care, and describe the various models currently in operation. Chapter 6 presents existing models that have integrated acute and long-term care in a managed care environment.

In Chapters 7 and 8, methods for providing more appropriate retiree- and employer-based services are examined. What businesses, corporations, employers, and employees and their families should know; what services should be provided; and who should pay for them—these are the key topics discussed. Chapter 9 describes and analyzes existing reform proposals regarding health and long-term care. Chapter 10 concludes with a vision for the future and makes recommendations for providing health and long-term care for the elderly in a cost-efficient and appropriate manner.

CYNTHIA POLICH
MARCIE PARKER
DEBORAH CHASE
MARGARET HOTTINGER

Minnetonka, Minnesota
December 1992

Acknowledgments

The authors wish to thank their friends, family, and colleagues who have supported and assisted them in completing this book. We would like to particularly acknowledge our former co-workers at InterStudy's Center for Aging and Long-Term Care whose research over four years contributed to much of the data and information presented in this book. Thanks to Laura Himes Iversen, Chuck Oberg, M.D., Suzanne Owens, Kris Korn, Judy Hale, and Laura Secord. Thanks also to Diane Cobb for preparing the manuscript.

About the Authors

Cynthia L. Polich is vice president of Managed Care for the Aged for United HealthCare Corporation. She is responsible for developing innovative programs for managing care of the elderly. Her career includes positions as President of InterStudy and with the State of Minnesota, the University of Minnesota's Center for Health Services Research, and as an independent consultant.

Ms. Polich received her bachelor of arts from the University of Texas and her master of arts from the University of Minnesota's Humphrey Institute of Public Affairs.

Marcie Parker is a manager within the Managed Care for the Aged division of United HealthCare Corporation. Her areas of research have included the financing and delivery of long-term care, HMOs and home health care, and private geriatric case management.

Ms. Parker has her master of arts degree and is currently doing work on her doctorate in family social science at the University of Minnesota.

Deborah Chase is a health policy analyst at United HealthCare Corporation where she focuses on health care reform issues involving the elderly. She received her bachelor of arts from Brown University.

Margaret Hottinger is vice president of The Long-Term Care Group, a subsidiary of United HealthCare Corporation, where she is responsible for developing managed long-term care programs. Ms. Hottinger holds a bachelor of science from William Jewell College, and is a certified public accountant.

About United HealthCare Corporation

United HealthCare Corporation has provided health care management services since 1974. The company's services include health maintenance organizations (HMOs), preferred provider organizations (PPOs), health plan management, pharmaceutical cost management, managed mental health and substance abuse services, utilization management, workers' compensation/management services, specialized provider networks, employee assistance services, Medicare and managed care programs for the aged, health care evaluation services, information systems, and administrative services.

Summary
Contents

Detailed Contents

One

Introduction—
The Shape of
America's Elderly

§ 1.1 OVERVIEW

This chapter provides a general overview of the elderly population. Current demographics and future projections are presented, and the general health care status and primary conditions of the elderly are described. This chapter also looks at trends in elderly persons' use of health and long-term care services and the effects a growing elderly population will have on the need for these services.

(a) DEMOGRAPHICS OF THE AGING POPULATION

The number of people over age 65 has increased faster than the rest of the population for several decades. Between 1950 and 1980, the number of those 65 years and older more than doubled—from 12.3 million in 1950 to 25.5 million in 1980, a 108 percent increase. The population under age 65 grew 65 percent over the same 30 years.[1] This growth is expected to continue for at least the next half-century. As shown in Figure 1.1, it is estimated that the elderly population will grow from 25.5 million in 1980 (11.3 percent of the total population)

1

Figure 1.1
The U.S. Elderly Population

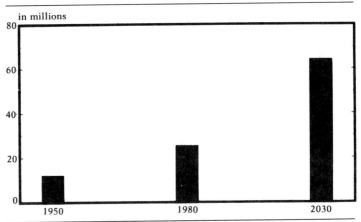

Source: National Research Council, *The Aging Population in the Twenty-First Century: Statistics for Health Policy.* Washington, DC: National Academy Press, 1988, p. 53.

to a projected 64.3 million in 2030 (21.1 percent)—a doubling of this group in 50 years.[2]

The number of the oldest old (those 85 years and older) has grown even faster than the overall elderly population—from 577,000 in 1950 to 2.2 million in 1980, a 281 percent increase—and its rate of growth will continue to escalate. It is estimated that the number of those 85 years and older will grow from 2.2 million in 1980 to 8.8 million in 2030 (see Figure 1.2). The number is projected to reach 16.1 million in 2050. The population over age 85 represented 1 percent of the total

Figure 1.2
The Oldest Old (85+) as a Portion of the Total Elderly (65+)

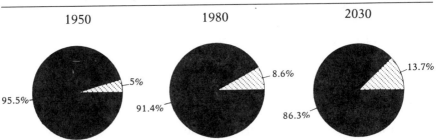

Source: National Research Council, *The Aging Population in the Twenty-First Century: Statistics for Health Policy.* Washington, DC: National Academy Press, 1988, p. 53.

population in 1980 and 9 percent of the elderly. By 2050, projections forecast that this group will increase to 5 percent of the total population and 24 percent of the elderly.[3]

This growth in the elderly population is attributable primarily to increased life expectancy. Most of the decrease in mortality among the elderly in the past decade has resulted from the substantial decline in the number of deaths from heart disease and cerebrovascular disease. Medical technology and treatment have improved, and many of the elderly can more easily obtain timely medical care.

The accuracy of these population growth rates is somewhat difficult to predict because of unknowns such as potential improvements in treatments for or prevention of acute and chronic conditions. For example, although the death rate from heart disease and cerebrovascular disease has declined, the death rate from cancer, particularly at older ages, continues to rise.[4] If a cure, prevention, or more effective treatment for cancer is found, the elderly population could grow at faster rates than are currently projected.

(b)   GENDER AND INFORMAL SUPPORTS

Within the elderly population, there are significantly more women than men, because of higher death rates for males and improvements in mortality rates for females. In 1980, there were 10.2 million elderly men aged 65 years and older, and 15.2 million elderly women, a ratio of 68 men to 100 women.[5] This ratio is expected to remain relatively stable over the next few decades. Among the oldest old, there are even fewer men than women, and this disparity is expected to increase. In 1980, there were 80 males per 100 females for those ages 65 to 74, and 44 males per 100 females for those aged 85 years and older. For the latter age group, the ratio is expected to fall to 36 men per 100 women by the year 2020.[6]

As with overall growth rates, the accuracy of future male-to-female ratios may also be difficult to predict. For example, men are much more likely to die from many types of cancer than women. They are five times more likely to die from lung cancer than women.[7] Therefore, cancer discoveries could dramatically affect gender differences in life expectancy.

Because there are so many more elderly women than men, there are and will continue to be many more women living alone. In 1983, half of all women 75 and older lived alone.[8] This statistic is significant because spouses are usually the first to provide care for elderly persons who are disabled or chronically ill.

(c) INCOME AND USE OF SERVICES

Although the number living in poverty has dropped substantially since the 1960s, many elderly persons, particularly among women and minorities, are close to or below the poverty line. In 1984, 5.9 million elderly lived below or near the poverty line. As Table 1.1 indicates, 46 percent of those 65 and older have income levels below $10,000, compared to 17 percent of those ages 15 to 64.[9]

In 1982, the median income for White men ages 65 to 69 was $11,900, and that of White women in the same age group was $5,700; the median income, in the same age group, of Black men was $5,900, and that of Black women was $3,900.[10]

Income level has been related to health status and level of disability as well as to the use and choice of long-term care services for the elderly. Those with low incomes have higher rates of disability brought on by chronic illness. They are less likely to be able to sustain themselves in the community, and thus are more likely to be institutionalized.[11]

(d) GEOGRAPHIC DISTRIBUTION AND LONG-TERM CARE NEEDS

As of 1980, America's elderly tended to be concentrated in eight states: California, Florida, Illinois, Michigan, New York, Ohio, Pennsylvania, and Texas. In 1980, Florida had the highest concentration of elderly— 17.3 percent of the state's total population. There are significant differences in the increase of the elderly by region. As Table 1.2 indicates, the elderly population is expected to increase 60 percent between 1980 and 2000 in the South and West regions of the country, compared to 12 percent in the Northeast and 16 percent in the North Central regions.[12]

Table 1.1
Comparison of Population Groups,
by Income Level and Age

Income Level	Ages 15 to 64	Age 65 and Older
$20,000 and up	58.9%	26.6%
$15,000 to 20,000	11.8	12.6
$10,000 to 15,000	11.6	18.2
Under $10,000	17.7	42.6

Source: William Oriol, *The Complex Cube of Long Term Care.* Washington, DC: American Health Planning Association, 1985, p. 44.

Table 1.2
Projected Growth in the Population
65 and Older (in thousands)

	1980	2000	Percent Change
Total	25,544	35,036	37.2
Northeast	6,072	6,828	12.4
North Central	6,691	7,763	16.0
South	8,484	13,582	60.1
West	4,298	6,864	59.7

Source: Charlene Harrington, Robert J. Newcomer, Carroll L. Estes, & Associates, *Long Term Care for the Elderly: Public Policy Issues.* Beverly Hills, CA: Sage Publications, Inc., 1985, p. 45.

This increase will have different effects on the demand for health and long-term care services in these regions. For example, in the Northeast and North Central regions, the number of nursing-home beds needed will escalate by 44 percent. In the South and West, the number of nursing-home beds needed will more than double.[13]

§ 1.2 HEALTH CARE STATUS AND CONDITION OF THE ELDERLY

As the demographic statistics reflect, the elderly are not a homogeneous group. Not only do they vary by age, gender, and income, but they also vary greatly in terms of health status, severity of illness, types of disabling conditions, need for acute and long-term care services, and availability of support systems.

(a) CARING FOR THOSE 65 YEARS AND OLDER

Caring for the elderly is not the same as simply caring for an older version of a younger person.[14] Health care needs can vary tremendously with age. For instance, many diseases have different symptoms in the elderly than they do in younger people, and an elderly person's condition can be much more complex.[15] Because the elderly often have a number of diseases or conditions, these can interact in ways that produce adverse effects not found in younger adults who have fewer ongoing conditions. Younger persons also seem to be able to ward off and minimize the duration of disease better than older persons. Changes in metabolism, immune response, and organ function, and the cumulative effects of multiple chronic conditions and diseases can negatively affect the makeup and course of disease in an older person. The elderly are also more likely to have multiple diseases, which can offset the normal course of any one particular condition, making treatments and cures all the more difficult. Lung cancer, breast cancer, isolated systolic hypertension, and diabetes are all harder to manage and treat in older persons.[16] The progress of disease in the elderly is also affected by overall condition. Nutrition, level of functional impairment, availability of social supports, economic condition, and environment can all play an interrelated role in the severity and progression of conditions or diseases. Health and functional status and quality of life are closely interrelated in the care of the elderly.

(b) PREVALENCE OF CHRONIC CONDITIONS

Almost all the reduction in health and functional status associated with increasing age originates from chronic rather than acute conditions. Of the elderly living in the community, approximately 50 percent of women and 35 percent of men have arthritis; 25 and 32 percent, respectively, have a hearing impairment; 43 and 31 percent have hypertension; and 28 and 26 percent have a heart condition.[17] The numbers are expected to increase substantially as the aging population grows. Studies estimate that the number of those with arthritis but not in nursing homes will increase from 11 million in 1979 to 14 million in 2000; those with hypertension, from 10 million to 13 million; and those with hearing impairments, from 7 million to 9 million.[18] Approximately 80 percent of the elderly report at least one chronic condition; on average, each elderly individual has three chronic conditions. These conditions often overlap, causing an elderly person to be faced with more than one impairment, many of which, singly or in combination, limit the activities of daily living. Activities of daily living are defined as the ability to perform the most basic functions, such as eating, bathing, dressing, and walking.

In 1980, the elderly experienced, on average, 39.2 days per year when they were restricted in their activities of daily living and 13.8 days in which they were bedridden. Eighty percent of these restricted days were related to chronic conditions.[19] Because the existence of chronic disease is so often linked to a diminished ability to carry out activities of daily living, these conditions can lead to increased functional impairment and dependency.[20]

(c) ASSISTANCE WITH ACTIVITIES OF DAILY LIVING

The results of several national surveys indicate that many of the elderly (ranging from 37 to 58 percent) report limited or complete inability to carry out activities of daily living.[21] The percentage of those needing such assistance increases dramatically with age. Approximately 10 percent of individuals ages 65 to 74 require assistance with activities of daily living; 50 percent require such assistance by age 85.[22, 23] Alzheimer's disease is estimated to increase ten- to twentyfold between the ages of 60 and 80, with a resulting loss of ability to carry out activities of daily living.[24]

The growing number of elderly, particularly the oldest old, will mean a major increase in the number of people with chronic conditions or limited functional ability, and therefore a growing number who require health and long-term care services. Based on projected growth rates for the elderly, it can be expected that, in 2030, approximately 9.5 million elderly will be impaired.

The elderly population is growing, and the numbers of those ages 85 and older are growing the fastest. The majority of the elderly are women. Many live alone, and many are poor. Because functional impairment is so common among the elderly, especially among the oldest old, increasing numbers of people will require help carrying out activities of daily living. As a result, many more people in the country will need care. Predominantly, they will need social support and help with basic functioning—a different type of care than our current health care system typically provides. Most of our health care resources—staffing, facilities, and funding—are geared toward institutional and acute care, not community-based care for chronic conditions.

§ 1.3 THE USE OF HEALTH AND LONG-TERM CARE SERVICES

Because of the elderly population's health status, described above, they use more health and long-term care services than younger individuals do. Compared to those under the age of 65, the elderly see a physician more often each year, have more and longer hospital stays, and greater use of long-term care services. The growth of the elderly population will result in ever increasing use of health care services.

(a) PHYSICIAN CARE

The elderly visit physicians more often than do those under age 65. People 65 years and older see a physician an average of 6.3 times per year, compared to 5.2 times per person for those ages 45 to 64, and 4.5 times per person for those ages 17 to 44.[25] As the elderly population continues to grow, overall visits to physicians will increase. Estimates foresee that total physician visits by the elderly will increase from 145 million in 1977 to 186 million in 2000.[26]

The portion of ambulatory medical practice devoted to caring for the elderly is substantial for many specialists. In 1985, almost half of all ambulatory visits to cardiologists were made by elderly persons. As Table 1.3 indicates, all specialists have seen an increase in the portion of their practice related to caring for the elderly.[27]

The need for physicians to care for the elderly will continue to increase as the elderly population grows. Because of the special health care needs of the elderly, they require physicians specially trained to address their needs. To adequately care for an older person, a physician

Table 1.3
Percentage of Total Ambulatory Visits to Various Medical Specialties by Persons 65 Years of Age and Over

	1978	1981	1985
All specialties	16.1	18.4	20.1
General practice/ Family practice	17.1	19.3	19.6
Internal medicine	31.1	34.4	39.2
Cardiology	39.1	46.1	47.2
Ophthalmology	30.0	39.3	43.8
Urology	29.9	37.6	39.6
General surgery	21.9	20.1	27.2
Neurology	13.2	17.7	21.0
Dermatology	12.2	13.4	18.3
Otolaryngology	14.1	16.9	17.0
Orthopedic surgery	10.9	13.7	13.9
Psychiatry	4.5	4.6	6.5
Obstetrics/Gynecology	2.2	2.6	3.3
Other	5.0	6.0	10.2

Source: National Ambulatory Medical Care Survey, National Center for Health Statistics, 1985.

should be aware of such unique problems as the interrelatedness of multiple conditions, the slower rate of rehabilitation, and the frequency of mental health needs. The overall physician supply is expected to be adequate in the future, but it is widely believed that there is a shortage of physicians trained in geriatrics and that this shortage will only intensify as the elderly population increases.

(b) HOSPITAL CARE

Hospital use increases with age. At present, the elderly use four times more days of hospital care each year than those under age 65,[28] and the use of hospital days is increasing as the aging population grows. Persons 65 years and older spent a total of 60 million days in the hospital in 1965; they had 105 million hospital days in 1980.[29] As the population continues to age, these figures will only grow more rapidly. By 2000, the elderly are expected to spend 273 million days in the hospital annually.[30]

As of 1986, the average national rate of days of hospital care for those 65 years and older was 3,120.8 per 1,000 population; the average rate of patients discharged was 367.3 per 1,000 population, and the average length of stay was 8.5 days. As Table 1.4 indicates, Nebraska has the highest rate of days of care (3,227), the highest discharge rate (377), and a length of stay of 8.6 days; Alaska's figures are the lowest: 2,891 days of care, 345.9 discharge rate, and an average length of stay of 8.4 days.[31]

(c) INFORMAL LONG-TERM CARE

Long-term care needs also increase with age. Frailty and functional impairment often accompany old age and are particularly prevalent among the very old. Many of the disabled or chronically ill elderly require assistance with activities of daily living (eating, bathing, dressing, toileting, and walking). The elderly, therefore, become increasingly dependent on some type of care provider to help them perform their activities of daily living. Friends and family are reported to be the major sources of long-term care for the elderly in the United States. Home health services, day care, transportation, and meal services are often provided through the unpaid, voluntary aid of friends and family. Such help is often referred to as informal support. Spouses are usually the first to provide informal support; other providers are close family members, friends, and neighbors. Informal

Table 1.4
Rate of Days of Care and Rate of Patients Discharged, Elderly Patients in Short-Stay Hospitals, by State: United States, 1986

State	Rate of Days of Care for Those 65 Years of Age and Over (per 1,000 population) Total	Rate of Patients Discharged for Those 65 Years of Age and Over (per 1,000 population) Total
United States	3,120.8	367.3
Alabama	3,105.3	365.8
Alaska	2,891.2	345.9
Arizona	3,050.1	360.7
Arkansas	3,135.0	368.6
California	3,105.2	365.8
Colorado	3,117.2	367.0
Connecticut	3,115.5	366.8
Delaware	3,074.9	363.0
District of Columbia	3,107.3	366.0
Florida	3,111.9	366.5
Georgia	3,078.9	363.4
Hawaii	3,035.7	359.4
Idaho	3,099.2	365.3
Illinois	3,124.0	367.6
Indiana	3,130.8	368.2
Iowa	3,211.2	375.7
Kansas	3,206.8	375.3
Kentucky	3,130.5	368.2
Louisiana	3,090.5	364.5
Maine	3,167.1	371.6
Maryland	3,078.7	363.4
Massachusetts	3,153.8	370.4
Michigan	3,099.5	365.3
Minnesota	3,196.8	374.4
Mississippi	3,130.7	368.2
Missouri	3,177.9	372.6
Montana	3,104.6	365.8
Nebraska	3,227.4	377.2
Nevada	2,938.3	350.3
New Hampshire	3,141.3	369.2
New Jersey	3,093.5	364.7
New Mexico	3,072.1	362.7
New York	3,140.9	369.2
North Carolina	3,071.0	362.6

Table 1.4 *(Continued)*

State	Rate of Days of Care for Those 65 Years of Age and Over (per 1,000 population) Total	Rate of Patients Discharged for Those 65 Years of Age and Over (per 1,000 population) Total
North Dakota	3,183.9	373.2
Ohio	3,111.6	366.4
Oklahoma	3,166.4	371.5
Oregon	3,117.0	366.9
Pennsylvania	3,100.3	365.4
Rhode Island	3,136.4	368.7
South Carolina	3,033.3	359.1
South Dakota	3,207.1	375.3
Tennessee	3,116.3	366.9
Texas	3,120.0	367.2
Utah	3,098.2	365.2
Vermont	3,173.5	372.2
Virginia	3,076.7	363.2
Washington	3,102.7	365.6
West Virginia	3,112.6	366.5
Wisconsin	3,164.3	371.3
Wyoming	3,106.8	366.0

Source: National Center for Health Statistics, *The National Hospital Discharge Survey,* 1986.

caregivers provide approximately 80 to 90 percent of the help needed by the elderly to perform activities of daily living. In fact, it is estimated that 80 percent of the noninstitutionalized, disabled elderly receive all needed services from informal supports.[32] The need for formal long-term care services usually only occurs after the informal caregivers are dead or incapacitated themselves.

As the elderly population increases in size and age, more women will be living without spouses, many of their children will be elderly and disabled themselves, and there will be fewer friends alive or able to provide care. Studies also report a tendency for parents not to have as many children and for children to live farther away, leaving fewer people available to provide care. As a result, fewer informal long-term care supports will be available for the elderly, especially the oldest old, who are usually the most functionally dependent.

(d)　FORMAL LONG-TERM CARE

Several factors may be used to predict the need for formal long-term care. Living alone, loss of functional independence, ability to carry out activities of daily living, and ability to pay for home care are prime indicators of the need for formal long-term care. Studies show that a person who requires assistance going to the bathroom or eating is 16 times more likely to live in a nursing home than the average person 65 years or older.[33] Approximately 20 percent of those living in nursing homes do not have living relatives, and more than 85 percent have no living spouse.[34]

Almost every person in a nursing home has at least one impairment, and the average is four impairments per resident.[35] The most recent and comprehensive survey of nursing home residents, the 1977 National Nursing Home Survey, identified the following as the leading primary diagnoses for nursing home patients:

- Circulatory disease (44 percent);
- Mental disorders (16 percent);
- Diabetes (6 percent);
- Arthritis and related diseases (5 percent);
- Hip and other fractures (3 percent).[36]

What most of these people need is chiefly support in carrying out activities of daily living.

The elderly are the predominant consumers of long-term care, and the need for this care tends to increase with age. Persons 75 years and older use 14 times more long-term care services per capita than those ages 65 to 69,[37] and nursing homes are currently the primary means of providing such services to the elderly. Nursing-home residents are primarily 85 years and older. In 1985, 45.2 percent of nursing-home residents were 85 years and older, compared to 38.7 percent ages 75 to 84 and 16.1 percent ages 65 to 74.[38] With the growing population 85 years and older, it can be expected that the need for nursing-home care will greatly increase in future years.

As mentioned earlier, nursing homes are already feeling the strain. Nationwide, the need for nursing-home beds is expected to increase significantly. In 1989, approximately 1.4 million elderly lived in nursing homes—2 percent (295,000) of those between ages 65 and 74, 7 percent (627,000) of those between ages 75 and 84, and 16 percent (489,000) of those over age 85.[39] Furthermore, one out of four women 85 and older lived in a nursing home compared to one in seven men.[40] There are expected to be 2 million nursing-home residents by 2000 and 5.2 million by 2040.[41] However, in 1985, the National Center for Health Statistics estimated there were 19,100 nursing homes with 1.6 million nursing-home beds.[42]

Given the increasing demand and limited availability of nursing-home beds, many more nursing homes will have to be built, or we will have to find alternative approaches for meeting the long-term care needs of the elderly. The total number of *new* nursing-home beds needed by 2000 is expected to reach 1.2 million, or nearly double the 1980 in-use total.[43]

Nursing-home staffing needs are also expected to escalate in the next several years. The Health Resources and Services Administration predicts that, by 2000, nursing homes will need 260,000 full-time equivalent (FTE) registered nurses and 300,000 other FTE licensed nursing personnel—approximately three times the staffing levels present in 1984. Other estimates call for even more nursing staff. An expert panel of nurses and representatives of several nursing and health care service associations reported, in the *Fifth Report to the President and Congress on the Status of Health Personnel in the United States,* a need for 838,000 FTE registered nurses, 339,000 other licensed nurses, and approximately 1 million nursing aides by 2000.[44] Will we be able to meet the staffing needs generated by an increasing elderly population, especially if their care is so heavily dependent on acute care, physicians' services, and nursing-home residency? Nursing shortages are already common, and there are no indications that the number of physicians trained in geriatrics will soon rise. Even if sufficient financing were available, it is uncertain whether there would be adequate staff to meet the need.

In the next 50 years, the elderly population will experience unprecedented growth. Overall, the number of those 65 years and older will increase greatly, and the number of those 85 years and older will grow in absolute size as well as in proportion to the total elderly population. The elderly, especially the oldest old, have more chronic conditions and limitations in performing the activities of daily living and so use significantly more health and long-term care services than the general population. Therefore, the expected growth of the elderly population, particularly the oldest old, will put increasing demands on health care services, which will increase overall health care costs. Chapter 2 discusses whether we will have the capacity or funds to provide this care.

NOTES

[1] National Research Council. *The Aging Population in the Twenty-First Century: Statistics for Health Policy* (p. 53). Washington, DC: National Academy Press, 1988.

[2] *Id.* at 54.

[3] *Id.* at 52, 54.

[4] Davis, K., and Rowland, D. *Medicare Policy: New Directions for Health Policy and Long-Term Care* (pp. 12–14). Baltimore: The Johns Hopkins University Press, 1986.

[5] National Research Council, note 1, at 54.

[6] *Id.* at 55.

[7] Harrington, C., Newcomer, R.J., Estes, C.L., and Associates. *Long Term Care of the Elderly: Public Policy Issues* (p. 45). Beverly Hills, CA: Sage Publications, Inc., 1985.

[8] Oriol, W. *The Complex Cube of Long Term Care* (p. 44). Washington, DC: American Health Planning Association, 1985.

[9] *Id.* at 48.

[10] *Id.* at 49; cited by U.S. Senate Special Committee on Aging.

[11] Hale, J. "Long Term Care: What Is It? Who Needs It? Who Uses It?" In *InterStudy's Long-Term Care Expansion Program: Issue Papers, Vol. II* (p. 35). Excelsior, MN: InterStudy, 1988.

[12] Harrington et al., note 7, at 55–56.

[13] National Research Council, note 1, at 56.

[14] *Id.* at 66.

[15] *Id.* at 72.

[16] *Ibid.*

[17] Hale, note 11, at 28–29.

[18] Davis and Rowland, note 4, at 17–21.

[19] *Ibid.*

[20] National Research Council, note 1, at 72.

[21] Davis and Rowland, note 4, at 17–21.

[22] *InterStudy's Long-Term Care Expansion Program: A Proposal for Reform* (p. 16). Excelsior, MN: InterStudy, 1988.

[23] Parker, M., and Polich, C.L. *The Provision of Home Health Care Services Through Health Maintenance Organizations* (p. 16). Excelsior, MN: InterStudy, 1988.

[24] Oriol, note 8, at 124.

[25] Davis and Rowland, note 4, at 22–23.

[26] *Ibid.*

[27] National Institute on Aging. *Personnel for Health Needs of the Elderly Through the Year 2020* (pp. 37–37A). Bethesda, MD: U.S. Department of Health and Human Services, 1987.

[28] Davis and Rowland, note 4, at 22–23.

[29] *Ibid.*

[30] *Id.* at 26.

[31] Furner, S.E., Brody, J.A., Levy, P.S., Mermelstein, R., Miles, T., Miller, B., Prohaska, T., Selker, L.G., Selma, T., Blesch, K.S., and Kernis, J. *Synthetic Estimation of State Health Characteristics for the Population 65 Years of Age and Over* (pp. 4–5). Chicago: University of Illinois, School of Public Health, 1992.

[32] Parker, M., and Iversen, L.H. "Informal Caregiving: Its Importance for Long-Term Care." In *InterStudy's Long-Term Care Expansion Program: Issue Papers, Vol. II* (p. 99). Excelsior, MN: InterStudy, 1988.

[33] Davis and Rowland, note 4, at 28.

[34] *Id.* at 17–21.

[35] *Id.* at 28.

[36] Hale, note 11, at 27.

[37] Oriol, note 8, at 57.

[38] Hale, note 11, at 7.

[39] Polich, C., Iversen, L.H., and Owens, S. "Rethinking Long-Term Care." *Compensation & Benefits Management* (Summer 1989): 276.

[40] Hale, note 11, at 8.

[41] *Id.* at 28–29.

[42] *Id.* at 2.

[43] *Id.* at 28–29.

[44] National Institute on Aging. *Personnel for Health Needs of the Elderly Through the Year 2020* (p. 113). Bethesda, MD: U.S. Department of Health and Human Services, 1987.

Two

Financing and Delivery of Health Care

§ 2.1 INTRODUCTION

Paying for elderly persons' health care is a constantly increasing financial strain. The strain is felt by society in general, but it is particularly heavy for providers, who receive low reimbursement under Medicare, and for the elderly, who must pay high out-of-pocket costs. As shown in Chapter 1, the projected growth in the older population over the next 50 years is expected to have a huge impact on health care costs. The elderly, who are more frail than the general population, use more health care resources—staffing, dollars, and facilities—than any other age group.

Because caring for the elderly can be extremely expensive, policymakers have increasingly focused their attention on how to contain the costs of such care. While not without some merit, the focused efforts to contain costs have not been as successful as expected. The reason lies in the architecture of the health care financing and delivery system for the elderly. In designing a plan of care for elderly patients, attention is often given to what will be covered by which payer, not what will be the best type, amount, and setting of care for the individual.

Financing of health care for the elderly is fragmented, and there is little coordination among funding sources and providers. In addition, the funding emphasis, particularly in the public sector, is geared toward acute and institutional care. The result has been a severely fragmented system that fails to appropriately meet the complex and unique needs of the elderly.

This chapter examines the costs of caring for the elderly, both now and in the future; the payers of this care; the fragmentation of services delivered to the elderly; and why inappropriate and inefficient services are often provided.

§ 2.2 HEALTH CARE EXPENDITURES

The elderly use more health care than any other age group. Although they made up only 12 percent of the overall population in the late 1980s, they accounted for approximately 36 percent of the nation's personal health care expenditures. The average per-capita amount spent on health care for all ages was $1,776; for those 65 and older, it was $5,360. As shown in Figure 2.1, in 1987, total personal health care

Figure 2.1
Portion of Total Health Care Costs (in billions)
Spent on the Elderly: 1987

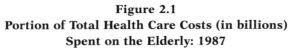

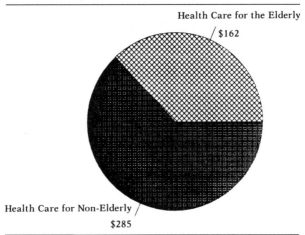

Health Care for the Elderly
/ $162

Health Care for Non-Elderly /
$285

Source: Daniel R. Waldo, Sally T. Sunnefeld, David R. McKusick, and Ross H. Amett III. "Health Care Expenditures by Age Group, 1977 and 1987." *Health Care Financing Review* (Summer 1989): 111.

spending reached $447 billion. Of this total, $162 billion was spent caring for the elderly.[1] Figure 2.2 shows the distribution of expenditures for such health care, and Table 2.1 indicates the high rate of elderly health costs versus those of the total population.

(a) ACUTE CARE

Of the $162 billion spent on health care for the elderly in 1987, $101.4 billion (62 percent) went toward acute care, including hospital and physician care. For both these services, Medicare was by far the largest payer. In 1987, hospital expenditures for the elderly came to $67.9 billion, of which 14.8 percent was paid privately, 69.6 percent was paid by Medicare, 4.8 percent by Medicaid, and 10.7 percent by other government programs (see Figure 2.3). In 1987, physician services for the elderly totaled $33.5 billion, of which 35.5 percent was paid privately, 60.6 percent was paid by Medicare, 1.5 percent by Medicaid, and 2.4 percent by other government programs (see Figure 2.4).[2]

(b) LONG-TERM CARE

Long-term care includes health, social, housing, transportation, and other supportive services that help people with physical, mental, or

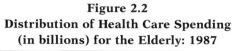

Figure 2.2
Distribution of Health Care Spending
(in billions) for the Elderly: 1987

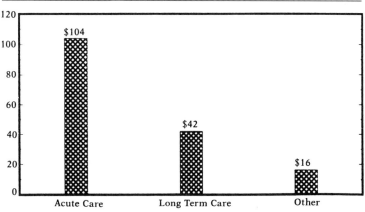

Source: Daniel R. Waldo, Sally T. Sunnefeld, David R. McKusick, and Ross H. Amett III. "Health Care Expenditures by Age Group, 1977 and 1987." *Health Care Financing Review* (Summer 1989).

Table 2.1
Personal Health Care Expenditures by Age, Source of Funds, and Type of Service: United States, 1987

Type of Service	All Ages					65 Years and Older				
	All Sources	Private	Public			All Sources	Private	Public		
			Total	Medicare	Medicaid			Total	Medicare	Medicaid
Aggregate Amount (billions)										
Personal health care	$447.0	$271.8	$175.3	$81.2	$49.4	$162.0	$60.6	$101.5	$72.2	$19.5
Hospital care	194.7	92.6	102.2	53.3	17.8	67.9	10.1	57.9	47.3	3.3
Physician services	102.7	70.9	31.8	22.3	4.4	33.5	11.9	21.6	20.3	0.5
Nursing-home care	40.6	20.6	19.9	0.6	17.8	32.8	19.2	13.6	0.6	11.9
Other care	109.0	87.6	21.4	5.1	9.4	27.8	19.5	8.3	4.1	3.7
Per-Capita Amount										
Personal health care	$1,776	$1,079	$896	$323	$196	$5,360	$2,004	$3,356	$2,390	$844
Hospital care	773	368	406	212	71	2,248	333	1,915	1,566	110
Physician services	408	282	126	89	18	1,107	393	714	671	17
Nursing-home care	16	82	79	2	71	1,085	634	452	19	395
Other care	433	348	85	20	37	920	644	276	135	123

Source: Health Care Financing Administration, Office of the Actuary, Data from the Office of National Cost Estimates. *Health Care Financing Review* (Summer 1989): 116–117.

Figure 2.3
Payers of Hospital Care for the Elderly: 1987

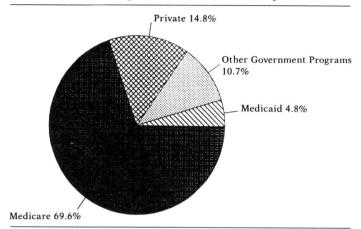

Private 14.8%

Other Government Programs
10.7%

Medicaid 4.8%

Medicare 69.6%

Source: Daniel R. Waldo, Sally T. Sunnefeld, David R. McKusick, and
Ross H. Amett III. "Health Care Expenditures by Age Group, 1977 and
1987." *Health Care Financing Review* (Summer 1989): 117.

Figure 2.4
Payers of Physician Services for the Elderly: 1987

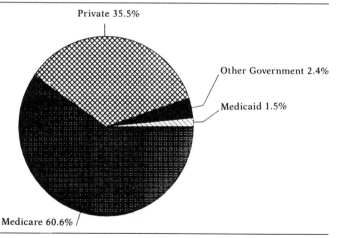

Private 35.5%

Other Government 2.4%

Medicaid 1.5%

Medicare 60.6%

Source: Daniel R. Waldo, Sally T. Sunnefeld, David R. McKusick,
and Ross H. Amett III. "Health Care Expenditures by Age Group,
1977 and 1987." *Health Care Financing Review* (Summer 1989): 117.

cognitive limitations that constrain their ability to live independently.[3] Like acute care costs, long-term care costs for the elderly are increasing rapidly: they totaled $42 billion in 1988—almost 9 percent of total health care expenditures that year—and are expected to reach approximately $120 billion by 2018 (in constant 1987 dollars). The majority of long-term care for the elderly is provided by family and friends. However, when formal long-term care is utilized, most of the funding goes toward nursing-home care.

In 1987, nursing-home care for the elderly totaled $32.8 billion, 20.2 percent of the elderly's total health care expenditures (see Figure 2.5). Of this amount, 57 percent was paid privately (excluding private long-term care insurance), 36.3 percent by Medicaid, 3.4 percent by other government programs, 1.8 percent by Medicare, and 1 to 2 percent by private long-term care insurance (Figure 2.6).[4] Nursing-home costs have been rising steadily at an annual rate of about 10.5 percent—a rate much faster than inflation. From 1988 to 2018, total nursing-home costs are expected to grow from $33 billion to $98.1 billion.

Nursing-home care is extremely expensive for individuals: a year in a nursing home now costs, on average, between $20,000 and $30,000; in some areas of the Northeast, the cost may be $50,000 a year. The average charge per day in nursing-home facilities was $86 in 1990, more than double the 1980 charge.[5] Home health care costs are also expected to increase. Home health care refers to services that provide assistance

Figure 2.5
Nursing-Home Care as a Portion of Total Health
Expenditures for the Elderly: 1987

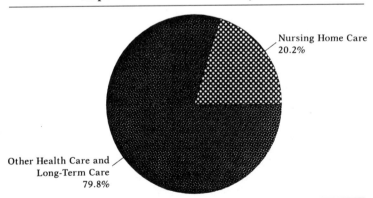

Source: Daniel R. Waldo, Sally T. Sunnefeld, David R. McKusick, and Ross H. Amett III. "Health Care Expenditures by Age Group, 1977 and 1987." *Health Care Financing Review* (Summer 1989): 117.

Figure 2.6
Payers of Nursing-Home Care for the Elderly: 1987

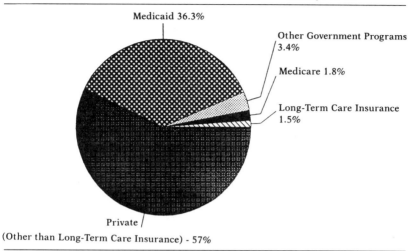

Medicaid 36.3%

Other Government Programs
3.4%

Medicare 1.8%

Long-Term Care Insurance
1.5%

Private
(Other than Long-Term Care Insurance) - 57%

Source: Daniel R. Waldo, Sally T. Sunnefeld, David R. McKusick, and Ross H. Amett III. "Health Care Expenditures by Age Group, 1977 and 1987." *Health Care Financing Review* (Summer 1989): 117.

to an individual in the home. Services can include medically oriented assistance, skilled nursing, personal care assistance (help with bathing, eating, and toileting), or housekeeping.[6] Costs for home health care are expected to rise from $8.6 billion in 1988 to $22 billion in 2018,[7] and the number of home care users is expected to increase from approximately 4 million in 1990 to 6.4 million in 2020.[8] This increase is due partly to the fact that federal funding policies have expanded slightly to include somewhat more coverage of home health care services. In 1986, the average charge per visit for home health care agencies under Medicare was $57.48.[9]

Services to the elderly may also be provided in the community, through senior centers, transportation, meals provided in the home or at congregate locations, adult day care, and visits from nurses or health aides. In 1990, about 1.5 million impaired older persons used community services at least once.[10] The Older Americans Act (OAA) funds a large amount of this care. In 1987, OAA provided $348 million in congregate meal services, $270 million for supported services and senior centers, and $74 million for home-delivered food services.[11]

Medicaid also supports community services. Under a special Medicaid waiver program, states can offer homemaker assistance, home health aid, personal care, adult day care, rehabilitation, and respite care to the poor elderly. As of 1986, 46 states were participating in the program; the cost of the program was $295 million in 1985.[12]

Like all long-term care, Medicaid and private, out-of-pocket payments are the chief financiers of community-based care. In adult day care programs, for example, funding sources include Medicaid, participant fees, the Older Americans Act, the Social Security Block Grant, Medicare, and private donations. However, only 2.4 percent of centers report receiving any Medicare funds, and about half of all contributions come from participants and Medicaid.[13]

§ 2.3   FUNDING SOURCES AND COVERED SERVICES

As we have seen, health care costs for the elderly are covered by several very different funding sources. In 1987, of the total health care expenditures for the elderly, 45 percent were paid by Medicare, 37 percent by private payments (out-of-pocket payments and some private insurance), 12 percent by Medicaid, and 6 percent by other government programs, primarily the Department of Veterans Affairs (see Figure 2.7).[14]

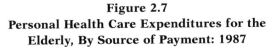

Figure 2.7
**Personal Health Care Expenditures for the
Elderly, By Source of Payment: 1987**

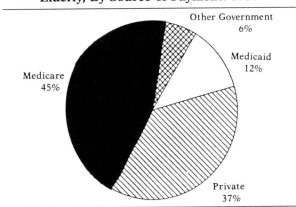

Source: Daniel R. Waldo, Sally T. Sunnefeld, David R. McKusick, and Ross H. Amett III. "Health Care Expenditures by Age Group, 1977 and 1987." *Health Care Financing Review* (Summer 1989): 117.

(a) MEDICARE

Medicare is funded entirely by federal funds, through payroll taxes on employed individuals, and is designed to protect those age 65 and older from the huge and unpredictable costs of medical care. Anyone receiving social security or railroad retirement benefits is also entitled to receive Medicare coverage. Approximately 95 percent of the elderly are covered by Medicare.[15]

Medicare is divided into two parts. Part A, which is financed through the mandatory hospital insurance (HI) payroll tax, pays for inpatient hospital services, posthospital skilled nursing services, home health care services, and hospice care. Participants must share the costs through deductibles and coinsurance. As Table 2.2 indicates, in 1992, the deductible for inpatient care was $652 for the first 60 days of care. For skilled nursing facilities (SNF), there was no deductible for the first 20 days; the charge was $81.50 per day for days 21 through 100.

Part B, the supplementary medical insurance (SMI) program, is voluntary and is paid for by participant premiums and general federal revenues. General federal revenues cover 72 percent of Part B costs, premiums cover 24.7 percent, and 3.4 percent come from interest and other income.[16] SMI covers physician services, outpatient hospital services and therapy, related physician supplies, and some home health care. The deductible for Part B was $100 in 1992, and the premium was $31.80 (see Table 2.2).

Currently, under Medicare Part B, the consumer pays coinsurance for each service provided. Medicare pays the provider 80 percent of a predetermined allowable charge. (In January 1992, Medicare, under Congressional mandate, implemented a new fee schedule that set new physician payment rates based on the time, skill, and intensity of the service as opposed to the previous system, which paid physicians based on an approved "reasonable" charge.) The patient is required to pay the other 20 percent either directly, through supplemental or Medigap insurance, or through Medicaid, if the patient is poor. In most states, where physicians are permitted to bill the patient more than the Medicare charge, the patient pays larger out-of-pocket fees. As of 1992, physicians were allowed to charge the patient up to 120 percent of the fee set by Medicare. This maximum allowable charge (MAC) will drop to 115 percent in 1993.

Medicare does not cover prescription or over-the-counter drugs, preventive services, dental care, routine eye exams, eyeglasses, hearing

Table 2.2
Medicare Allowances, 1986–1992

Terms of Medicare	1986	1987	1988	1989	1990	1991	1992
Inpatient Care (Part A)							
1–60 days	$492 Ded*	$520 Ded	$540 Ded	$560 Ded/year	$592 Ded	$628 Ded	$652 Ded
61–90 days	$123/day	$130/day	$135/day	Unlimited hospital	$148/day	$157/day	$163/day
91–150 days**	$246/day	$260/day	$270/day	days	$296/day	$314/day	$326/day
SNF Care							
First 20 days	No charge	No charge	No charge	$25.50 daily for first 8 days***	No charge	No charge	No charge
21–100 days	$61.50/day	$65/day	$67.50/day		$74/day	$78.50/day	$81.50/day
Outpatient Care (Part B)							
Deductible	$75	$75	$75	$75	$75	$100	$100
Coinsurance	80/20%	80/20%	80/20%	80/20%	80/20%	80/20%	80/20%
Medicare Beneficiaries (Part B monthly premium)	$15.50	$17.90	$24.80	$31.90	$28.60	$29.90	$31.80

* Ded = Deductible.
** 60 lifetime reserve days (nonrenewable).
***During 1989, a Medicare beneficiary had 150 days of SNF care each calendar year.
Source: Health Care Financing Administration, Office of the Actuary, 1992.

aids, or long-term institutional services, as many Americans incorrectly assume.[17]

Medicare pays primarily for hospital and physician care. In 1990, Medicare expenditures for personal health care benefits totaled $108.9 billion, an 8.6 percent increase over 1989. Of this amount, $68.3 billion was spent on hospital care (63 percent of all Medicare benefits and a 9.9 percent increase over 1989), $30.0 billion on physician services (27 percent of the total), $2.9 billion on home health care, and $2.5 billion on nursing-home care (see Figure 2.8).[18] Total Medicare spending for Parts A and B is projected to reach $187.7 billion in 1995 and $320.1 billion in 2000.[19] If Medicare's funding priorities remain the same, over 90 percent of this money will continue to pay for hospital and physician care.[20]

(b) MEDICAID

Low-income elderly persons are covered by Medicaid, which pays Medicare premiums, deductibles, and coinsurance fees, as well as services not covered by Medicare. Medicaid is funded jointly by federal, state, and local governments. The federal government sets minimum requirements for eligibility and services, and each state designs the scope of

Figure 2.8
Distribution of Medicare Expenditures (in billions): 1990

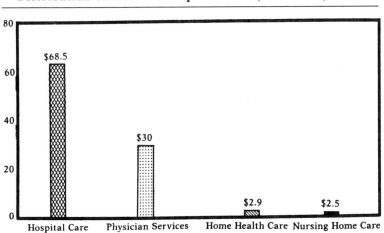

Source: Katharine R. Levit, Helen C. Lazenby, Cathy A. Cowan, and Suzanne W. Letsch. "National Health Expenditures, 1990." *Health Care Financing Review* (Fall 1991): 39–40.

the program to meet the confines of its own budget. States are required to cover inpatient and outpatient hospital care, physician services, rural health clinic services, laboratory and x-ray services, skilled nursing facility services, and home health services. They may then choose to cover, with matching federal funds, additional services such as prescription drugs, eyeglasses, dental care, private duty nursing, and intermediate care facility services. However, many states choose to limit these services.[21]

Medicaid expenditures are primarily geared toward institutional care, with 39.9 percent spent on hospital care and 33.8 percent spent on nursing-home care in 1990. Medicaid, the largest third-party payer of long-term care, paid for a total of 45.4 percent of all nursing-home care in 1990.[22]

Half of all nursing-home residents are poor and qualify for Medicaid. In 1985, Medicaid was the primary source of payment for 50.4 percent of nursing-home residents.[23] However, many are not poor until shortly after they enter a nursing home. They are either forced into poverty because they do not have enough money or adequate insurance to pay for the tremendous costs of the health and long-term care services received prior to admission to a nursing-home, or they become poor after entering a nursing home and paying for this very expensive form of care. Furthermore, in order to qualify for Medicaid nursing-home coverage, the consumer must deplete his or her income and assets and become impoverished.

Medicaid covers the poor for nursing-home care and some home care, but the elderly near-poor have almost no access to long-term care coverage. Community-based services are extremely limited and poorly funded by Medicare and therefore are largely unavailable to low-income people who do not qualify for Medicaid. Often, the only option for a near-poor (or even middle-class), chronically ill older person is to go to a nursing home, pay out-of-pocket until personal resources are depleted, and then qualify for Medicaid. This process is costly and humiliating.

(c) PRIVATE-SECTOR FINANCING

Medicare, Medicaid, and Medigap policies do not cover the total costs of providing health care services for the elderly; the difference is paid either by the individual directly or by additional private insurance coverage. Many of the elderly are limited in their access to services because of the heavy out-of-pocket expenses they would be forced to incur and cannot afford, particularly for nursing-home and home health care services.

(1) Out-of-Pocket Payments

In 1991, elderly Americans spent about 18 percent of their annual incomes on health care.[24] The amount of care that the elderly are responsible for covering has increased dramatically, at a rate far exceeding growth in their income. Between 1977 and 1988, the elderly consumer's per-capita spending for out-of-pocket health expenses, Medicare premiums, and private insurance premiums rose approximately 226 percent. This increase was 67 percent greater than the average income growth from social security payments, pensions, and investments. Overall, estimated out-of-pocket spending as a percentage of personal income rose from 9 percent in 1977 to 13 percent in 1988.[25] In 1991, the average elderly person used 4.5 months of social security checks to cover medical expenses.[26] In 1985, 44 percent of all long-term care expenditures and 94 percent of private expenditures (those costs not covered by the government) were funded directly by consumers.[27]

Out-of-pocket payments go primarily toward nursing-home care (42 percent), services not covered by Medicare (e.g., drugs, home care) (31 percent), and physician care (21 percent). Another 6 percent is used to cover hospital care.[28] Private payments account for the majority of nursing-home expenditures. Of the total $54.5 billion spent on nursing-home care in 1990, $28 billion (51.3 percent) came from patients and their families, and $22.1 billion (40.6 percent) came from state Medicaid programs.[29] Most home health care is similarly funded. In 1987, over half of all home health care was funded solely by private payments,[30] although this ratio has changed somewhat because of some expanded public funding of home care.

(2) Medigap

For those who can afford additional coverage, private health insurance is available to supplement Medicare. In addition to Medicare Part B (supplementary medical insurance), the elderly can purchase Medigap insurance policies to cover out-of-pocket expenditures resulting from Medicare deductibles, coinsurance, and uncovered benefits such as private nursing and drugs.[31] Medigap coverage rarely requires cost sharing by the consumer. Of the elderly living in the community, approximately 65 percent have private policies that supplement Medicare, 10 percent are covered by Medicaid, 20 percent are covered by Medicare only, and 4 percent have some other form of coverage.[32]

(3) Retiree Plans

Postretirement health benefit (PRHB) plans are another option. Some employers provide this coverage to retired employees to help cover the costs of health care after retirement. Benefits under PRHB plans range from payment for limited coverage to supplement Medicare (such as deductibles and coinsurance) to comprehensive benefits resembling the plan for active employees.[33] In 1988, 43 percent of individuals aged 40 and over (39 million) had some form of PRHB coverage through their own or their spouse's current or former employer.[34]

(4) Long-Term Care Insurance

Recently, private long-term care insurance has become available for purchase by the elderly. Long-term care insurance provides the elderly with the security of knowing they will avoid bankruptcy if they ever need extensive long-term care. Policies vary, but, typically, long-term care insurance covers all levels of nursing-home care, home care, and sometimes adult day care, with benefits ranging from $20 to $100 per day. Half the daily benefit is usually available for home care. Long-term care insurance is primarily purchased by persons 55 years and older, although, as more employer-sponsored programs emerge, younger individuals are also buying plans.

Currently, long-term care insurance accounts for 2 percent of total long-term care financing,[35] with less than 4 percent of the elderly and 1 percent of the total U.S. population covered by long-term care policies. However, long-term care insurance is growing. According to the Health Insurance Association of America, the number of employer-sponsored plans increased from 54 to 81 in 1990. The number of Americans who have purchased this insurance has risen from 815,000 in 1987 to 2 million in 1990, according to a report issued by the Employee Benefit Research Institute.[36]

The relatively low demand at this point for long-term care insurance is attributable to several factors—the misperception by the elderly and their families that Medicare covers long-term care costs; conservative pricing by insurers, resulting in premiums not being affordable to large segments of the market; a residual lack of consumer confidence in earlier products and carriers; and a hostile regulatory environment. Nonetheless, industry experts estimate that, even if this environment does not improve, annual growth in long-term care policies sold will be between 20 and 30 percent.[37] This prediction is based partly on two facts: (1) products are expected to improve and better meet the diverse needs of the elderly, and (2) eligibility for government programs is expected to be related more to lack of income than to age, in the future.

(d) COVERAGE FOR VETERANS

The Veterans Administration (VA) is the largest single provider of health services in the United States, with 172 hospitals and 226 outpatient clinics as well as other services nationwide. The VA provides hospital and outpatient care, when needed, for all *service-connected* medical care, and, on a space-available basis, to all veterans over age 65.[38] The VA also provides some dental care. Health care accounts for about one-third of the total VA budget.[39] In 1990, the VA health care budget totaled $11.4 billion. Of this, $9.5 billion was spent on hospital care, $100 million on physician services, and $1 billion on nursing-home care.[40] It is estimated that 46 percent of these services go toward providing care for the elderly.[41] In 1991, nearly 53 percent of VA patients received long-term care; by 1993, because of the growing elderly veteran population, it is expected that 57 percent will receive such care.[42] It is estimated that, by 2000, 9 million veterans will be aged 65 and older, accounting for 65 percent of the elderly male population.[43]

§ 2.4 THE IMPACT OF FINANCING ON UTILIZATION OF SERVICES

The above description of funding sources shows the basic problems with the health and long-term care financing system for the elderly. Funding is extremely fragmented: one elderly person can have his or her care financed by three or four sources, sometimes simultaneously. As the previous discussion shows, financing is biased toward acute and institutional care, with 80 percent of all health and long-term care funding going toward hospital, physician, and nursing-home care. Furthermore, as shown in Chapter 1, utilization of services by the elderly is skewed toward acute and institutional services, although the elderly suffer primarily from chronic, not acute conditions. This situation leads to the question of whether the decision of which services to use is based on actual health needs or on what service is funded. We believe it is the latter. The results of this situation are misallocation of resources, inappropriate care, fragmentation that leads to confusion, and unnecessarily high costs.

If service use is motivated by availability of funding, then the decision of what types of care to seek becomes heavily shaped by funding priorities. In our current system, resources are misallocated: priority is given to technology-intensive acute care and nursing-home care. As a result, many services that would greatly help the overall condition of the elderly are underfunded and underutilized. Preventive care is an example of such a service.

(a) PREVENTIVE CARE

America's current health care financing system puts little or no emphasis on preventive or early treatment services for the elderly. Medicare does not pay for routine physical exams, eye exams to prescribe or fit eyeglasses (except after cataract surgery), or dental care. The focus is largely on technology-intensive treatment directed at specific illnesses. As a result, Medicare patients generally use the services of medical specialists rather than general practitioners. In 1986, the largest share of Medicare-allowed physician charges for professional services was for surgical specialists (37 percent). In contrast, general practice accounted for only 8.6 percent of total allowed charges.[44]

Medicare also places heavy emphasis on technology-intensive procedures. In 1986, Medicare paid for 98,000 coronary artery bypass and autogenous grafts, at an average allowed charge of $3,709 per procedure. Total charges for that procedure increased $63 million (21 percent) from 1985 to 1986 alone. Half of the increase was attributable to increased volume and half to increased approved charges per procedure. In 1986, Medicare also covered 737,000 cataract lens surgeries at a total cost of $1.2 billion in allowed charges.[45]

By utilizing preventive and early treatment services, it is possible that many serious and expensive conditions could be avoided. For example, if an elderly person with high blood pressure had regular annual visits to a primary care provider, the condition would be identified and monitored, a plan of nutrition would be developed and recommended, medication prescribed, and potential serious illness avoided. However, without regular checkups, the patient may not be aware of the condition and may allow it to deteriorate into an eventual heart attack or stroke, resulting in a great deal of pain and the need for very costly hospitalization and/or nursing-home care.

With proper prevention and early treatment, many elderly can maintain good health and even improve their condition. Debilitating conditions can be stabilized, and the elderly can return from a temporary illness to good health.

The health system's bias toward acute and institutional care does not encourage the regular use of these types of services. Medicaid and Medicare do not provide for monitoring of blood pressure, education on the proper way to treat chronic conditions, or transportation to help the elderly get proper food and medicine. Each of these services is far less expensive than bypass surgery or nursing-home care, and each goes a long way toward improving the health and quality of life of the elderly. Nonetheless, these services are not covered by most insurance payers and, consequently, are underutilized.

Overall, payment priorities seem to have a significant effect on health care utilization. A study of health care usage by the elderly found that more than 80 percent of respondents had seen a physician during the past year, nearly 20 percent had been to the hospital, and only 2 percent had used dental or home care services. The study also found that (1) use of the two health services not covered by most health insurance (dental and home care) was influenced by level of income and (2) cost of these services appeared to be a significant barrier to use by the low-income elderly.[46]

(b) INAPPROPRIATE CARE

The current emphasis on care for the elderly is not consistent with either the needs or preferences of the elderly. Medical services—not supportive services—are given priority. With Medicare largely biased toward acute care and Medicaid biased toward institutional care, little financing is provided for community- or home-based care. As a result, the system does little to meet the needs of those with chronic disease or functional loss.

Home care, although it is largely preferred by the elderly and may allow a higher quality of life for the recipient than institutional care, receives only minimal public funding. In 1986, only 2.8 percent of Medicare's budget and 3.1 percent of Medicaid's budget was spent on home care.[47] The care that is financed is for acute, illness-related conditions. Medicare-financed home care is restricted to medically oriented services and is usually only provided after hospitalization for an acute illness or condition. In 1986, the most frequent principal diagnosis for all persons using home health services under Medicare was acute, ill-defined cerebrovascular disease. The second ranking diagnosis was heart failure.[48] Between 60 to 100 percent of a home health care agency's clients are Medicare patients; home health care agencies therefore usually model their benefits and services after Medicare's.[49]

In addition, Medigap, which is available to supplement Medicare financing, is based on the medical model because it is designed to pay physician and pharmaceutical costs. It is not focused on providing social support services or assistance with the activities of daily living.

The medical model bias underpinning public financing sources can, in many instances, result in inefficient and inappropriate service provision and use. Evidence shows that living in an institution may be risky to one's health,[50] and a common result is overutilization of services. Nursing-home care is needed for some patients, but it is not the preferred type of care for those who need help with daily activities. Furthermore, not all people with chronic illnesses are functionally disabled. If support services were available, many could avert a nursing-home stay. If the elderly had help with activities such as eating, bathing, toileting, and shopping, many would be able to remain in their homes. However, both Medicaid and Medicare reimburse minimally for social supports, and the current role of long-term care insurance is limited. Therefore, many people enter a nursing home inappropriately because it is the only long-term care option for them that is financed.

Because of the priority placed on medical care, treatment for chronic conditions is often pursued in acute care settings, often with inappropriately trained personnel. A longitudinal study of elderly high users of health care services found that elderly high users of medical care most frequently sought care for chronic conditions (over 40 percent of total contacts) and that high users tended to have chronic conditions and multiple problems. The study concluded that more nonmedical support services and better integration of mental health services with ongoing primary care could lead to more appropriate care and could possibly reduce the use of general medical care overall.[51]

(c)   FRAGMENTED SERVICES AND LACK OF CONTINUITY OF CARE

The provision of health care services for the elderly is extremely fragmented. Three or four funding sources may be paying for care at one time, with no one responsible for coordinating the various services, funders, providers, and care sites.

The system lacks a continuum of social and medical services. Social support is largely informal or privately paid; medical care is largely publicly funded and administered by professionals. One reason why social services are not funded as well is that the need for social services is much harder to evaluate than the need for medical services.

For example, a course of care for mental illness is much more ambiguous than one for cancer. Providers of social and medical services have different philosophies, perspectives, and educational backgrounds, which may make collaboration difficult. Nonetheless, the need for medical care may often be reduced through the use of social support services. The importance of this symbiotic relationship has often been overlooked.

Coordination between informal and formal care is also lacking. Informal services are necessary for many people but are not supported by current programs. Sometimes, formal long-term care services displace informal supports when they should be enhancing informal care. Such a supportive relationship could allow an impaired elder to remain in the community for a longer period of time. For instance, if an elderly person receiving care in the home from a relative were also to receive care two days a week in an adult day care center, this time away from the home may enable the relative to tend to her or his own life and to receive a respite from continuous care. Often, this approach can allow the relative to continue to provide informal care for a longer period of time. The elderly person benefits from the physical and social activities, friendships, and social services that the center provides. A combination of informal and formal care can often result in the impaired elderly person's remaining in the community longer, with nursing-home placement postponed or avoided all together.

There is also a lack of coordination among acute, ambulatory, and long-term care. Specialists tend to have little experience or interest in other settings, and they tend not to communicate among themselves or to work together as a team. Providers often lack an understanding of how the different parts of the health care system can work together (for example, how an elderly person can benefit from adult day care after being stabilized in an acute care setting such as a hospital). They are often unaware of the existence of many services, especially those that are community-based.

(1) Fragmented Funding and Delivery

Public financing and delivery is extremely fragmented. Federal, state, and local governments all fund portions of care for the elderly. Many of the same services can be funded by many entities, each of which has different qualifications and variations of the services offered. For example, at the federal level, Medicare, Medicaid, Social Service Block Grants, the Veterans Administration, and the Older Americans Act all fund some home care for the elderly. Each has its own eligibility requirements, benefit coverage, regulations for providers, administrative structure, and service delivery mechanism.[52] In such an environment, it is extremely difficult to find the appropriate services to meet the needs of a potential recipient.

The two largest public funding sources are very segregated in what they cover. Because the majority of Medicare funds go toward hospital and physician care and the majority of Medicaid funds for the elderly go toward nursing-home care, with private insurance or out-of-pocket payments filling in the gaps in coverage, it is difficult to integrate acute and long-term care benefits. Often, the care needs of an elderly person are best serviced by a mix of services, and the consumer must juggle a myriad of different agencies and providers.

To complicate matters further, the elderly usually need to use more than one type of care. Because over 40 percent of all admissions to nursing homes are for 90 days or less,[53] in most cases, the elderly person requires some other form of care. However, most funding sources do not pay adequately for more than one type of care. As a result, the recipient can be moved from one funding source to another (if he or she has any outside funding at all), each with different rules and requirements. Thus, it is extremely difficult to coordinate different funding sources in order to develop a comprehensive plan of care.

(2)   Lack of Continuity of Care

The fragmented and complicated health care financing and delivery system makes it difficult for the elderly and their families to select appropriate services. Because of the multiple conditions many elderly persons have, it is difficult for their families to define their problems and needs. If they do manage to identify the needs, they are often unaware of the services available (such as adult day care or meals service) and where they can be obtained. In a complex system with multiple payers and provider organizations, no single coordinating agency or provider can be consulted to define the full scope of needs, produce an adequate plan of care, and then locate needed services.

Even if an elderly person locates a coordinated course of care, it may not be appropriate for his or her particular needs; furthermore, he or she may have chosen it largely because it was financed. It is widely believed that, even though the elderly would rather stay at home, nursing-home care has been overutilized in the past.[54] It is also the only long-term care service that receives significant third-party funding. The health care system should provide a mix of services that will best meet the unique needs of the elderly. As described in Chapter 1, the elderly are not a homogeneous group. The presence of multiple, chronic conditions makes the progression of any particular disease or condition different for many elderly persons, depending on the inter-relatedness of other conditions present. Within this environment, co-ordination of services becomes necessary in order to locate and ensure the best plan of care for the individual.

Because the elderly often require care in multiple settings, care may become duplicative and inappropriate in the absence of coordination. For example, it is important that providers in different settings know the person's basic level of functioning prior to treatment. Hospitaliza-tion may result in deterioration, which reduces the person's normal level of functioning. Dehydration, the shock of moving into a new envi-ronment, and certain drugs may cause disorientation in the elderly. If the provider is not aware of the patient's basic level of functioning, the disorientation may be perceived as permanent or irreversible. Further-more, the use of multiple care settings, providers, and funding agen-cies often requires that the elderly duplicate exams, procedures, and forms. The resulting overlap of services is not only inefficient but also can be dangerous to the patient's health.

(3) Public Policy Implications

Public policy priorities seem disjointed as well. The system sends con-flicting messages. Even within the federal government, there does not seem to be a consensus on what type of care is needed or how best to fund it. Medicare emphasizes acute care and seems to place little im-portance on long-term care. Medicaid is biased toward nursing-home care. The consumer prefers informal community or home care. The political consensus, leadership, and strong political vision that are necessary to address the needs of the health care system are lacking.

Rapidly escalating overall health care spending, especially by fed-eral and state governments, has motivated government-run health care programs for the elderly to focus largely on cutting costs. The result has been an effort by each program at every level to shift costs (and patient care) out of its jurisdiction as much as possible. Hospitals, heavily subsidized by Medicare, are motivated to discharge patients as quickly as possible. However, when the patient is discharged, he or she often needs additional care. If another provider and another fund-ing source (with its own rules) cannot be found, the person must pay out-of-pocket or go without additional care. Many patients and their families are forced to make these decisions alone because no knowledgeable adviser is available to coordinate the various options and services. A patient may jump from one funding source to another, and from one course of care to another, without any evaluation or monitoring of his or her ongoing condition and care needs. In addition, those patients who do not have the money to pay for or the ability to locate appropriate care may be forced to use inappropriate care because they cannot afford or locate other options.

Provision of care for the elderly is extremely expensive, and costs are expected to continue to escalate as the elderly population grows. Because of the health system's funding priorities, the services most available in this high-priced system are largely focused on technology-intensive medical care and institutional care. However, these services are often inappropriate to the actual needs of the elderly.

It is not surprising that, under a cost-generating system, cost containment efforts have failed. Chapter 3 discusses one approach to dealing with this problem: the application of managed care to the funding, organization, and delivery of health and long-term care for the elderly.

NOTES

[1] Waldo, D.R., Sunnefeld, S.T., McKusick, D.R., and Amett, R.H., III. "Health Care Expenditures by Age Group, 1977 and 1987." *Health Care Financing Review* (Summer 1989): 111, 116–118.

[2] *Ibid.*

[3] Harrington, C., Cassel, C., Estes, C.L., Woolhander, S., and Himmelstein, D.V. "A National Long-Term Care Program for the United States." *Journal of the American Medical Association* (December 1991), *266:* 3023.

[4] Waldo, et al., note 1.

[5] Levit, K.R., Lazenby, H.C., Cowan, C.A., and Letsch, S.W. "National Health Expenditures, 1990." *Health Care Financing Review* (Fall 1991): 36.

[6] Parker, M., and Polich, C.L. *The Provision of Home Health Care Services Through Health Maintenance Organizations* (p. 11). Excelsior, MN: InterStudy, 1988.

[7] Rivlin, A.M., and Wiener, J.M. *Caring for the Disabled Elderly: Who Will Pay?* (p. 11). Washington, DC: The Brookings Institution, 1988.

[8] *Id.* at 41.

[9] Ruther, M., and Helbing, C. "Use and Cost of Home Health Agency Services under Medicare." *Health Care Financing Review* (Fall 1988): 108.

[10] U.S. Senate Special Committee on Aging, American Association of Retired Persons, Federal Council on the Aging, and U.S. Administration on Aging.

Aging America: Trends and Projections, 1991 Edition (p. 168). Bethesda, MD: U.S. Department of Health and Human Services, 1991.

[11] Hale, J. "Long-Term Care: What Is It? Who Needs It? Who Uses It?" In *Inter-Study's Long-Term Care Expansion Program* (pp. 15–17). Excelsior, MN: Inter-Study, 1988.

[12] *Ibid.*

[13] Zelman, W.M., Elston, J.M., and Weissert, W.G. "Financial Aspects of Adult Day Care: National Survey Results." *Health Care Financing Review* (Spring 1991): 29.

[14] U.S. Senate Special Committee on Aging, note 10, at 136.

[15] Davis, K., and Rowland, D. *Medicare Policy: New Directions for Health Policy and Long-Term Care* (pp. 35–38). Baltimore: The Johns Hopkins University Press, 1986.

[16] Personal communication with the research office of the Health Care Financing Administration, April 8, 1992.

[17] Davis and Rowland, note 15.

[18] Levit et al., note 5, at 39, 52.

[19] Health Care Financing Administration, Office of the Actuary. Data compiled in 1989.

[20] Levit et al., note 5, at 40–42.

[21] Davis and Rowland, note 15, at 50.

[22] Levit et al., note 5, at 40–42.

[23] National Center for Health Statistics. *Health, United States, 1990* (p. 196). Hyattsville, MD: Public Health Service, 1991.

[24] Harrington et al., note 3, at 3024.

[25] Employee Benefit Research Institute. *EBRI Issue Brief* (March 1991): 21.

[26] Harrington et al., note 3, at 3024.

[27] Polich, C., and Korn, K. "The Role of Private Financing in Long-Term Care." In *InterStudy's Long-Term Care Expansion Program* (p. 50). Excelsior, MN: Inter-Study, 1988.

[28] Polich, C., Iversen, L.H., and Owens, S. "Rethinking Long-Term Care." *Compensation & Benefits* (Summer 1989): 276.

[29] Buchanan, R.J., Madel, P., and Persons, D. "Medicaid Payment Policies for Nursing Home Care: A National Survey." *Health Care Financing Review* (Fall 1991): 55.

[30] Polich et al., note 28, at 276.

[31] Davis and Rowland, note 15.

[32] National Research Council. *The Aging Population in the Twenty-First Century: Statistics for Health Policy* (p. 156). Washington, DC: National Academy Press, 1988.

[33] de Lissovoy, G., Kasper, J.D., Di Carlo, S., and Gabel, J. "Changes in Retiree Health Benefits: Results of a National Survey." *Inquiry* (Fall 1990): 291–292. (Chicago: Blue Cross and Blue Shield Association.)

[34] Employee Benefit Research Institute, note 25, at 17.

[35] General Accounting Office. *Long-Term Care Insurance: Risks to Insurance Should Be Reduced* (pp. 2–3). Washington, DC: Author, December 1991.

[36] American Hospital Association. *AHA News,* September 2, 1991, p. 3.

[37] Greenberg, J. *Long-Term Care Group.* Presentation at Executive Enterprises, New York City, May 1992.

[38] Veterans Benefits Administration. *Summary of Department of Veterans Affairs Benefits* (pp. 12–15). Washington, DC: Department of Veterans Affairs, 1991.

[39] Polich, C.L., Parker, M., Iversen, L.H., and Korn, K. *Case Management for Long-Term Care: A Review of Experience and Potential* (p. 54). Excelsior, MN: InterStudy, 1989.

[40] Levit et al., note 5, at 53.

[41] Conversation with Department of Veterans Affairs representative, February 6, 1992.

[42] *Health Legislation and Regulation,* February 5, 1992, p. 2. (Newsletter published by Faulkner and Gray, Washington, DC.)

[43] Veterans Benefits Administration, note 38.

[44] Fisher, C.R. "Trends in Medicare Enrollee Use of Physician and Supplier Services, 1983–1986." *Health Care Financing Review* (Fall 1988): 12–14.

[45] *Ibid.*

[46] Branch, L., Jette, A., Evashwick, C., Polansky, M., Rowe, G., and Diehr, P. "Towards Understanding Elders' Health Service Utilization." *Journal of Community Health* (Winter 1981): 89.

[47] Iversen, L.H. "Utilization Control: What's Appropriate for Long-Term Care." In *InterStudy's Long-Term Care Expansion Program* (p. 115). Excelsior, MN: InterStudy, 1988.

[48] Ruther and Helbing, note 9, at 107.

[49] Parker and Polich, note 6.

[50] Oriol, W. *The Complex Cube of Long Term Care* (p. 173). Washington, DC: American Health Planning Association, 1985.

[51] Freeborn, D.K., Pope, C.R., McFarland, B.H., and Siegenthaler, L. *Consistently High and Low Elderly Users of Medical Care* (pp. 5–8). Washington, DC: National Center for Health Services Research, 1988.

[52] Rivlin and Wiener, note 7, at 9.

[53] *Id.* at 13.

[54] Iversen, note 47, at 115.

Three

Managing Care

§ 3.1 INTRODUCTION

Never before has there been so much concern about how to finance and deliver health and long-term care services to the elderly. The escalating number of older persons in the population, the growing awareness of the unique needs of the elderly, and the high costs associated with geriatric care have led policymakers and providers alike to question the effectiveness of the current health and long-term care system. The flaws of the current system are numerous and have a profound impact on the well-being of the elderly population.

The service delivery and financing system is tremendously fragmented and confusing. The system discourages coordination of services and offers no incentives to integrate acute and long-term care benefits. Moreover, there is a clear institutional and acute care bias, with limited long-term care financing. The system is especially inadequate for near-poor and frail individuals.

In the midst of concerns about how to best meet the needs of the elderly, health maintenance organizations (HMOs) and other managed care organizations (MCOs) have emerged as significant providers of health care to Medicare beneficiaries. As of January 1992, there were over 1 million older persons enrolled in HMOs to receive complete Medicare benefits. Some advocates have argued that MCOs can significantly improve the overall delivery of health services to the elderly by coordinating care, reducing overall costs, and emphasizing preventive services. Critics have suggested that managed care plans are not the preferred method of delivering care because of their emphasis on cost containment and acute care.

The purpose of this chapter is to consider the appropriateness of MCOs as providers of health and long-term care services to the elderly. First, the chapter defines what is meant by managed care and what type of organizations fall under the rubric of MCOs. Next, MCOs are examined as providers of health and long-term care to the elderly. This section includes a discussion of the unique needs of the elderly and how case management within the MCO structure can best meet those needs. The chapter concludes with a discussion of why health care for the elderly is so difficult to manage.

§ 3.2   MANAGED CARE AND MANAGED CARE ORGANIZATIONS*

The term "managed care" suggests the careful planning and delivery of health care services. Although the term is relatively new, the concept is not. Early proponents of prepaid group practice plans believed that patient care conducted in a group setting through a prepaid financing mechanism facilitated not only preventive care and early treatment of illness, but also the effective, efficient management of members' acute and chronic health conditions. A managed care plan is one that:

- Offers one or more products that integrate financing and management with the delivery of health care services to an enrolled population;
- Employs or contracts with an organized provider network that undertakes the responsibility to deliver services and (as a network or as individual providers) either shares financial risk and/or has some incentive to deliver efficient services;
- Uses an information system capable of monitoring and evaluating patterns of utilization and financial outlays.

Managed care also refers to plans that are prospectively reimbursed for the services delivered and are then financially "at risk" for the services used. The organizations receive the same prepaid reimbursement

---

* This section contains information from an InterStudy report: J.H. Hale and M.M. Hunter, *From HMO Movement to Managed Care Industry: The Future of HMOs in a Volatile Healthcare Market.* Excelsior, MN: InterStudy, 1988.

per enrollee, regardless of the actual cost of services used by the enrollee. At present, the most common type of managed care is conducted in HMOs.

Managed care has become an extremely strong force in the health care field and will continue to have a tremendous impact on both the health care industry and the buyers of health care. In the future, it may be expected that managed care organizations will become increasingly important in the provision of long-term care as well. This section reviews the emergence of the HMO industry and the proliferation of the various other managed care systems.

(a)   THE HMO: THE FIRST DEPARTURE FROM INDEMNITY INSURANCE

When HMOs came into existence, they represented a major departure from indemnity health insurance, the dominant method for financing medical care in the United States. As an entity that integrates financing and service delivery in a single organization, the HMO accepts the responsibility for the quality of care delivered and for influencing the behavior of doctors and other providers. Traditional indemnity insurers have not historically demonstrated such an interest in "managing" the medical care they have financed.

Health maintenance organizations and indemnity health insurance plans, therefore, have historically represented different approaches to financing and delivering medical care. HMOs' primary interest has been the *delivery* of affordable, comprehensive medical services; insurance companies have viewed themselves as a mechanism for *financing* health care. As a result, each had different philosophies, different organizational structures, and, most importantly, different methods for controlling the payer's financial risk.

Another difference between traditional indemnity insurance and HMOs is that, with insurers, the relationship between the third-party payer and the providers is very indirect. When a patient covered by indemnity insurance receives medical services, he or she pays the provider directly and then submits a claim to the insurer for reimbursement. Insurers typically have no responsibility for the quality of care delivered and no influence over medical providers' behavior.

HMOs, however, provide comprehensive medical services—with limited cost-sharing requirements for consumers—designed to ensure that a person who needs medical care will seek it promptly and will receive appropriate and timely treatment. The integration of providers with the payment system creates the opportunity—and incentives—for decisions about allocation of resources to be linked with decisions about the most appropriate and effective style of medical care.

(b) THE MANAGED CARE CONTINUUM

The emergence of HMOs has had far-reaching effects on the health care field. There has been a tremendous growth in the HMO industry; today, over 35 million HMO members are enrolled in nearly 600 HMOs. A major consequence of this growth has been a blurring of the distinctions between HMOs and indemnity insurers. HMOs and insurers alike have moved to develop intermediate products that might enhance their market share and/or profit. Thus, these two very distinct products and approaches to the delivery and financing of health care have now become endpoints on a continuum (see Figure 3.1).[1]

A variety of new managed care organizations have emerged in recent years. These include the traditional HMO, open-ended HMOs, exclusive provider organizations (EPOs), and preferred provider organizations (PPOs). These are described briefly below.

(1)   Health Maintenance Organizations

An HMO is a health plan that offers prepaid comprehensive health coverage for both hospital and physician services. In exchange for a predetermined monthly fee, HMO members are guaranteed access to all basic health services with only limited additional out-of-pocket expense, such as nominal copayments for office visits. Comprehensive benefit coverage, as prescribed by federal and (most) state law, requires HMOs to cover preventive services such as physical exams, eye exams, and well-baby care. Members are required to use participating providers and are enrolled for specified time periods. Figures 3.2 and 3.3 and Table 3.1 comprise an aggregate growth trend analysis for the expansion of HMOs and their enrollment from December 1981 to January 1991. In 1988, the first decrease in the net number of HMOs occurred.

(2)   Open-Ended HMOs

An open-ended HMO removes one of the key requirements of HMOs—that enrollees must receive services only from HMO providers (sometimes known as a lock-in). The lock-in feature is viewed by many as the most significant barrier to broader HMO enrollment. In the open-ended

Figure 3.1
The Managed Care Continuum

Plan Feature	"Pure" Indemnity	Modified Indemnity	PPO	Open-Ended HMO	EPO	IPA HMO	"Pure" HMO
					Managed Care Plans		
Utilization review	No utilization review	Preadmission certification, concurrent review, second surgical opinion	MIS Physician profiling			Formal peer review	Informal peer review protocols
Provider panel	No provider selection		Selected providers				Staff providers
Consumer choice of provider	Total freedom of choice		Incentives to limit choice		Lock-in		
Benefit structure	Varied coverage—deductibles, coinsurance routine, preventive care uncovered		Waive deductibles, reduce coinsurance			Comprehensive coverage including preventive; limited copayments	
Provider payment	FFS payment					Withholds capitation	Salary
Rating method	Experience rated					Community rated	
Practice setting	Independent practice						Group practice

Hybrid—takes characteristics from each end of the continuum.

Source: InterStudy, 1988.

Figure 3.2
Growth in HMO Enrollment

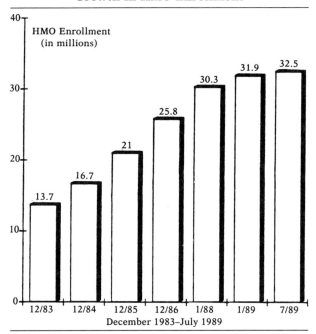

Source: InterStudy, 1990.

model, enrollees are covered if they choose, without referral, to receive services outside of the HMO provider network. Coverage is offered under a financing mechanism similar to traditional indemnity insurance and is available at any time service is desired. Benefits for services received outside the HMO network are typically less comprehensive than the HMO benefit and usually include deductibles, copayments, and/or coinsurance.

(3)   Exclusive Provider Organizations

Some health plans that are otherwise similar to PPOs restrict enrollees to the panel of preferred providers. These plans, sometimes referred to as exclusive provider organizations (EPOs), may, depending on their structure and benefits, operate almost exactly like HMOs. However, they typically have more flexibility in benefit design and pricing structure than do HMOs. Although still few in number, EPOs may become more prevalent, especially in the self-insured portion of the market, where they are subject to no regulation.

Figure 3.3
Growth in Number of HMOs

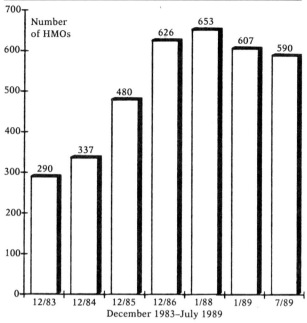

Source: InterStudy, 1990.

(4) Preferred Provider Organizations

Preferred provider organizations (PPOs) are a type of health plan that may be offered by an insurance company or a Blue Cross and Blue Shield plan, or may be arranged by a self-insured employer. An HMO could (and, in fact, frequently does) also offer a PPO product.* Because they are not subject to the same kind of regulation as HMOs, PPO plans vary considerably in organization, financial arrangement, and benefit structure.

* Unlike HMOs, PPOs are not organizations legally established for the business of insuring and financing health services. Often, the term PPO is used to refer to a preferred provider *network*—a legally constituted entity comprised of a hospital or group of hospitals, or a group of physicians, or a group of hospitals and physicians, that offers the providers' services on a contractual basis to a financier, usually but not necessarily at a fee-for-service price lower than usual charges. The network may also offer administrative services such as utilization review and development of benefit plans.

Table 3.1
Growth in HMOs: 1981—1991

	12/81	12/82	12/83	12/84	12/85	12/86	12/87	1/89	1/90	1/91
No. of plans	260	269	290	337	480	626	650	607	575	556
Annual percentage change	—	3.5	7.8	16.2	42.4	30.4	3.8	-7.1	-5.3	-3.3
Enrollment (1,000s)	10,497	11,606	13,643	16,743	21,052	25,777	29,286	31,940	33,093	34,072
Annual percentage change	—	10.6	17.6	22.7	25.7	22.4	13.6	9.1	3.6	3.0

Source: InterStudy Edge, 1989, 1990, 1991.

Nevertheless, PPO plans are generally considered to share the following features:

- *Enrollees are offered incentives to limit their care givers to the panel of preferred providers.* Incentives include lower copayments and deductibles, or coverage of more services, when the enrollees use preferred providers.
- *Services are provided by participating providers at negotiated rates; usually, the normal charges are discounted.* Although interest in sharing risk with providers is growing, PPOs are still considered to be primarily fee-for-service arrangements.
- *The PPO network does not bear insurance risk.* In a PPO plan, the risk must be borne by an insurance company, a Blue Cross and Blue Shield plan, an HMO, or a self-insured employer.
- *The PPO network may be organized by groups of hospitals and physicians, by independent brokers, by self-insured employers, by commercial insurance companies, or by health service corporations.* Broker-sponsored and provider-sponsored networks are typically marketed to self-insured employers.

PPO plans' benefits for using preferred providers may closely match HMO benefits. Especially where HMO market penetration is high, PPOs may offer comprehensive coverage with only minimal copayments, and may cover the same preventive care required of HMOs. PPO benefits may offer the promise of no claims and no paperwork; the difference is that PPOs are not required to do so by law. In most markets, PPO benefits look more like insurance plans with sizable deductibles, copayments, and coinsurance.

§ 3.3 MEDICARE HMOs

The federal government has promoted enrollment of the elderly in HMOs for over a decade, because of the belief that HMOs are effective in reducing health care costs and utilization. When Medicare was enacted in 1965, it contained some limited provisions that allowed beneficiaries to enroll in HMOs. The 1973 HMO Act and subsequent amendments went a step further and encouraged HMOs to enroll the elderly. Most importantly, however, the 1982 Tax Equity and Fiscal Responsibility Act (TEFRA) modified reimbursement arrangements to provide incentives to HMOs to enroll Medicare members. Figure 3.4 and Table 3.2 show the overall growth trends and the total Medicare enrollment in HMOs.

There are four types of programs through which Medicare benefi-ciaries can receive services from HMOs: cost contracts, risk contracts, health care prepayment plan (HCPP) contracts, and supplemental ben-efits packages. In cost contracts, HMOs receive enrollee per-capita prepayments that are later adjusted to reflect actual costs. In risk con-tracts, HMOs receive enrollee per-capita payments of 95 percent of the

Figure 3.4
Growth in TEFRA Risk HMOs, 1985–1992

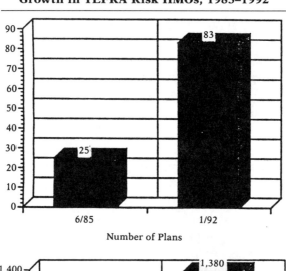

Number of Plans

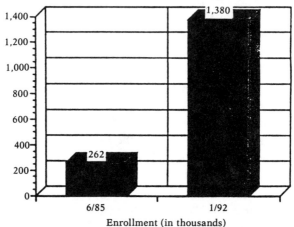

Enrollment (in thousands)

Source: Health Care Financing Administration, 1992.

Table 3.2
Total Medicare Enrollment in HMOs, 1982–1989

	6/82	6/83	6/84	6/85	6/86	6/87	6/88	1/89
Total Medicare enrollment	430,936	492,035	671,186	848,464	1,256,389	1,555,112	1,581,054	1,560,516
Annual change	—	14.2%	36.4%	26.4%	48.1%	23.8%	1.7%	−1.3%
Number of HMOs	70	80	105	102	175	179	162	136
Annual change	—	14.3%	31.3%	−2.9%	71.6%	2.3%	−9.5%	−16.0%

Source: L.H. Iversen, C.L. Polich, S. Owens, and K. Korn. InterStudy's Report to the Prospective Payment Assessment Commission, 1989.

average adjusted per-capita cost (AAPCC). The AAPCC is an estimate of what the federal government would spend to care for an enrollee if he or she had remained in the Medicare fee-for-service program. These payments are not adjusted for actual costs. In HCPP contracts, the HMO contracts with the Health Care Financing Administration (HCFA) to provide Medicare beneficiaries with certain Medicare Part B benefits only. HCPP contracts are cost-based and have been allowed since Medicare was enacted. Supplemental benefits, also known as Medigap coverage, are not provided through any contract with HCFA because the coverage does not include Medicare benefits.

By far, the most common mechanism is the TEFRA risk contract. In January 1989, two-thirds of all Medicare HMO enrollees were enrolled through TEFRA risk contracts. Between December 1986 and January 1992, the number of TEFRA risk enrollees rose from 797,000 to 1,380,000; the number of risk HMOs dropped from 111 to 83 (see Table 3.3).

TEFRA risk contracts are so named because they were established under the Tax Equity and Fiscal Responsibility Act. Medicare risk contracts with HMOs existed before TEFRA, but were subject to retrospective adjustments based on the actual costs of providing care to Medicare members. Under TEFRA, however, HMOs receive a fixed, prepaid amount for each enrollee regardless of the actual costs incurred. These risk contracts accommodate the payment system HMOs use for younger enrollees, and offer HMOs a greater opportunity to save (or lose) money based on their ability to manage care. HMOs are paid 95 percent of what the federal government estimates it would have spent to care for the enrollees if they had remained in the Medicare fee-for-service program. By paying 95 percent, the federal government, in theory, saves 5 percent for every individual who joins an HMO. The HMOs presumably can save additional money by cost-effectively managing the enrollees' care. The amount paid to the HMO varies by the age and sex of the enrollee, by whether the enrollee is eligible for Medicaid, by whether he or she resides in a nursing home, and by the county of residence.

Table 3.3
Number of TEFRA Risk HMO Enrollees and Plans, 1985–1992

	1985	1986	1987	1988	1989	1991	1992
Enrollees	262,000	797,000	896,000	942,143	1,037,000	1,375,000	1,380,000
Plans	25	111	117	105	93	93	83

Source: Health Care Financing Administration.

(a) SCOPE OF SERVICES

TEFRA risk HMOs vary dramatically in the scope of services they provide to their enrollees. The most limiting plans are TEFRA risk HMOs that provide only the services presently covered under Medicare. All TEFRA risk HMOs are required, at a minimum, to provide the services covered under Medicare: basic acute care coverage for hospital and physician services, and "medically necessary" short-term home care and nursing-home care following a hospital stay. Other TEFRA HMOs offer somewhat more extensive acute and long-term care services, including case management.

(1) Limited Acute and Long-Term Care Benefits

Medicare TEFRA risk HMOs often go beyond Medicare to offer added benefits, such as extended hospital days, preventive care, and eye care. The percentage of HMOs offering various types of extended coverage can be seen in Table 3.4. Most plans include these services as part of their "basic" Medicare package. Other HMOs (11 percent) have both high- and low-option plans. (Low-option plans have lower premiums

Table 3.4
Benefits Provided Over and Above Medicare-Covered Services in TEFRA Risk HMOs and CMPs,* July 1988

	Percent of Plans Offering Benefits in Either Basic or High-Option Package
Routine physicals	97%
Unlimited hospital days	93
Immunizations	92
Eye exams	77
Health education	73
Ear exams	67
Outpatient mental health	59
Outpatient drugs	31
Extended skilled nursing-home days (beyond 100 days)	27
Dental care	17

*CMPs are "competitive medical plans"—certain prepaid plans that, like HMOs, can enter into risk contracts. The vast majority of risk contracts are with HMOs.

Source: Health Care Financing Administration, 1988.

and fewer services that exceed Medicare.) In November 1991, the average monthly premium per person for a basic package was $42.06; the highest premium charged was $108.69. In exchange for these premiums, the enrollee receives not only the extra benefits, but also coverage for Medicare deductibles and copayments. With this similarity to the coverage provided through Medigap plans, HMOs are integrating Medicare and Medigap coverage.

As shown in Table 3.4, the additional benefits provided in HMOs are primarily related to acute and preventive care. Long-term care benefits that are provided are generally similar to standard Medicare-provided services, in that they emphasize care related to medical need. A survey of 41 large, experienced TEFRA risk HMOs showed, for example, that skilled nursing-home care and medically necessary home care were offered by all 41 plans, while custodial nursing-home care was not provided by any plan.[2] A significant minority of plans (27 percent), however, did provide other supportive home care services (e.g., homemakers) that are not covered under standard Medicare. Plans providing this care generally reported that it was not a formally provided or marketed benefit, but that it would, on a case-by-case basis, be used as a lower-cost alternative to institutional care. Supportive home care services might also be provided if desired by the enrollee, as long as the expense did not exceed the expected cost of institutional care.

In a later survey of 103 Medicare HMOs and their provision of home health care, similar findings were reported: a minority of plans (33 percent) offered supplemental home health services not covered under Medicare. These services included help with meals, housework, laundry, transportation, chore services, and respite care. Respite care was the supplemental service offered most frequently.[3]

The survey of 41 plans also showed that HMO coverage of nursing-home and home health care exceeded standard Medicare benefits by allowing additional days of care and/or by not requiring copayments or prior hospital stays. Two-thirds of the 41 HMOs provided 100 days of nursing-home coverage per benefit period, and 31 percent provided more than 100 days. In all plans, coverage of home care was not limited by a specific number of days or visits, but by determinations of medical necessity or cost effectiveness. None of the HMOs reported that they required copayments for nursing-home or home care benefits. A prior hospital stay was required by only 17 percent of the HMOs for a skilled nursing-home stay, 2 percent for medically necessary home care, and 0 percent for other home care. Again, measures of medical need and probable cost effectiveness were used as eligibility criteria in place of a prior use requirement.

(2)   Case Management in HMOs

Case management within managed care systems contains several characteristics that are unique to HMOs. First, the financing and delivery structure of managed care organizations gives them flexibility to deliver care that is especially able to meet older persons' health and long-term care needs. Second, HMOs contain significant cost containment incentives inherent in a capitated risk-sharing arrangement to help facilitate cost consciousness.[4]

The flexibility afforded by the way in which HMO services are financed and delivered can be seen by comparing Medicare HMO benefits with Medicare benefits provided in the fee-for-service sector. Fee-for-service Medicare providers are restricted by specific Medicare provisions that dictate when services are and are not authorized. Moreover, the vast majority of persons receiving these benefits do not receive any level of case management—benefits received are not coordinated or integrated. This can result in an inappropriate service/treatment mix or in costly duplications in services.

In Medicare HMOs, however, the HMOs receive a fixed, prepaid amount for each enrollee, to provide that enrollee with the mix of necessary services. At a minimum, the HMO must provide all services covered under Medicare. However, there are no unauthorized services. The HMO can use the capitated amount to finance whatever services it feels are appropriate. For example, the HMO could use part of the capitated amount to provide an air conditioner to a member with a respiratory problem, if that air conditioner (rather than repeated hospital stays) would improve the individual's health. The HMO's primary physician would be in a position to coordinate, or at least monitor, the various health and long-term care services the member is receiving through the HMO. The fact that the HMO network includes a wide variety of acute and long-term care providers gives the HMO the flexibility to choose providers known to be qualified to deliver appropriate care.

It is important to note that the structure of HMOs and other managed care systems provides them with the potential to manage care in this way. In reality, however, HMOs vary substantially in the degree to which they provide case management. Nearly all HMOs at least coordinate care through a primary care physician. A 1987 InterStudy survey of 41 large Medicare HMOs showed that 34 percent of the plans had a geriatric case management program or were developing one.[5] A later study (also conducted by InterStudy) of 103 Medicare HMOs found that Medicare HMOs generally are more flexible in providing nonmedically necessary home health services than traditional Medicare. Again, however, there was considerable variation among the HMOs.[6]

(b) MANAGEMENT OF COSTS

In addition to encouraging flexibility in order to appropriately meet needs, HMOs have financial incentives to conduct case management so that the cost of care is carefully monitored. As noted, HMOs receive the same fixed amount per enrollee, regardless of the actual cost of services used. This means that the HMO must absorb the loss if costs exceed the reimbursement level, or will accumulate savings if costs are lower than the reimbursement amount.

To maximize its profits and minimize its losses, the HMO will attempt to modify utilization patterns. This may be accomplished by reducing inpatient hospitalizations and promoting the utilization of less costly preventive home- and community-based services. The HMO may also control costs by providing preventive care and promptly and effectively treating known conditions before they become more serious.

The rewards of cost containment strategies are realized not only by Medicare and the HMO, but also by the beneficiary of the care. The Medicare beneficiary in the traditional Medicare program is faced with a confusing and, often, difficult-to-manage array of deductibles, copayments, and uncovered costs for the various services provided. Enrollment in HMOs can help to minimize these out-of-pocket expenditures and facilitate the budgeting of limited resources by the reducing payments to a monthly predetermined premium. This may be particularly beneficial for low- and moderate-income older persons.

There are several potential disadvantages to the HMO model. Because HMOs are reimbursed on a fixed, capitated basis, there is a potential to underserve and promote the underutilization of care. Numerous studies have documented that the quality of care rendered in HMOs is equal or superior to the care delivered in the traditional fee-for-service sector for traditional HMO enrollees who are young, healthy, and employed. Studies of Medicare HMOs have generally shown that Medicare HMO enrollees receive care that is equal or superior in quality to fee-for-service care. However, as yet, few studies of this type have been conducted. As HMOs continue to expand into care for the elderly, appropriate quality assurance systems will need to be implemented to protect this more vulnerable and less healthy population.

§ 3.4 DIFFICULTIES OF MANAGING HEALTH CARE

HMOs have made significant progress in managing health care, particularly acute care, for the elderly. Their results have been impressive, particularly in utilization of hospital care. Nationally, the elderly use 3,100 hospital days for every 1,000 individuals. This includes approximately 350 admissions per 1,000 and an average hospital stay of nearly 9 days. HMOs with risk contracts have reduced their enrollees' use of hospital care by about one-third. Most HMOs have achieved under 2,000 hospital days per 1,000 persons. Some have further reduced utilization to under 1,500 hospital days per 1,000. Length of stay has been similarly affected, with HMOs managing stays of 5 to 6 days instead of the typical 8 to 9 days seen in the Medicare fee-for-service program. HMOs achieve these results through selected provider networks, provider financial incentives, and proactive, focused care management.

Another reason HMOs have been successful in managing costs and length of stay in acute care is that they have integrated virtually all acute care needs of the elderly into one package. In other words, they are responsible for all aspects of acute care for their enrollees. Conversely, one of the main reasons that health care for the elderly is so difficult to manage in the broader system is the fragmentation of funding and service delivery, described in Chapter 2. With such fragmentation, no one funder or provider has sufficient incentive or control to manage all aspects of care for a patient. Without integrated funding and service delivery, effective management of the costs and utilization of health care for the elderly will continue to be difficult.

Two additional characteristics of the health and long-term care system for the elderly also inhibit effective management of care and appropriate provision of services: the social/medical dichotomy and the chronic/acute dichotomy.

The system currently in place to serve the needs of the elderly is medically oriented and biased toward acute and institutional care. Unfortunately, the needs of the elderly are as often social in nature and relate to chronic conditions. While 80 percent of the elderly experience at least one chronic condition (and the average elderly individual has three), nearly 70 percent of the funding for health and long-term care is for acute care services. The vast majority of the elderly prefer home- and community-based care, but two-thirds of the funding for health and long-term care is for institutional care. We have a very basic mismatch of current funding and services compared to the elderly's needs and preferences.

A fundamental requirement of an appropriate system for providing health and long-term care for the elderly is the integration and management of services across a broad continuum of acute and chronic care. At present, this integration is made difficult by a fragmented and confusing financing system. Yet, many efforts have been made to appropriately and cost effectively manage care for the elderly. The following chapters provide examples and descriptions of these efforts to manage long-term care, to manage acute care, and to integrate acute and long-term care services in a managed care setting.

NOTES

[1] Hale, J.H., and Hunter, M.M. *From HMO Movement to Managed Care Industry: The future of HMOs in a Volatile Healthcare Market* (p. 13). Excelsior, MN: InterStudy, 1988.

[2] Iversen, L.H., Oberg, C.N., and Polich, C.L. *Health Services Provided to Medicare Beneficiaries in HMOs.* Excelsior, MN: InterStudy, 1987.

[3] Iversen, L.H., Oberg, C.N., and Polich, C.L. "The Availability of Long-Term Care Services for Medicare Beneficiaries in Health Maintenance Organizations." *Medical Care* (1988), *26*(9): 14.

[4] Spitz, B. "Medicaid Lessons for Business." *Business and Health* (February 1985), *2*:21.

[5] Iversen et al., note 2.

[6] Iversen et al., note 3.

Four

Case Management for Long-Term Care

§ 4.1 INTRODUCTION*

Case management for long-term care became popular in the 1970s because of growing concern about the impact of a fragmented and institutionally biased long-term care system on the well-being of the elderly. Prior to this time, elderly persons in need of long-term care were predominantly cared for in nursing homes. Widely reported research cited astounding levels of inappropriate placement in institutions, indicating that as many as 40 percent of persons in nursing homes could be living in the community. It was strongly believed that the problem of overinstitutionalization was caused by a lack of coordination among services and programs as well as inadequate assessment of patient need. Consequently, case management services were developed to provide the chronically ill elderly with adequate access to appropriate and reasonably priced community-based services, with the case manager acting as client advocate and care coordinator.

This concept captured the imagination of long-term care researchers and providers and became an instrumental part of the nation's first community-based long-term care demonstration projects.[1]

*This chapter contains information from an InterStudy report: C.L. Polich, M. Parker, L.H. Iversen, and K. Korn, Case Management for Long-Term Care: A Review of Experience and Potential. Excelsior, MN: InterStudy, 1989.

The SITO (Services Integration Targets for Opportunity) demonstration projects, among the first to provide case management for elderly persons in need of long-term care, were followed by the Triage program in Connecticut, On Lok in San Francisco, and ACCESS in New York, to name but a few. Within these demonstration projects, case management was used to assess the physical, functional, emotional, and financial status of the chronically ill and functionally disabled elderly; to develop and implement their care plan; to regularly monitor their condition; and to identify any needed changes in their care plan.

During the 1980s, case management shifted away from the client advocacy approach of the 1970s and evolved into a gatekeeping mechanism for containing escalating health care expenditures. This change in the role and use of case management paralleled similar changes in our nation's health care system. Spurred by skyrocketing health and long-term care expenditures, a growing elderly population, and increasing demand for home- and community-based services by the aged, the focus of case management shifted from care coordination toward cost containment.

Further demonstration projects (Channeling, for example) were begun, aimed at determining whether case management was an effective tool for containing the cost and use of long-term care. In these projects, the assumption of appropriate placement in nursing homes was challenged by examining the extent to which individuals at risk of nursing-home placement could be diverted to a community-based setting. Further, the demonstrations were expected to prove that case management was an effective vehicle for identifying these at-risk elderly, assessing their needs, and arranging care that would be less costly than nursing-home care.

Today, the debate continues regarding the value of case management in long-term care. This debate can be framed by one simple question: What is the goal of case management? The answer to this question varies tremendously according to who is responding. Consumers, providers, public policymakers, and long-term care financiers all have different perspectives on case management and, as a result, seek to develop a system that tries to satisfy conflicting goals.

§ 4.2 DEFINITIONS OF CASE MANAGEMENT

Many terms are used to describe case management. Some of these include care management, case coordination, continuing care coordination, service integration, continuity coordination, and service coordination. Case management is often confused with other services that include some of its elements, such as geriatric consultation, utilization review, preadmission screening, discharge planning, or social casework.

Some definitions of case management highlight the following aspects:

- A systematic process of assessment, planning, service coordination and/or referral, and monitoring through which the multiple service needs of clients are met.[2]
- A negotiation of systems by one person on behalf of another, to deliver the greatest number of available services.[3]
- [A system in which] the best possible match between available service responses and the identified needs of individual clients [is arrived at], with care tailored to need in a way that, to the extent possible, meets both the fiscal requirements of the system and the preferences of the particular client.[4]
- A system of assessment, treatment planning, referral, and follow-up that ensures the provision of comprehensive services and the coordination of payment and reimbursement for care.[5]
- A method of assessing comprehensive, unified, coordinated, and timely services to disabled elderly in need of those services through the efforts of a primary agent who, together with the client and family, develops goals and objectives, and takes responsibility for accessing or procuring the services needed to enhance the disabled older person's ability to function productively and independently.[6]
- A set of logical steps and a process of interaction within a service network which assure that a client receives needed services in a supportive, effective, efficient, and cost-effective manner.[7]

What is striking about these definitions is that they are extremely broad, and, as already discussed, are often inconsistent regarding the goals that case management services are expected to achieve.

Although long-term care case management has many goals, they can be narrowed down to the following three basic objectives:

- To control long-term care expenditures by providing less costly alternatives to institutionalization and easier access to community-based and in-home care;
- To contain costs and control utilization by targeting those in greatest need of long-term care services;

- To help elderly persons and their families negotiate a fragmented and often confusing long-term care system and to arrange for the most appropriate type of services.

§ 4.3 COMPONENTS OF CASE MANAGEMENT

Although definitions vary, most experts agree that case management is comprised of seven basic components: identifying and attracting the target population, screening/intake and eligibility determination, assessment, care planning, service arrangement, monitoring or follow-up, and reassessment.[8,9] These components are described in the sections that follow.

(a) IDENTIFYING AND ATTRACTING THE TARGET POPULATION

In order for an organization that provides case management to reach all elderly persons who are in need of the services it offers, it must define a target population and devise an outreach mechanism for attracting this population to its program. The need for an outreach component in case management stems from the fact that many elderly persons and their families are overwhelmed by the vast array of long-term care services that are available, or feel helpless because they are unaware of the long-term care services that exist, or do not know how to use and coordinate these services themselves.

Although case management alleviates many of these problems by educating elderly individuals and their families about the various types of long-term care services that are available and by coordinating their care, a case management program is utterly ineffective if its outreach component does not attract the individuals who need its services. Outreach is also important because it makes case management known to other service providers and helps ensure proper referrals and coordination of care.

There are several ways in which a case management agency can reach out to other agencies and the general public. For example, in order to maintain visibility with other service providers, a case management agency can establish a network of organizations and people who have contact with the target population (e.g., hospitals, nursing homes, home care agencies, attorneys, physicians, religious institutions, and caregiver support groups). In order to inform the public, a case management organization can disseminate printed materials describing what case management is, which services are provided, where case management is available, and how much it costs.[10]

(b) SCREENING/INTAKE AND ELIGIBILITY DETERMINATION

Once an organization has established its target population and attracted a group of clients, it must then determine which of these individuals need and are eligible to receive the case management services it offers. This identification can be achieved by devising a mechanism for screening out those individuals who do not match the criteria of the organization's target population.

Both the target population and the screening and intake mechanisms will vary for each provider of case management, depending on its goals and objectives. The scope and depth of the screening will also vary for each program. Some screening procedures may only involve filling out a form; others may involve more extensive, in-depth, or even in-home evaluations conducted by case management staff.

(c) ASSESSMENT

After a client is admitted to a case management program, a case manager or a case management team assesses the client before developing a care plan. The assessment involves a much more extensive evaluation than is performed during client screening and intake. Client assessment typically includes a comprehensive evaluation of the individual's physical, cognitive, emotional, social, and economic status, as well as his or her self-care capacity.[11] The assessments vary among different programs according to emphasis, method of evaluation, and staff mix. Client assessments may be conducted by one case manager, or by a multidisciplinary team.[12]

(d) CARE PLANNING

After the assessment is complete, case managers develop a care plan to meet the needs of clients and their families. The care plan should appropriately meet the physical, functional, and emotional needs of the client, and should be compatible with his or her financial status. Because it is often difficult to find an ideal balance between the most appropriate and the most cost-efficient services, case managers must understand the unique needs of the elderly as well as the long-term care system.

(e) SERVICE ARRANGEMENT

After creating a care plan for a client, a case manager is responsible for arranging services and coordinating the different components of the client's care. The case manager (or case management team) contacts various providers and often negotiates a price for the care. Coordination of services is a very important component of case management, because many elderly persons and their families simply do not have the time, energy, knowledge, or capability to arrange for services themselves. In addition, many individuals do not understand the intricacies of the long-term care system well enough to develop and arrange for an appropriate and cost-efficient care plan.

(f) MONITORING OR FOLLOW-UP

When the care plan is implemented and the client begins to receive the services arranged by the case management team, the case managers are responsible for monitoring the patient in order to verify that the original care plan is appropriate, identify any changes in the client's condition, and/or make necessary modifications in the care plan. An individual's physical and emotional state is dynamic and requires continual observation in order to identify problems or necessary changes in the care plan.

(g) REASSESSMENT

Many case management systems include a reassessment component in their program. Reassessment differs from client monitoring in that it is more involved and comprehensive. Client monitoring is ongoing; reassessment occurs at specific time intervals. Under many case management programs, client reassessment involves the same procedure that was initially used to assess a client's condition and establish the original care plan. Reassessing a client's physical, functional, emotional, mental, and economic status is imperative if appropriate care is to be provided to the client on an ongoing basis.

§ 4.4 OBJECTIVES AND PHILOSOPHIES OF CASE MANAGEMENT

Although there is a general consensus regarding the basic components of case management, the goals and objectives of case management often conflict among different constituencies. Differing opinions as to why there is a need for case management, and what the ideal case management system should be, are rooted in two basic philosophies. These two philosophies are best explained by examining the two basic types of case management system: client-oriented and system-oriented case management.[13]

Client-oriented case management focuses more on the needs of the individual, emphasizing the importance of providing appropriate care; *system-oriented* case management focuses more on the need to reduce unnecessary spending for long-term care and to provide care in the most cost-efficient manner. "Gatekeeping" is a term commonly associated with system-oriented case management.

Table 4.1 lists the goals of case management, distinguishing between those that are primarily client-oriented and those that are primarily system-oriented.[14] This is not to imply, however, that client-oriented and system-oriented case management systems have *fundamentally* different objectives. Both case management systems strive to reduce costs, prevent inappropriate institutionalization, and support the right of the client to be in the least restrictive setting. It is the degree of emphasis given to each of these objectives that varies between client-oriented and system-oriented case management programs.

Table 4.1
Goals Associated with Case Management

Client-Oriented Goals

   To ensure that services given are appropriate for the needs of a particular client.
   To follow clients, to guarantee continued appropriateness of service.
   To improve client access to the continuum of long-term care services.
   To support the client's informal caregivers.
   To serve as a bridge between institutional and community-based care systems.

System-Oriented Goals

   To facilitate the development of a broader array of noninstitutional services as substitutes for nursing-home care.
   To promote quality and efficiency in the delivery of long-term care services.
   To enhance the coordination of long-term care service delivery.
   To target individuals most at risk for nursing home placement, in order to prevent inappropriate institutionalization.
   To contain costs by controlling client access to services, especially high-cost services.

For example, the reduction of unnecessary institutionalization is accepted as one of the objectives of case management. In achieving this objective, client-oriented systems put a greater emphasis on the rights and needs of the individual to be in the least restrictive setting; system-oriented systems focus more on the need to reduce spending for long-term care by limiting costly institutionalization. Likewise, although cost containment is a fundamental objective of case management, client-oriented systems tend to focus more on reducing costs for the individual, and system-oriented case management emphasizes the importance of reducing public (or system) expenditures.

Although these different philosophies of case management may appear subtle, they are very important when considering how case management should evolve, and in determining how and whether to include case management in future long-term financing reform.

§ 4.5 DIFFERENCES IN CASE MANAGEMENT SYSTEMS

Case management systems differ not only in philosophy, but also in organizational structure. Organizational differences among case management systems include: composition of case management staff, total versus partial provision of case management services, total versus partial provision of community-based services, organizational auspices, and degree of financial control over the care plan.

(a) COMPOSITION OF CASE MANAGEMENT STAFF

Under some case management systems, all case managers are professionals and hold advanced degrees (i.e., MA, MSW, or PhD) in a field directly applicable to case management and the elderly; under other case management systems, only some of the case managers hold advanced degrees.

Some programs maintain that it is not necessary for all case managers to hold advanced degrees, particularly when some individuals are involved with aspects of case management that do not require extensive knowledge or expertise about the needs of the elderly. For example, a case management program may have a very straightforward and objective method for screening potential clients, one that does not require an extensive, in-depth analysis. In this type of program, some argue, it is unnecessary to use a highly trained staff member to ensure that the work is done in a competent and appropriate manner.

Others, however, are strong advocates of *professionalization*, in which a case manager with an advanced degree and considerable experience is responsible for performing all aspects of case management. Generally speaking, there is some agreement that case managers who perform the assessment and care-planning aspects of case management should hold advanced degrees.

The degree to which the different components of case management are dispersed among case managers is referred to as *specialization*. Under a highly specialized case management system, each staff member has a specific task. As a result, each client may see as many as six or eight different staff members. In less specialized case management systems, one staff member is responsible for performing all components of case management.

Some observers believe that case management systems should be highly specialized; others argue that it is better for one case manager to be responsible for performing all case management services. Advocates of the latter type of system maintain that having one case manager perform all aspects of case management helps prevent the fragmentation and confusion that tend to occur under a more specialized case management system; older persons and their families may find it easier to relate to one case manager.

In addition to professionalization and specialization, the *disciplines* of those who complete client assessments and create care plans vary among case management programs. Some organizations believe that client assessments should be completed by persons working in the medical field (i.e., nurses); others believe that it is more appropriate for persons in social service positions (i.e., social workers) to do client assessments. Still others believe that client assessment and care planning should be completed by a multidisciplinary team of individuals involved in both medical and social services occupations. At the heart of this issue is whether case management is primarily a medical or social service. Advocates for the use of interdisciplinary teams maintain that case management serves both the medical and social needs of elderly persons, and that using only persons in the medical field, or only those in social service positions, fails to take into account the multiple needs of elderly individuals.

(b) TOTAL VERSUS PARTIAL PROVISION OF CASE MANAGEMENT SERVICES

Some case management agencies provide all case management services; others offer only some components of case management. The provision of case management services can be divided into the following three patterns.[15]

(1) Total Provision, Single Agency

The provision of the case management function may be based entirely within one agency. Under this type of system, all components of case management (e.g., outreach, screening/intake, client assessment, care planning, service arrangement, monitoring, and reassessment) are provided by a single agency. Total provision of case management should not be confused with total provision of actual services, however; many case management agencies provide all the components of case management but coordinate the actual care plan with outside providers in the community.

(2) Partial Provision, Single Agency

Case management may be located in one agency, but one or more of the component functions may be delegated to other organizations or agencies in the community. Under this type of program, the majority of case management services are provided by a single agency, but the agency delegates one or more of the components to an outside agency or organization. For example, a case management agency may provide all case management components except client assessment.

(3) Total Provision, Multiple Agencies

The authority for the case management function may originate from a single source, but the provision of the entire case management function may be delegated to a set of agencies through a contract or formal agreement. Under this model, a central agency (such as an Area Agency on Aging) organizes the system and sets policies and procedures, reporting and staffing requirements, and rules for establishing provider relationships. The central agency, however, provides no case management services; it delegates this responsibility to other local agencies and organizations.

(c) TOTAL VERSUS PARTIAL PROVISION OF COMMUNITY-BASED SERVICES

Some case management organizations provide all community-based services needed by their clients; others simply coordinate services with other providers in the community. The degree to which an agency provides community-based services to its clients is, to a large extent, determined by its degree of financial control. Agencies that have the authority to purchase services typically provide more direct services than agencies that have little authority to purchase services.

The degree to which a case management agency provides community-based services can be divided into three models: the brokerage model, the combination model, and the direct services model.[16]

(1) Brokerage Model

Under the brokerage model, a case manager coordinates the different services of a client's care package, but the case management agency itself does not provide any services. Hence, the terms "brokering" or "linkaging" evolved, reflecting the emphasis given to coordinating and negotiating under this type of system.

(2) Combination Model

Under the combination model, a case management organization provides a limited number of services for the client, and coordinates the remainder of the needed services with external agencies.

(3) Consolidated Direct Services Model

Under the consolidated direct services model, the case management agency directly provides services to clients. Services are either provided by the organization itself or delivered through a contract. Typically, this type of organization has a single pool of funds from which it pays for both the services it directly offers and those provided through contracts.

(d) ORGANIZATIONAL AUSPICES

Case management can be provided through many different organizational structures. Among these are public social service agencies, Area Agencies on Aging, hospitals, private case management agencies, home health agencies, and HMOs. In addition, case management may be centrally delivered at the state level, provided in the community at a local level, or offered somewhere in between the two at a regional level. The organizational auspices of case management may be categorized into four groups: public, nonprovider case management systems; private, nonprovider case management systems; acute provider-based systems; and long-term care provider-based systems.

(e) FINANCIAL CONTROL

Case management organizations with the greatest degree of financial control are those with "statutory authority, and the power to requisition, terminate, and authorize payment for services."[17] This type of case management is often mandated by the state or insurer; the case manager has complete financial authority over all aspects of the program, including all components of case management and the delivery of services.

Case management systems with the second degree of control are those with no statutory authority, but with forceful monetary incentives and the ability to offer waivered services or contracts for service. This type of case management program is not mandated by the state, but does have a certain degree of financial authority. Case managers can receive financial authority, and the freedom to purchase certain services that are normally unavailable, through waivers of Medicare and Medicaid payments and through clients who give case managers the financial authority to purchase long-term care services.

The case management systems with the least control are those that are based on goodwill and staffed by volunteers. This type of case management system has the least degree of financial authority, and basically coordinates care with existing providers in the community.

In summary, case management systems for long-term care vary dramatically. Some of the dimensions in which case management systems differ include:

- The extent to which the case management services are client-focused or system-focused;
- The extent to which the services are professionalized;
- The extent to which the system is specialized in its provision of the components of case management;
- Whether the system has a medical, social service, or multidisciplinary emphasis;
- The organizational auspice (public, nonprovider; private, non-provider; acute, provider-based; or long-term care, provider-based);
- Total versus partial provision of case management services;
- Coordinated versus direct provision of community-based services;

- The degree of financial control over the provision of long-term care services.

§ 4.6 MODELS OF LONG-TERM CARE CASE MANAGEMENT

(a) CASE MANAGEMENT IN AREA AGENCIES ON AGING

(1) Definition and Background*

The Area Agencies on Aging (AAAs) are part of a large network of aging-related agencies funded through the Older Americans Act (OAA) and administered through the federal Administration on Aging (AoA). Part of this network includes 10 regional offices of the AoA, 57 State Units on Aging (SUAs), and 673 AAAs.

The AoA is mandated to be the chief advocate for the elderly at the national level and to coordinate federal efforts on their behalf. The AoA provides grants to states to plan and develop a comprehensive and coordinated system of social and nutrition services to assist older persons in living at home. AoA regional offices help states to develop programs for supportive services, such as nutrition services and multipurpose senior centers. These regional offices must approve plans submitted by state agencies. They also try to ensure statewide program effectiveness.[18]

SUAs, usually designated by the governor, have been established in each of the 50 states and the District of Columbia, the Commonwealth of Puerto Rico, the Virgin Islands, Guam, American Samoa, the Northern Mariana Islands, and the Trust Territory of the Pacific Islands. SUAs are responsible for state activities and programs funded by the Older Americans Act. SUAs must divide their states into planning and service areas and must designate an AAA to develop and administer the OAA programs in each area. The SUAs must also approve plans submitted by the AAAs and incorporate them into statewide plans. These plans are submitted to the AoA for review, approval, and funding.

Thirty-two SUAs function as independent, single-purpose agencies that report directly to the governor, and 25 SUAs are organized as units within multipurpose human service agencies.[19]

---

*Information for this section on AAAs comes from unpublished background papers for a publication by the Office of Technology Assessment on information and referral services and case management services for Alzheimer's patients; *Confused Minds, Burdened Families: Finding Help for People with Alzheimer's and Other Dementias* (1990).

Area Agencies on Aging are locally controlled and operated agencies designated by each state and designed to address the needs and concerns of older Americans at the local level. Every area of the country is covered by an AAA. The AAAs plan, coordinate, and advocate for the development of comprehensive community-based long-term care services that assist older persons to remain independent in their homes and communities. The National Association of Area Agencies on Aging (NAAAA) is a national nonprofit organization representing the interests of AAAs across the country.[20]

AAAs now number 670 nationally and are located in 44 states. Six states and the seven territories have designated their entire geographic area as a single planning and service area in which the SUA performs the AAA functions; this single designation reflects either small geographic area or small population size. An AAA can be a unit of county, city, or town government, or a private nonprofit agency.

A 1984 survey of 121 AAAs indicated that approximately 53 percent were single-purpose agencies and 47 percent were located in multipurpose agencies. The survey also found that 34 percent were private, nonprofit agencies; 33 percent were either regional planning or economic development agencies; 30 percent were county agencies; and 2.5 percent were city agencies. When designating an AAA, states are required to give preference to an existing office of aging operating within an area.[21] New York has the largest number of AAAs at 58.

(2) History

The AAAs were created under the 1973 Comprehensive Service Amendments to Title III of the Older Americans Act (OAA) of 1965. They form a national network developed to meet the social service needs of persons aged 60 or over.

Originally, the OAA established a state agency on aging in each state, to develop community projects that would provide social services for older Americans. In 1972, funds were provided to develop nutrition services. In 1973, states were required to designate planning and service areas, and local AAAs. Amendments to the OAA in 1978 consolidated the social services, nutrition services, and multipurpose senior center programs under Title III. Amendments in 1984 mandated particular attention to the needs of low-income, minority older persons and required AAAs to promote coordination of community-based long-term care services. Amendments in 1987 further defined, reinforced, and expanded the functions of the AAAs.

(3) Services

In addition to providing information and referral, advocacy, and comprehensive service delivery, AAAs are required "to develop an area plan and to carry out, directly or through contractual or other arrangements," a program of supportive services, nutrition services, and, where appropriate and needed, multipurpose senior centers.[22]

SUAs and AAAs have some choice in the supportive services they provide. Such services may include transportation, short-term counseling, legal assistance, and in-home services. Priority has been given to in-home services for the frail elderly. These services include homemaker and home health aides, visits and telephone reassurance, chore maintenance, in-home respite care and adult day care, and minor home modification (not to exceed $150 per client).

Although Title III funding for supportive and in-home services is relatively small (compared to Medicare and Medicaid expenditures), the SUAs and the AAAs can provide services otherwise unavailable to the elderly population, thereby helping persons who may be ineligible for services elsewhere.[23] For example, some state agencies have chosen to develop case management and assessment systems through the area agencies.[24] It is difficult to know for certain how many AAAs either provide or contract out for case management services. Not only is there a great deal of state-by-state variation in the AAAs' service packages but, for political reasons, different states use different labels (such as "advocacy") for case management activities. However, in 1986, AAAs contracted with more than 26,000 service providers nationwide for community-based services for the elderly. A 1987 NAAAA survey showed that 153 AAAs were providing case management services, including information and referral, screening, case conferencing, care plan development, follow-up monitoring, and reassessment.

(4) Clients

The OAA requires that all services be available to anyone aged 60 and over. Persons under 60 are usually not eligible for services. Furthermore, Title 45 of the Code of Federal Regulations (C.F.R. 1321.67) prohibits the use of means testing to determine eligibility for OAA services, and specifies that any contributions to cover the cost of services be on a voluntary basis. Cost sharing may be permitted for some programs that receive only state funding.[25]

Currently, OAA programs serve approximately 9 million older persons annually. The OAA specifies that older individuals with the greatest economic or social needs (low-income minority individuals) are to receive preference in obtaining OAA services. AAAs are required to give priority to serving frail, homebound, or isolated older persons. "Frail" is defined as having a physical or mental disability, including having Alzheimer's disease or a related disorder with neurological organic brain dysfunction, which restricts an individual from performing normal tasks or which threatens the capacity of an individual to live independently.[26]

(5) Costs and Reimbursement

For fiscal year 1988, the OAA appropriation for services was $834 million. Of this, $561 million was appropriated for nutrition services, $268 million for supportive services and senior centers, and $4.8 million for in-home services for the frail elderly. Congress makes separate appropriations for supportive services, congregate nutrition services, and home-delivered nutrition services. The law allows SUAs and AAAs some flexibility to transfer funds (up to 20 percent) among the three service categories.[27]

OAA funding is allocated to the states via grants based on a formula representing a state's portion of the national population aged 60 or older. SUA budgets vary significantly, depending on the size of the state's elderly population and the roles and responsibilities assigned to each SUA by the respective governors and state legislatures. States may combine OAA funding with other federal and state moneys and may coordinate programs with other health and social service agencies.

Title III funds make up 50 to 80 percent of the budgets of most SUAs; only 38.5 percent of the SUAs derive more than 50 percent of their funding from other sources.[28] For 1984, the total SUA budget was made up of 48.3 percent OAA funding, 26.5 percent state funding, 5 percent Title XX Social Services Block Grant funding, 14.9 percent of funding from other federal sources, and 5.3 percent from private and in-kind sources.[29] Depending on the size of the planning and service area and the number of older residents served, individual AAA budgets vary from slightly less than $100,000 to $14 million. Twenty-five percent of AAA funds were allocated to in-home services,[30] and approximately 50 percent of this allotment went for home-delivered meals. The rest was used for in-home services such as housekeeping, personal care, and chore services.[31]

(6) Case Management

Within the past few years, case management in the AAAs has become an extremely controversial subject. The OAA specifically forbids SUAs and AAAs from *providing* rather than *contracting for* services except where, "in the judgment of the state agency, provision of such services by the state agency or an area agency on aging is necessary to assure an adequate supply of such services, or where such services are directly related to such state or area agency on aging's administrative functions, or where such services of comparable quality can be provided more economically by such state or area agency on aging." The National Association of Area Agencies on Aging is seeking to persuade Congress that case management should not be defined as a direct service, that is, that AAAs should not be barred from providing case management.[32]

Many AAAs report that they provide case management, but there is much confusion about what constitutes "case management." Some AAAs consider case management to be an administrative function essential to ensuring access to community-based long-term care services. Other AAAs view case management as a direct service to the client and believe that AAAs are, and should be, prohibited from providing it. In 1987, the NAAAA proposed establishing the nation's 670 AAAs as specialists in elder care case management. This would create a nationally promoted and marketed program available to the general public on a fee-for-service basis. The proposal has sought to establish the AAAs as the recognizable access point nationwide—the point where the public could seek a case management assessment, the development of a care plan, brokering of services needed to fulfill the care plan, and monitoring of the care plan.

Through letters and testimony to Congress, the NAAAA has attempted to build the case that elder care management is simply a "newer, enhanced information and referral system," an integral part of the AAA's advocacy function, and "a very practical way of assessing both what the client needs and the community can provide."[33]

The proposal by the NAAAA to establish a nationwide fee-for-service case management service has been extremely controversial and has resulted in a sharp schism between the NAAAA and NASUA (National Association of State Units on Aging). The controversy centers around the federally mandated role of the AAAs as *contractors* rather than providers of service. The AAAs that were providing case management services before the controversy, and those planning to do so, have gone forward with this service provision.

(b) HOME HEALTH CARE AND CASE MANAGEMENT

(1) History

Until 1965, home health care services were not well known or widely available in the United States; they were not reimbursed by the federal government or by private insurers. In 1965, Medicare was enacted with a home health care (HHC) provision. Because no one at the time had extensive home health care experience, the federal government relied on the testimony of medical experts to develop a home health care model for implementation. The result was a Medicare HHC provision that was quite restrictive; over time, with more experience and history with home health care, these restrictions have been eased.

To be eligible to receive Medicare payments for HHC services, agencies must meet Medicare's certification requirements; that is, the agencies must primarily provide skilled nursing and other therapeutic services. Agencies that provide HHC services may include hospital-based HHC programs, freestanding private organizations, a variety of state and local agencies, and public health nursing and visiting nurse associations.

Since 1965, when the Medicare program was enacted, there has been tremendous growth in the number of HHC agencies. For example, in 1963, there were 1,163 HHC agencies in the United States, only 141 of which met later Medicare requirements that home health agencies provide at least one other therapeutic service in addition to skilled nursing care. By 1987, there were 5,877 HHC agencies nationwide that met Medicare certification requirements.[34]

In 1980, the Omnibus Reconciliation Act introduced major revisions of the Medicare HHC benefit, by eliminating the 100-visit limit and the 3-day prior hospitalization requirement (for Medicare Part A coverage) and the deductible and the 100-day visit limit (for Medicare Part B coverage). At the same time, the bill made it easier for proprietary HHC agencies to become Medicare-certified, opening the way for a sharp increase in the number of those types of HHC contractors and changing the proportion of proprietary/nonproprietary agencies dramatically.

In addition, recent studies indicate that the number of hospital-based HHC agencies is rapidly increasing.[35] The first hospital-based HHC program was established in 1947 at Montefiore Hospital in the Bronx, New York City. The primary purpose of hospital-based HHC has been to refer clients to the most appropriate home care services in a timely and well-coordinated fashion.[36] More recently, hospitals have attempted to offset some of their financial losses incurred after the implementation of Medicare's prospective payment system by developing such services. For instance, a 1985 American Hospital Association survey found that 75 percent of those hospitals responding had plans either to add or expand a hospital-based HHC program.[37]

(2) Services

Medicare's HHC benefit is basically an acute care benefit, based on the medical model; reimbursement occurs only for what the physician finds to be medically necessary. For example, Medicare HHC benefits are limited to those defined as homebound, needing intermittent (as opposed to chronic) skilled nursing services and/or physical therapy. Other services, such as occupational therapy, home health aide, and medical social work, are also Medicare-reimbursable if they are ordered by the physician to start in conjunction with the skilled nursing and physical therapy services outlined above. The actual care must be provided by or contracted by the HHC agency; fiscal intermediaries contract with the Health Care Financing Administration (HCFA) to provide the actual administration of the Medicare HHC program.

A survey conducted in 1983 by the House Aging Committee, and published by the U.S. Congress in 1985, outlined the typical services provided by the average Medicare-certified HHC agency.[38] The survey found that the average agency provided 13,530 annual visits (51 percent by registered nurses (RNs), 5 percent by licensed practical nurses (LPNs), less than 1 percent by physicians, 2 percent by medical social workers, and 14 percent by physical therapists). The average RN (or 1 full-time equivalent (FTE)) made 353 HHC visits per year, and the average home health aide (or 1 FTE) made 590 home visits per year. The HHC agencies received about 48 percent of their referrals from hospitals, 26 percent from physicians, and less than 6 percent from community service agencies. The survey also found that 46 percent of patients receiving HHC services were terminated from Medicare coverage because of "no further need," 26 percent because they were admitted to an institution (e.g., a hospital or nursing home), and 20 percent because they lacked insurance.

Home health care is a required service for state Medicaid programs. In addition, the Omnibus Budget Reconciliation Act of 1987 allowed a waiver program that has substantially increased the range of HHC services available to the elderly. These increased benefits include homemaker, personal care attendants, adult day care, and respite care services specifically for those who might otherwise be admitted to a nursing home.

(3) Staffing

Nurses do most of the case management in home health care; to a much smaller degree, it is done by social workers.[39] The House Aging Committee's 1983 survey outlined the staffing mix in the average Medicare-certified home health care agency and found that the average agency employs 45 employees (or 27.9 FTEs on a full- or part-time basis). An additional 7.67 FTEs are employed to provide direct care under contracts. Of these employees, 12.4 are RNs, 1.2 are LPNs, 0.4 are physicians, 2.9 are physical therapists, 0.7 have a Masters degree in social work, 0.9 are occupational therapists, 0.2 are bereavement counselors, and 9.7 are homemaker/home health aides. Of all the agency's employees, 74 percent are in direct care services and 26 percent are in administrative or clerical services.

The agencies usually contract for the services of physical, occupational, and speech therapists and they typically hire the RNs, LPNs, medical social workers, bereavement and other counselors, and homemaker/home health aides. The average agency also uses 8 volunteers, most of whom volunteer 20 hours a week or less. These volunteers split their time equally between direct patient services and administrative/clerical services.[40] The same survey found that, for the average Medicare-certified home health care agency, 73 percent of the clients are over 65 years of age and nearly 66 percent are women. The average agency delivered 13,530 home health care visits per year, or 9.6 visits per client. The average HHC agency reported serving many clients with diabetes, high blood pressure, heart and circulatory problems, stroke recovery, and cancers of various kinds.[41]

(4) Costs and Reimbursement in Home Health Care

Home health care services are reimbursed through several sources, including such public programs as Medicare, Medicaid, Title XX of the Social Services Block Grant Program, Title III of the Older Americans Act, and a variety of state aging programs. In addition, HHC agencies are reimbursed on a private-pay basis by home care clients and by a number of private third-party payers (e.g., insurance companies). Home health care agencies (particularly visiting nurse associations and public health nursing agencies) also offer provider services to those who are uninsured and from whom no payment or reimbursement can be expected.

It is difficult to calculate the actual cost to an agency of providing case management services within home health care. The calculation of cost varies by the time spent on selected activities, the personnel required, and the agency resource–overhead consumption. The costs also vary according to the scope of the HHC agency's case management services. A Veterans Administration study, cited by Cary, indicated that case management constitutes 27 to 29 percent of the cost of services for home care clients.[42] Other HHC agencies may report a smaller or greater percentage, based on the complexity of care for a particular client or the restrictions on access to community resources. Cary also pointed out that, as a rule, case management is not "unbundled" as a chargeable service that is billable to Medicare by HHC agencies serving older patients.

According to the 1983 survey by the House Aging Committee, the average client cost per visit to a Medicare-certified HHC agency was $37.95, or $364.32 per case. Typically, the agency was reimbursed by Medicare, on average, $26 to $45 for RN visits, $26 to $40 for physical therapy visits, and $20 or less for visits by homemaker/home health aides.[43]

Currently, Medicare is the largest third-party payer of HHC services in the nation. Medicaid's HHC reimbursements have also grown dramatically within recent years. In addition, HHC coverage has increased greatly in the private sector, with many insurance companies providing reimbursement for HHC in an attempt to contain the costs of hospitalization.

(5) Case Management in Home Health Care

As noted earlier, nurses have been predominantly responsible for case management within home care. The actual implementation of case management in home care depends on each HHC agency's philosophy, management objectives, productivity, quality assurance standards, and clients' service needs.

Home care agencies define and operationalize case management in at least two ways. The first definition focuses on the delivery *and* coordination of services for clients who are admitted to the agency. Activities included under this case management definition include:

- Preadmission—assessment of the referring provider's orders and the client's current and predicted health status; determination of the client's health care, financial, psychosocial, and environmental needs; determination of reimbursement resources; assessment of agency and community support systems to maintain the client optimally with home care services; the client's expectation and willingness to accept home care services; and interagency and interdisciplinary coordination meetings.

- Admission—intake; admission assessment of physical, mental, and social functioning; reimbursement resources; environmental and caregiver support sources; assessment of agency and community resources to respond to a plan of treatment orders and the client's emerging needs; planning of resource allocation requirements for care delivery; care coordination and continuity of care conferences; care delivery; evaluation of utilization, process, outcomes, and quality measures; assessment of patient/provider satisfaction and community perspectives.

- Continuity of care planning—assessing client needs and resources for optimal functioning upon termination of service; planning and arranging for service/informal care support upon discharge; advocating for clients' needs among community services; validating that transitional services are in place for clients who need them; communicating with providers and agencies offering postdischarge services; evaluating postdischarge outcomes.

Although preadmission, admission, and continuity of care planning are described as three separate processes, in actual practice they often occur simultaneously and reiteratively.

The second definition of case management in home health care focuses on the coordination of services for clients admitted to the agency. This definition of case management may include all of the activities previously listed under preadmission, admission, and continuity of care planning, but does not include the actual delivery of in-home services. An example of this type of case management is the demonstration project awarded to the Visiting Nurse Association of Texas by the Robert Wood Johnson Foundation. In this case, the care coordination is predominantly for non-health care services such as grocery shopping, personal care, errand service, household maintenance, and financial management.[44]

Many home health care agencies see care management as basic to their mission. Some have RNs whose primary function is to visit area hospitals on a routine basis. Their goals are to educate medical staff and social workers on the general principles of home care and private duty care and to coordinate services for specific patients. In discussions between these HHC RNs and the hospital staff, the RNs sometimes suggest sending a patient home earlier than originally planned, based on the needs and abilities of the patient and family.[45]

Case management, however, now ends once the patient no longer needs skilled nursing or physical therapy at home because, to comply with Medicare/Medicaid and private insurance guidelines, the case must be closed. Often, the HHC agency refers the patient and family to another resource to keep them connected to the health care delivery system. If and when the patient requires further skilled care at home, the active HHC status resumes. Thus, there is a loose and informal system of continuity of care between community services.

Another type of case management beginning to be provided by home health agencies is catastrophic case management following a major illness or accident. One such catastrophic case management program was designed and implemented in May 1988 as the Visiting Nurse Association Large Case Management (VNA/LCM) Program in St. Louis, Missouri. This program defines catastrophic case management as a process carried out by RNs to assess a patient and his or her current mode of care; to design the optimum treatment plan considering the patient's needs and monetary resources, and the available resources of the community; to recommend exceptions to the patient's current benefit plan, in order to achieve a treatment plan without additional expense to the patient or his or her insurance carrier; and to create a system in which someone coordinates all aspects of care for as long as the patient will benefit from such intervention.

The VNA/LCM Program has a national network of VNAs to do on-site reviews; to work directly with patients, family, and staff; and to give advice about local resources. Clients in the VNA/LCM Program are identified at the time of precertification for hospital admission. The VNA nurses work closely with utilization review firms that have computers programmed to print out a weekly list of patients whose admitting diagnosis requires screening for case management.

The VNA/LCM Program charges $400 for the initial assessment and recommendation, which is completed within five days of accepting the referral. To implement and maintain a care plan, the program charges $50 an hour. VNA/LCM is reimbursed either by the utilization review firm requesting the service or by the self-insurer.[46] The VNA/LCM Program does a final cost analysis to evaluate its effectiveness at maximizing the health care dollar. In the final report, the program evaluates how well the stated goals for the patient have been achieved.

The strengths of the VNA/LCM Program are its emphasis on patient advocacy and on developing a cohesive plan involving home care, after-care, day care, and self-help groups to provide wide support for the patient. However, the program suffers from some communication problems among various providers of care. Care plans are difficult to implement unless there is ongoing input from family members, benefit managers, and physicians.

(c) ADULT DAY CARE AND CASE MANAGEMENT

(1) Definition

Adult day care has come to occupy a small but important niche in the continuum of health and long-term care in the United States. Adult day care is difficult to define because it serves a wide variety of needs and clients, from frail and isolated elderly with minimal support needs to rather severely disabled or demented persons who need virtually total support.[47] Most centers serve clients whose needs fall between these two extremes.

The National Institute on Adult Daycare (NIAD), a constituent unit of the National Council on Aging, defines adult day care as:

> A community-based program designed to meet the needs of functionally impaired adults through an individual plan of care. It is a structured, comprehensive program that provides a variety of health, social, and related support services in a protective setting during any part of a day but less than 24-hour care. Individuals who participate in adult day care attend on a planned basis during specified hours. Adult day care assists its participants to remain in the community, enabling families and other caregivers to continue caring for an impaired member at home.[48]

It is important to differentiate adult day care from the senior center and the nursing home. Both adult day care centers and senior centers provide socialization, recreation, meals, and transportation, but the staff at the senior center do not establish a care plan for participants. In contrast, establishing treatment goals is important in adult day care. While adult day care centers may serve severely impaired persons and use a care plan, they actually provide care for a limited number of hours during each day, and most participants attend 2 or 3 days a week. One goal of adult day care is to help keep participants in the community and living at home. In contrast, people who use nursing homes actually live in the facility full-time, 7 days a week.[49]

According to NIAD, the goals for adult day care include:

- Promoting the individual's maximum level of independence;
- Maintaining the individual's present level of functioning as long as possible, preventing or delaying further deterioration;
- Restoring and rehabilitating the individual to his or her highest possible level of functioning;
- Providing support, respite, and education for families and other caregivers;
- Fostering socialization and peer interaction;
- Serving as an integral part of the community service network and the long-term care continuum.[50]

Adult day care centers are sponsored by a wide variety of organizations—private, nonprofit agencies (74 percent) and public agencies or joint public/private sponsorship (16 percent). Recently, for-profit agencies (10 percent) have also been setting up adult day care centers.[51] Sponsoring groups include corporations, local governments, schools, churches, senior centers, nursing homes, hospitals, home health care agencies, rehabilitation centers, and others. Day care centers may be located in the sponsoring organization's own facility or in some other suitable and convenient location, such as a local church. Recently, some new adult day care centers have been housed in facilities specially designed and constructed for them.[52]

There are many models of adult day care (because the population served is so diverse), but the main models at this time are adult day health care (the medical model, which emphasizes medical supervision and care), the social/recreational model (which emphasizes the social stimulation and recreational benefits of adult day care), and adult day care designed especially for persons with Alzheimer's disease.[53]

(2) History

Adult day care first started in the former Soviet Union in the form of day hospitals for psychiatric patients.[54] These psychiatric day hospitals, designed to help patients stay at home while receiving intensive outpatient therapy, developed to alleviate a shortage of hospital beds by allowing for earlier discharge of patients.[55] Day hospitals developed in the United States between 1945 and 1949 in Massachusetts, Kansas, and Connecticut.[56] In an evolving form of the psychiatric model, Great Britain began to develop day hospitals for disabled elderly adults. The first British geriatric day hospital used nurses and occupational therapists as staff and provided physical therapy, social work and geriatric services, transportation, and meals. Adult day care, as we know it today, did not arrive in the United States until the 1960s, when the first center was established in North Carolina.

By 1973, there were fewer than 15 adult day care programs in the United States. By 1978, there were 300 centers, and by 1980 the number had grown to 618.[57] By 1986 estimates, there were 1,200 adult day care centers in the United States.[58] The average enrollment was 37, and these centers served more than 44,000 families at any given time.[59]

(3) Services

Adult day care centers provide a specially designed setting for the daytime care of frail, disabled adults who do not need 24-hour nursing-home care but who do need regular professional supervision. Not only do adult day care centers provide exercise, activities, and a social life for participants, but they also give a respite break for caregiving family members.

Most adult day care centers are open 5 days a week, and 50 percent are open 8 hours or more a day. Some centers are open 2 or 3 days a week, and some are open on Saturdays. The average center serves 19 participants a day, with a total caseload of 37.[60]

Although there is great diversity in terms of services, target populations, funding, and staffing, adult day care centers share certain basic components. These components include individual care plans for participants; supervision or assistance with the activities of daily living (walking, eating, bathing, dressing, and toileting); written policies and procedures for dealing with medical emergencies or environmental disasters such as fires; planned activities; health screening/monitoring/education; nutrition services (a noontime meal and morning and afternoon snacks); dietary counseling; and transportation to and from the center as needed. Emotional support for participants and their families, information and referral services, and advocacy on behalf of participants are other basic components. Other services that may be available in adult day centers include:

- Distribution and/or supervision of medications;
- Skilled nursing;
- Physical, occupational, and speech therapy;
- Physician services;
- Podiatry, audiology, ophthalmology, and dentistry;
- Homemaker, home health, or chore services;
- In-home respite care (sitters and companions);
- Art, poetry, or music therapy;
- Sheltered workshop;
- Specialized services for particular patient populations (such as persons with Alzheimer's disease, Parkinson's disease, head trauma, and stroke).[61]

(4) Staffing

Nurses, social workers, and recreational therapists are the most commonly reported paid professional staff in adult day care centers. These staff members often direct the center. Physicians, psychiatrists, or dentists may be available as part-time consultants. Other professionals and laypersons may volunteer their services as needed.[62]

(5) Clients

Adult day care centers serve a wide variety of clients of various ages and conditions. A study by the NIAD has indicated that the average adult day care center participant is a 73-year-old white woman who lives with friends or relatives and has an average monthly income of $487.[63] Half of adult day care clients require some degree of supervision; one-fifth require close, constant supervision; one-fifth use canes or walkers; and one-eighth need help to transfer from their wheelchairs. Problems with incontinence and disruptive behavior are not uncommon; one in 13 clients needs changing during the day because of incontinence of bowel or bladder, and one in 13 has a behavioral problem and is disruptive.

Webb has stressed that adult day care serves to help both the participant and the caregiver:

> Adult day care participants are a severely impaired population. It is often difficult to care for them within the day care center. Care at home may be even harder—in that home care is most often provided by family or friends who have no special training to do what they must do. At the

same time, if the home situation breaks down, all the work the day care staff has done with the participant may be for naught. For this reason, adult day care centers take on the large task of serving not only the participant, but also attending to the needs of the participant's family. The extent of involvement with families varies among centers. . . . All adult day care centers, however, must somehow determine that the care provided at home is adequate to support the goals of the center. And that involves caring for families. Adult day care services, then, have a dual nature—focused both toward the participant and the family. Because of this, the term client [often refers] to the whole family unit. This terminology is one way of recognizing a basic fact of day care: as [adult day care] providers, we must work in concert with the participants' families, and in attendance to their needs.[64]

(6) Costs and Reimbursement

Fees and donations from clients are the major funding base for adult day care; however, most clients cannot afford to pay the full cost of adult day care. This means that many adult day care centers try to develop fund-raising activities or seek government or foundation grants or contracts to supplement client fees. The average daily cost for adult day care services is $27.[65] Unless the participant is eligible for Medicaid benefits, adult day care services are usually paid for out-of-pocket. Currently, neither Medicare nor private insurers reimburse for adult day care services.[66] However, there are bills before Congress to make adult day care services eligible for Medicare coverage or to establish it as a separate Medicare service.[67] Twenty-one states currently have Medicaid reimbursement. Thirty-six states have opted to request "2176 waivers" permitted under Section 2176 of the Omnibus Reconciliation Act of 1984, which allowed adult day care payment through Medicaid. Other programs receive Title III money from the Older Americans Act, Title XX of the Social Security Act, United Fund, miscellaneous grants, and private pay. According to the Office of Technology Assessment:

> States pay for adult day care with funds from Title III of the Older Americans Act, the Social Services Block Grant, and Medicaid Home and Community (2176) Waivers. Approximately two-fifths of the funds come from nongovernment sources such as participants' fees, foundations, donations, fund raising, private insurance, and United Way. Funding sources may influence the types of services a program offers. For example, programs using Medicaid funds have a health care orientation whereas programs using Social Services Block Grant funds offer only social services. Where possible, programs use multiple sources of funding to provide both social and medical services.[68]

The Veterans Administration also provides reimbursement for adult day care services. The VA is funding the entire cost of 15 health model programs that are operated out of VA medical centers. The VA also has allocated $2 million to be spent on adult day health care (ADHC), which is provided to veterans by their local community ADHC centers under contract with the VA. The average cost per patient per day in the VA programs is $50, including primary medical care. Average daily cost in the VA contract programs in the community is $35.[69]

(7) Case Management in Adult Day Care

When they design a program, adult day care staff must decide which services to offer, which populations to target, and what eligibility requirements to develop for participants.[70] After clients are admitted to the center, case management services in adult day care should include the basic components of any good case management system—assessment, planning, service coordination and referral, monitoring, and reassessment.

Generally speaking, participants at adult day care centers live in the community and are frail elderly persons. Many of them have been involved with other agencies for varying lengths of time, and some are receiving other services in addition to adult day care. It is the policy of most adult day care centers to perform case management services if they are the primary sources of assistance to the participant. If another agency (such as the County Nursing Service or Social Services) is already involved, the adult day care staff usually cooperate in planning services but do not necessarily take over the planning. As the adult day care center moves toward the medical model, case management becomes more important and is more emphasized.[71]

In most adult day care centers, case management has routinely been performed, almost as a given, when a plan of care is developed. In Ohnsorg's opinion, there are few settings where the staff know so much about an individual who is still living in the community. The staff have privileged access to a great deal of information about the client's medical, health, emotional, financial, environmental, family and support network, past history, and current situation. Staff are involved with assisting families in many ways, but the help often stops short of a thorough case management system, for two reasons: (1) there may be a lack of staff with appropriate expertise, and (2) the staff may lack authorization for new services and payment for services.[72]

(d) CASE MANAGEMENT IN STATE NURSING-HOME PREADMISSION SCREENING PROGRAMS

(1) Definition/Background

One type of case management that has been developed in a majority of states over the past decade is state-administered preadmission screening (PAS) programs. These programs are designed to screen applicants prior to nursing-home admission, to ensure that nursing-home care is needed and appropriate. In most cases, PAS attempts to control costs and utilization by identifying those at risk for nursing-home placement and substituting less expensive home- or community-based care for costly nursing-home care.

Cost control, particularly the reduction of Medicaid expenditures, is the primary goal of many of these state programs. Medicaid expenditures have risen tremendously over the past decade, in large part because of increases in nursing-home costs. Many states limit screening programs to Medicaid-eligible persons, often as a prerequisite to receiving Medicaid-funded nursing-home or in-home services. Cost control is not, however, the only goal. PAS also attempts to improve the quality of life for older persons and their families by assisting them in making appropriate long-term care decisions and in maintaining independence.

These programs vary tremendously from state to state.[73] Generally, however, applicants receive a comprehensive in-home assessment of their needs, and then are offered a recommendation concerning what long-term care services are needed and where they should be provided—in the home or in an institution. Assessments generally include an evaluation of the client's physical and mental health, functional status, and formal and informal social supports. In some cases, home care services are then provided to those at risk for nursing-home placement, in order to prevent or delay institutionalization.

The number and scope of PAS programs have increased considerably in the past decade. A 1986 study indicated that 31 programs were operational in 29 states and the District of Columbia.[74] Twenty-one (68 percent) of these programs operated on a statewide basis, and 10 (32 percent) were partial state programs. Six states were also found to conduct a two-level screening process in which an initial screening was used to determine which participants required a more extensive assessment. These are referred to as "screen-to-screen" programs.

Programs were operated through a large variety of state agencies: Department of Health Services, Department of Human Resources,

Department on Aging, and Department of Medical Assistance. Local administration was conducted through public agencies in 25 programs (51 percent); 6 programs (19 percent) subcontracted at least a portion of their services to private agencies.

(2) Scope of Services

Comprehensiveness of Screening. An important aspect of PAS, affecting its cost and effectiveness, concerns the comprehensiveness of the screening. The comprehensiveness of the screening varies by state program, and may also vary by client origin—whether the person being screened originates from a community setting (usually his or her own home), a hospital, or a nursing home (as a nursing-home transfer) (Table 4.2).

Physical health, mental health, and functional status are assessed in all PAS programs, regardless of client origin.[75] Informal social supports (e.g., nonpaid assistance from family and friends) are another frequently assessed aspect of a client's status. Ninety-one percent of programs screening community or hospital clients assess informal social supports, as do a large majority (70 percent) of programs screening nursing-home transfers.

The assessment of formal social supports (e.g., paid services from an agency or individual) shows similar variation by client origin. Over 85 percent of programs screening community and hospital clients assess formal supports, compared to 60 percent of programs screening

Table 4.2
Components of Assessments

	Client Origin		
	Community	Hospital	Nursing-Home Transfer
Total*	23	22	10
Physical health	23 (100%)	22 (100%)	10 (100%)
Mental health	23 (100%)	22 (100%)	10 (100%)
Financial resources	15 (65%)	15 (68%)	7 (70%)
Formal social support	20 (87%)	19 (86%)	6 (60%)
Informal social support	21 (91%)	20 (91%)	7 (70%)
Functional status	23 (100%)	22 (100%)	10 (100%)
Other	9 (39%)	10 (45%)	2 (20%)

*Number of states reporting assessment data for this client origin group (with 31 states reporting programs).

Source: Adapted from L. Iversen, *A Description and Analysis of State Pre-Admission Screening Programs.* Excelsior, MN: InterStudy, 1986.

nursing-home transfers. The screening of transfers may exclude these factors because these clients have fewer supports, or their status is already known, or they have a smaller chance of returning to the community.

An evaluation of financial resources is included in approximately two-thirds of the programs' assessments, regardless of client origin. All states evaluate some aspect of their clients' financial status, but this evaluation may not be part of the screening process; that is, it may constitute a separate evaluation.

Other aspects of client status are evaluated in a number of states. Community and hospital client evaluations may include living arrangements, family motivation, medication and treatments, cognitive functioning, and the overall ability to remain in the community.

Services Funded, Provided, or Coordinated in Conjunction with PAS. In many states, screening is just one component of a more comprehensive case management system. These states believe that screening cannot be effective without an accompanying system for funding, providing, and coordinating community-based services. Screening and recommendations for home care may be meaningless, for example, if necessary services are not available and affordable. Other states argue that service provision and service coordination are unnecessary because they duplicate family efforts to arrange care. More frequently, the costs associated with case management services deter states from offering them. How states balance these issues and decide whether to fund, provide, and coordinate services in addition to PAS is important in evaluating the cost, significance, and effectiveness of PAS.

Survey data from the 1986 study of PAS indicate that a majority of states do arrange, fund, or provide community services.[76] Seventeen of the 25 programs (68 percent) providing the data reported that they fund, provide, or coordinate community services in conjunction with PAS.

The most frequently *coordinated* services—those coordinated in at least 11 programs—included skilled nursing at home, personal care, transportation, home-delivered meals, homemaker/housekeeper, and home health aide services. Chore/homemaker services were also arranged in 10 programs. Adult day care and respite care were coordinated in 8 programs; congregate meals, in 7 programs; and "other" services, in 6 programs. "Other" services included counseling and occupational therapy; mental health and rehabilitation services; physical, speech, and occupational therapy; nursing home and other referrals;

and, in Wisconsin's program, "any service the client needs as long as the county maintains average caseload costs within the allocation."

Personal care services, home health aide services, and homemaker/ housekeeper are the most frequently *funded* services. Adult day care is funded in 8 programs, chore/home maintenance services and transportation services, in 7 programs, and respite care, in 6 programs. Less commonly funded services include skilled nursing and home-delivered meals (5 programs each) and congregate meals (2 programs).

Few states report that they provide services in conjunction with their PAS program. Personal care, homemaker/housekeeper, chore/ home maintenance, and adult day care are provided in 3 programs. Services provided by 1 or 2 programs include skilled nursing, transportation, home health aide services, congregate meals, home-delivered meals, respite care, and counseling/occupational therapy.

(3) Staff

Overall, RNs are most frequently involved in the PAS screenings. In the 1986 survey of 31 programs, all programs that screened nursing-home transfers used RNs, as did the vast majority of programs screening clients from hospitals (95 percent) or the community (91 percent). These high rates indicate that the medical status of applicants is perceived to be a primary factor affecting whether the applicant will receive home care or nursing-home care.

Social workers are also included in a large number of programs: 91 percent of programs screening community clients and 83 percent of programs screening hospital clients utilize social workers. Social workers are used to screen nursing-home transfers in 70 percent of the programs.

Physicians and others (such as mental health/retardation professionals and case managers) participate in the screening process in fewer than half the programs. They are most likely to screen community clients (43 percent of community screening programs involve physicians and 35 percent involve "others") and least likely to screen nursing-home transfers.

About a quarter of all programs use RN/social worker teams to conduct PAS. Larger teams are more often used to assess community and hospital clients than nursing-home transfers. Forty-eight percent of the programs screening community clients and 41 percent of those screening hospital clients report that their teams are comprised of an RN, a social worker, a physician, and/or an "other" professional. These larger teams conduct nursing-home assessments in 40 percent of the programs.

(4) Clients

States vary significantly in the types of clients they serve. Medicaid eligibility is often used to determine who receives PAS. As of 1986, 10 programs (32 percent) screened only those eligible for Medicaid, and 6 (19 percent) screened Medicaid-eligible persons and those expected to soon become eligible for Medicaid. Fifteen programs (48 percent) reported that all nursing-home applicants may or must be screened, regardless of income and resources. Generally, this means that Medicaid-eligible persons are required to be screened to receive Medicaid funds, and private-pay clients may request a screening. In 3 states, all nursing-home applicants are required to be screened, regardless of income or resources.

As noted previously, program participants may also vary by client origin (e.g., whether clients are from the community or a hospital, or are nursing-home transfers). Of the programs reporting these data in the 1986 survey, a large majority (92 percent) screened clients coming from the community, and 88 percent screened hospital clients. Nursing-home transfers were screened in only 40 percent of the programs.

A third way in which some programs determine who receives PAS is by conducting a two-level screening process. Six "screen-to-screen" states relied on initial functional and health information in 1986, to determine whether a client required a more comprehensive screening. The purpose of "screen-to-screen" programs is to ensure that the state's limited resources are used to conduct comprehensive screenings only for those clients who want or need it.

States may also limit the coordination, funding, and provision of community services to a subgroup of those being screened. There is considerable variation among states regarding these eligibility criteria. In the 13 states reporting these data in 1986, 4 programs required that participants be older persons (age 60 or 65), and some type of means test was used to limit services in 7 programs. Other eligibility criteria are used to ensure that persons receiving home care would probably be institutionalized if they were not receiving the services. "At risk" for nursing-home placement in most cases is defined as meeting Medicaid level-of-care criteria for nursing-home placement or having applied for nursing-home care. Screening and a recommendation for community placement are prerequisites to receiving services in one program; in another, services are provided only if care plan costs are less than 60 percent of the Medicaid cost of nursing-home placement.

The number of persons screened varies greatly among states. In the 1986 survey, numbers ranged from 275 screened in Delaware's demonstration project (February to October, 1985) to 18,000 in Indiana's statewide program (fiscal year 1985).

(5) Cost and Reimbursement

Overall Funding Sources.   Perhaps the most important factor affecting any PAS program is its funding source: the amount of funding often determines the scope and significance of the program. The type of funding (e.g., state, federal, or local) may also affect program flexibility and the types of services that are required or appropriate. Regulations regarding the use of local funds, for example, are often more flexible than regulations governing state or federal funds.

Medicaid is the primary funder of PAS. In 1986, Medicaid funded all or a portion of 20 of the 23 PAS programs reporting these data. In 13 of these programs (57 percent), Medicaid funded the entire program. Other payment sources included state appropriations, Title XX Social Services Block Grants, state general revenues, and client fees. Not surprisingly, PAS payment sources vary according to whether the program serves Medicaid clients, other income-tested clients, and/or private-pay individuals. In most cases, federal Medicaid moneys fund at least half of the program.

Cost and Reimbursement per Screening.   Limited data show tremendous variation among states in the amounts they spend to conduct screenings, and in how much reimbursement they receive per screening. In 1986, reported costs per screening ranged from $28 to $148, and reimbursements ranged from $28 to $160. No data are available for a direct comparison of reimbursement to costs.

(6) Evaluation of Effectiveness—Past Research

At present, a conclusive quantitative analysis of the effectiveness of PAS programs is not possible because few studies in this area have been completed. One reason for the lack of research is that most programs are relatively new; another reason is that states rarely have the time and staff to conduct comprehensive data analysis. In addition, PAS programs vary greatly from state to state, making comparisons difficult.

Finally, results of studies that have been conducted must be viewed cautiously because of the complex and constantly changing nature of the long-term care system. Determining what effect PAS has had on long-term care admissions and costs in the midst of these changes is extremely difficult.

The few studies that have been conducted regarding PAS do not allow many generalizations because of the tremendous variation, among states, in how and why PAS is implemented. In some states, for instance, PAS is only one component of a comprehensive home- and community-based case management system in which services are funded, provided, or coordinated. In other states, there are no formal linkages between PAS and community-based programs. Even in these instances, however, programs may vary in the amount of informal contact they have with health and long-term care providers.

Another important variation among states that makes evaluation difficult is whether the screening teams' recommendations are binding or advisory. Given the limited data and the variations, therefore, it is likely that current studies at best only hint at the effect PAS can have on overall utilization of long-term care services.

The few studies that have directly or indirectly addressed the question of whether PAS and other case management programs can control costs or utilization show mixed results and reflect the limited data and analysis that are available for PAS at this time.[77-82] There is some evidence, however, that PAS and related home care programs increase the use of community-based services without reducing nursing-home utilization.

Mixed results have also been reported in a more subjective study of the perceived impact of PAS on long-term care. In the 1986 study of PAS programs, Medicaid directors and PAS program were asked to report how they felt PAS had affected community services, nursing homes, and the overall long-term care system.[83]

Eighty-six percent of the respondents felt that the utilization of community services had increased because of PAS, and 33 percent felt that PAS had increased community service costs. None of the respondents felt that PAS had decreased the utilization or cost of community services. As for the effect on nursing homes, respondents most frequently reported that the costs and utilization of nursing homes had not been affected. Nearly half (43 percent) of the respondents, however, felt that PAS had reduced the cost of long-term care, with 10 percent perceiving an increase, and 48 percent believing that there was no change or they "didn't know."

These mixed results show the need for additional research on PAS, to more accurately determine its effect on costs and utilization of long-term care services. These studies also indicate, however, that PAS may be increasing, rather than decreasing, the overall cost of long-term care, because it is increasing the cost and use of home and community services without a corresponding reduction in nursing-home utilization. (PAS could, however, be slowing the increase in long-term care costs.)

(7) Strengths and Weaknesses of State-Administered Preadmission Screening Programs

A major advantage of PAS for the elderly and their families is that, because the programs are connected to the Medicaid system, all persons seeking Medicaid-financed nursing-home coverage are linked to the PAS system. This means that a large number of older persons have access to the services and that long-term care services are coordinated for them. Compared to programs offered by other providers, a state-administered, nonprofit program may be (or is perceived to be) more concerned with meeting client needs. In short, PAS staff may offer the most objective screenings possible. Further, most PAS programs provide a fairly comprehensive evaluation of an individual's needs and assist persons in seeking and funding alternative services as available. As such, PAS services are generally both comprehensive and funded.

PAS may have important advantages for public policymakers because it provides a mechanism for potentially controlling costs and/or offering the most appropriate services possible.

It is also important to note, however, that PAS policymakers are not at all a homogeneous group. Some policymakers may have cost control as the major or only goal of PAS; others may have a great commitment to expanding services. One weakness of PAS is that, because it is state-administered, it is subject to changing, and possibly inconsistent, directives at the state level. At the same time, balancing comprehensive coverage and cost control in a legislative process may help ensure an appropriate balance between these often conflicting goals.

The major disadvantage of PAS is that, for several reasons, it simply may not be effective in controlling utilization. One reason is that basic assumptions underlying the programs may be invalid. Specifically, most programs are developed under the assumption that there are many people at risk for nursing-home placement who could be diverted to less expensive home care. This assumption may be erroneous: it may well be that few persons applying for nursing-home admission can be diverted. Because older persons generally prefer home care to nursing-home care, it is likely that many nursing-home applicants and their families are aware of available options and have considered the nursing-home placement option only after all other alternatives have been exhausted. Diversion might be more likely if PAS could be conducted well before nursing-home admission was applied for or considered.

Diversion may also be difficult if home- or community-based services are not available (in rural areas, for example). Some individuals may not have family or friends willing or able to assist them in living at home. In some areas, the supply of community services may be inadequate to meet the needs of the older population. The implementation of diagnosis-related groups (DRGs) and other prospective payment arrangements has resulted in shorter hospital stays. Reportedly, a greater number of individuals now need home care services, and many communities apparently have not been able to meet this increased demand. Formal community assistance may be unavailable to some persons because overall demand in the community is too low to warrant the development of a service network. Some rural areas, for example, may not have agencies that provide home health care, adult day care, or other supportive services.

A second problem that may hinder the cost effectiveness of PAS is that it must be assumed that only those persons at risk for nursing-home placement are receiving PAS-related services. PAS generally provides clients with both a comprehensive assessment and information about alternatives to nursing-home placement. It may also provide home care services, to prevent institutionalization. These valuable services may be sought out by many persons, not only those at immediate risk for nursing-home placement. It is possible that considerable resources are being spent on assessing and advising persons who are not at risk for institutionalization. In short, PAS may be inefficient in that services are not well-targeted to the population most at risk and in need. This is an especially important factor for programs that coordinate and fund services in conjunction with the screening.

Although important to the success of PAS, the evaluation of who is at risk for institutionalization is not easily done. Numerous studies have suggested that age, gender, medical health, functional and psychological status, and informal support systems may be indicators of risk. However, these variables may interact with one another, and their relative importance appears to vary considerably from study to study. Moreover, several of the factors, such as informal support systems, are very difficult to measure or predict consistently.

Although each of these issues is important, the ability of PAS to control long-term care utilization is perhaps most adversely affected by the fact that PAS policymakers, administrators, and screening personnel perceive and emphasize different, and sometimes conflicting, program goals. Policymakers are likely to be pressured by shrinking state and federal budgets and escalating long-term care costs. Line staff, however, encounter the pressures of individual clients and families with long-term care needs. To them, home care may be seen as a benefit for frail older persons in general, rather than only for those persons who are at immediate risk for institutionalization. If PAS staff view home care services only as a substitute for institutional care, they may be forced to deny time and services to persons who are not at immediate risk for nursing-home placement, but who may still need home care services to improve their quality of life.

In a recent national survey, PAS administrators were asked to indicate what they felt various groups perceived to be the primary purpose of PAS. Considering all groups, "improving the quality of life for the elderly" was perceived to be the most important reason for implementing PAS. Government policymakers, however, were perceived to regard containing or reducing the cost of long-term care as the most important reason. Differences in goals at the policy level versus goals at the implementation level may also explain the previously discussed finding that almost no respondents felt that nursing-home costs had decreased as a result of PAS, and none felt that community costs had decreased; yet, 43 percent felt the overall cost of long-term care had been reduced. Respondents may have felt that PAS is supposed to reduce general costs, but when specific costs were considered, they perceived no reduction. Open-ended responses to the survey also strongly indicated that PAS administrators felt that there was a need to provide more funding and more community services. These results again indicate that policymakers may see PAS as a way to control utilization of services, while PAS administrators see screening as a way to expand the provision of services.

In addition to disadvantages related to the political nature of PAS and its questionable effectiveness in controlling utilization, PAS may be viewed by health care and case management providers as interference and competition. Many hospitals and nursing homes, for instance, already feel they provide adequate case management services and see PAS as duplicative and unnecessary. More importantly, some providers may feel that PAS actually interferes with the client/provider relationship if clients experience PAS in addition to the provider's case management. Finally, PAS may be viewed as a competitor by case management firms, if persons are choosing to be served by the public program rather than seeking private services.

(e) PRIVATE GERIATRIC CASE MANAGEMENT

(1) History and Definition

Case management for older persons and their families has been an important part of the long-term care continuum for almost two decades. As the complexity of the service system has grown, so too has the need for assessment, planning, service coordination, and ongoing support in negotiating the system. Private case management firms seek to meet those needs for individuals who either do not qualify for publicly funded programs or who seek a different type of service than they would receive in the public sector.

The emergence of private case management as a distinct field is the result of many factors, including a rapidly growing older population; increasing concern over the cost of services; growth in the number and types of services targeted at the elderly and thus the complexity of the system; the entrepreneurial spirit of a number of human service professionals; and a realization that public programs cannot meet the care coordination needs of all older persons and their families.

(2) Organizational Aspects

Private case management is a relatively new phenomenon and is performed primarily by small firms that have been in business for 5 years or less. A 1987 study found that a majority (70 percent) of these firms are independent and self-managed; those reporting formal affiliation with another organization are predominantly affiliated with hospitals, social service agencies (both public and private), and nursing homes.[84] Almost 65 percent of private case management firms operate on a for-profit basis. Interestingly, the vast majority (75 percent) of the nonprofit providers are affiliated with another organization.

(3) Services

Most private case managers provide four components of the case management process: assessment, planning, service coordination/referral, and monitoring. A few firms, however, provide only the first three components; their involvement in a case ends after referral. Some case managers indicate that it is not uncommon for clients to request only an assessment and referral. For some clients, this may be enough. For other clients, particularly those without informal support systems, the complete process is considered essential. Almost universally, a multidimensional assessment is completed by the case manager, although the medical assessment is often performed by a physician. Planning generally includes both short- and long-term strategies and involves family members or other informal supports in addition to the elderly client. Service coordination often includes contacting direct service providers, assisting with form completion, arranging services from other agencies, and obtaining nursing-home or housing placement. The monitoring process is usually ongoing, with reassessment provided as needed.

In addition to the basic components of case management, many private case managers provide client and/or family counseling. More than 25 percent of private case management firms provide psychotherapy, retirement planning, support groups, and financial counseling to their clients. Relatively few firms provide direct home care services, transportation, chore services, or respite care. The types of direct services provided by private case management firms vary somewhat, depending on the types of staff employed. Firms employing at least one case manager who is a registered nurse (RN) or whose highest level of education is a bachelor's degree (BA/BS) tend to directly provide homemaker, home health aide, home health care, and companion services slightly more often than do firms only employing case managers with the master's degree in social work (MSW) or other specialities. Firms employing case managers with MSW degrees, other master's degrees, or more advanced degrees, tend to provide direct psychotherapy and counseling services more often than do firms employing case managers with less advanced degrees.

Controversy surrounds the issue of whether case managers should provide direct services. The concern is that case management firms that are also direct service providers will limit the service choices of their clients to only those the firm has available. It is argued that a case manager who is also a direct service provider will not be able to be a true advocate for the client but rather will have an allegiance to the needs of the firm. There is particular concern about situations in which the case manager has control of a client's funds, as is often true when guardianship services are provided.

The opposing belief is that there is no more conflict of interest for a case manager providing direct services than there is for an attorney acting as a guardian or a banker providing financial counseling. The code of ethics and practice principles of the profession should provide the necessary safeguards to prevent manipulation of the client and his or her funds. It is also argued that a case management firm that provides direct services can have far greater control over the quality of service provision than a firm that only makes referrals to outside providers; in addition, families sometimes prefer to work with one person who can access all services rather than with several different individuals.

Referral Sources.   Private case managers coordinate and refer their clients to a wide variety of services. The number and types of services enlisted are affected by five primary factors: (1) client needs, (2) client resources, (3) services provided directly by the case management firm, (4) services available in the community, and (5) client eligibility.

The majority (75 percent or more) of private case management firms refer their clients to home health aides, homemaker services, home health care, legal services, in-home meals, transportation, adult day care, respite care, companion services, senior centers, and nursing homes. Referrals to housing placement, financial counseling, psychotherapy, and client or caregiver counseling occur less often, probably because these services are often provided directly by private case management firms.

Personalized Service.   The types of services provided and coordinated by private case managers do not set them apart from other providers of case management. Rather, their personalization of service seems to be their distinguishing factor. Private case managers, who enjoy smaller caseloads, greater flexibility, and more autonomy than case managers in agency settings, have the freedom to customize the services they provide to a much greater degree.[85] The personalization of services can be done in a number of ways; perhaps most frequently cited is their availability on nights, weekends, and holidays—times when most agency offices are closed. Private case managers make themselves available at the convenience of the client or the client's family. They are often able to act more quickly on behalf of a client than are agency case managers, who have large, prioritized caseloads. As a result, private case managers are in a position to be proactive—the client need not be in crisis to seek services (although crisis status is common). They are also able to provide the personal touches that place the case manager in the role of "surrogate adult child" rather than merely "service provider."

(4) Staffing

More than 65 percent of private case management firms employ only one or two case managers, usually individuals with postgraduate degrees (often in social work). Caseloads for private case managers are small (1 to 20 cases per month). Many case management firms have limited administrative or secretarial support; just over 45 percent employ part-time administrative or secretarial personnel.

(5) Clients

The clients served by private case managers fit the description of the general population of older persons in need of supportive services. Typically, they are in their late 70s or early 80s, female, widowed, living alone, and have annual incomes of $35,000 a year or less (most often, $5,000 to $15,000 per year). Low-income clients usually have friends and family members who pay for the services of the private case manager. Private case managers also work with attorneys, bankers, corporations, and insurance and disability companies to help employees and clients find needed services.

(6) Cost and Reimbursement

Fees for private case management are generally set in five different ways: hourly rate, set rate per session, set rate for a "package" of services, set rates that vary according to the case management function provided, and sliding fee scales.

Over 57 percent of private case management firms use an hourly rate in setting fees for some, if not all, of their clients; 31 percent use a sliding fee scale; 26 percent use a set rate that varies according to the services provided; 19 percent use a set rate per session; and 9 percent use a set rate for a package of services. Many firms use more than one fee-setting method in establishing rates.[86]

Hourly rates charged for private case management ranged from $13 to $100 in 1987. However, just over half (51.5 percent) of private case management firms charged $41 to $60 per hour, and more than half of those (53 percent) charged $50 per hour.[87] In 1989, the range of hourly charges was $50 to $150, with the average hourly charge between $80 and $100.[88]

(7) Payment Sources

Payments for private case management come from five sources: (1) client (out-of-pocket); (2) family/caregiver (out-of-pocket); (3) private insurance; (4) Medicare; (5) Medicaid.

A variety of sources are reportedly used by clients to pay for case management services, but most payments are privately paid out-of-pocket by the client or the family/caregiver. Nearly all private case management firms (91 percent) report that at least some of the payments they receive are paid out-of-pocket by the client,[89] and 77 percent report that at least some of their fees are paid out-of-pocket by the family/caregiver.

(8) National Association of Private Geriatric Care Managers (NAPGCM)

The purpose of this association of private practitioners is ". . . the development, advancement, and promotion of humane and dignified social, psychological, and health care for the elderly and their families through counseling, treatment, and the delivery of concrete services by qualified, certified providers."[90] NAPGCM seeks to work toward the highest quality of care for the elderly and their families through education, advocacy, and ethical standards of private practice. The NAPGCM was founded in 1986; in 1991, it had 460 members located in 40 states, had developed a code of ethics, and was working to develop an accreditation procedure to ensure the quality of services provided by its members.[91]

The NAPGCM defines a private geriatric care manager as a professional with a graduate degree in a field of human services (social work, psychology, gerontology), or a substantial equivalent (i.e., RN), who is certified or licensed at the independent practice level of his or her state or profession and is trained and experienced in the assessment, coordination, monitoring, and direct delivery of services to the elderly and their families.

Services provided by private geriatric care managers may include some or all of the following:

- Assessment;
- Counseling;
- Home care: assessment, implementation, long-term monitoring;
- Crisis intervention;
- Placement;
- Care management;
- Entitlements;
- Advocacy;

- Psychotherapy;
- Education;
- Consultation;
- Information and referral.

Private geriatric care managers receive referrals from families (especially those living at a distance from their elders), attorneys, hospitals, physicians, trust departments of banks, conservators, community agencies, employee assistance programs, and the general public.

Full membership in the NAPGCM is open to individuals only. In Fall 1992, the NAPGCM expanded its membership to include individuals who meet the educational and experiential requirements, regardless of the setting in which they are employed. To avoid any conflict of interest, the NAPGCM accepts individuals only in situations in which remuneration is not offered or accepted either in moneys or in kind for referral to an agency. In addition, the client must be informed of the nature of the relationship of the private geriatric care manager to the agency.

Members of the NAPGCM are committed to protect their customers by:

- Setting standards of practice and ethics;
- Accepting for membership only those professionals who meet these standards;
- Developing a national network of professionals for the purposes of reliable cross-referral and the exchange of ideas;
- Providing locations, occasions, and instruments (national and local meetings, publications, etc.) for ongoing professional in-service education;
- Acquainting the public with member services and qualifications;
- Advocating/lobbying on local and national issues important to their client group and to the members of their association.

(f) FAMILIES AS CASE MANAGERS

Much of the recent literature about long-term care services for the elderly begins with the assumption that older persons should remain at home in their communities—if necessary, with supportive services. Ideally, these supportive services should allow for a social support system that permits socialization with a degree of regularity and for crisis intervention as it is needed. In many cases, this support system is the older person's family. Family members may provide a wide range of assistance, particularly as the older person becomes functionally disabled. A great deal of both formal research and anecdotal evidence suggests that most families have a strong commitment to providing for the welfare of older relatives. In fact, studies document that as much as 80 percent of the care provided to functionally disabled elderly persons is given by family, friends, and other volunteers.[92] This role requires taking an active, ongoing interest in arranging for and overseeing the services used by frail older family members and providing a significant amount and range of direct services. This section looks at families that act as case managers on behalf of frail, vulnerable elderly relatives.

Families must confront a number of realistic and unrealistic fears as they arrange services for a loved one. Several major researchers in the field have pointed out that families are not only concerned about the quality of services, but they fear that no one will take care of the patient as well or as lovingly as a family member. Families are also concerned that providers may not have specialized training in caring for clients with cancer, diabetes, or Alzheimer's disease.[93]

Family members who act as case managers get information on services from many different sources—other family members, friends, relatives, acquaintances, provider organizations, caregiver support groups, information and referral services, hospital discharge planners, and professional case managers.[94]

They may, however, need some training in how to seek out information and access services. One function of a professional case manager might be to train family members as case managers—showing them how to find and evaluate services and when and where to use a formal case manager as a back-up expert.[95]

There are a number of costs for families who act as case managers and provide informal services for elderly family members. Aside from the financial costs of caring for an older relative, family members may pay a great price in terms of their own health, well-being, finances, and emotional reserves.[96] They may face a restricted social life, difficulties in continuing to hold down a paying position in the marketplace, and the stresses of caring for dependent children at the same time. Acting as case manager can be upsetting for family members who find it difficult to be assertive with providers or who have ambivalent feelings about arranging for services or nursing-home placement for the older person.[97]

Despite these difficulties, families often work against great odds to serve as both case managers and service providers for older family members. To do a good job as a case manager, a family member must:

- Be able to obtain information on services available;
- Know which community providers offer the services;
- Have the time and skills to assess and evaluate the services offered;
- Have a substitute caregiver to take care of the older person while the family member makes phone calls, visits providers, and arranges services.

That families can serve effectively as case managers for older family members was shown in at least one study, which attempted to develop a closer partnership between the formal and informal networks for the betterment of the elderly.[98] In this study, elderly persons (mean age, 83 years) were randomly assigned to either an experimental group in which family members participated in a case management training program or to a control group. After case management training, family members in the experimental group performed a significantly greater number of case management tasks on behalf of their elderly relatives than family members in the control group. Furthermore, the study found that the formal services were needed for a significantly shorter period of time for elderly persons in the experimental group.

Studies such as this are leading to a growing realization on the part of researchers and formal providers that it may be appropriate to expand supportive services to include formal case management training for competent, willing family members.

In sum, for family members to act as effective case managers for their frail elderly, they need complete and accurate information about the availability, appropriateness, and quality of services in the community.

(g) CASE MANAGEMENT IN THE ACCESS PROJECT

(1) Introduction

ACCESS is the case management unit of the Monroe County Long Term Care Program, Inc. (MCLTCP, Inc.), located in Rochester, New York. MCLTCP, Inc. was initiated in 1975 to develop a community-wide, population-based model for the organization, delivery, and financing of long-term care for the adult disabled and aged. The primary goal of MCLTCP, Inc. was to develop a long-term care system that provides more cost-effective and better quality services than those offered under the existing system. MCLTCP, Inc. sought to demonstrate the feasibility and utility of a freestanding community-based organization for planning and managing long-term care. ACCESS (Assessment for Community Care Services) was the program that evolved.[99] The specific objectives of ACCESS are as follows:

- To encourage persons needing long-term care to choose home care in preference to institutionalization when it is an appropriate and less costly alternative;
- To provide coordination and continuity of case management for long-term care clients;
- To improve long-term care assessment and review procedures;
- To collect data about the needs, service utilization, and appropriateness of placement of persons requiring long-term care, to facilitate future planning and evaluation for clients;
- To minimize inappropriate utilization of long-term care resources;
- To reduce the number of Monroe County residents who inappropriately wait in acute care hospital beds for placement in a long-term care facility;
- To reduce Medicaid expenditures for individuals needing long-term care (including expenditures for long-term care and for alternate care days spent in acute care hospitals while waiting for long-term care arrangements).

(2) History

Discussions leading to the development of MCLTCP, Inc. began in 1974, a time when efforts to reduce long-term care expenditures first began to receive attention in our society. Prompted by rising long-term care expenditures, Rochester area and other state officials met to discuss means for creating a more cost-effective and efficient long-term care system in Monroe County. In 1976, MCLTCP, Inc. was formed under the joint efforts of the New York State Department of Social Services (NYDSS) and Monroe County. MCLTCP, Inc. was a freestanding, non-profit organization governed by a board made up of equal numbers of consumers, health professionals (providers), and public officials.

ACCESS began program operations in December 1977, and the program was fully implemented by June 1978. In 1980, ACCESS received a grant to offer and pay for an expanded package of services for Medicare beneficiaries, in addition to Medicaid enrollees.[100]

(3) Clients

ACCESS serves adults who are at risk of needing extended long-term care (defined as over 90 days in duration). Any adult in Monroe County who is incapable of self-care, needs social and health services to remain at home, or has a physical or psychosocial handicap that interferes with home functioning, is eligible for the preadmission assessment and care planning process. Patients of hospitals and other health facilities who need another form of institutional care, or who might be discharged if home services were available, are also eligible. The majority of clients—approximately 85 percent—are over age 65.

(4) Staff

ACCESS has a multidisciplinary staff: case managers, nurses, physicians, social workers, and community health nurses.

(5) Services

ACCESS offers a wide range of long-term care services, including:

Nursing home care;

Friendly visiting;

Home nursing and home health aide services;

Heavy chore services;

Medical equipment and supplies;

Respite care;

Physical therapy;

Housing assistance;

Speech therapy;

Moving assistance;

Personal care;

Social transportation;

Medical transportation;

Housing improvement;

Preadmission assessment;

Adult foster family care;

Case management services.

(6) Case Management

All services offered by ACCESS are provided through its case management process. ACCESS's case management program consists of five basic components: casefinding, assessment, determination of level of care, service plan development, and monitoring and reassessment.

Casefinding. ACCESS receives referrals from community sources (e.g., families, physicians, community health nurses, and agencies) and from hospital discharge planning staff. ACCESS tries to reach the public through brochures and public relations materials, through interaction between ACCESS staff and professionals in the community and hospital, and through a consumer-oriented outreach program funded in large part by a grant from the Administration on Aging.

Assessment. Potential clients receive either community or hospital assessments. Assessments are based on a four-page form, called the Preadmission Assessment Form (PAF). The PAF is used to record objective data about the patient, including demographic information, medical data, functional status, family support information, and a description of the client's required therapies. Inpatient clients receive assessments from the hospital's discharge planning and nursing staffs, and a one-page medical summary from their physicians. For nonhospital clients, an ACCESS staff member arranges for assessments. If a patient is in a long-term care facility, the assessment is completed by a member of the facility's nursing staff. When the client is in a domiciliary care facility or at home, a community health nurse employed by either the Monroe County Health Department or the Visiting Nurse Service performs the nursing evaluation; the medical evaluation is performed by a physician who is reimbursed upon completion of the document.

Other reimbursable assessment services include financial counseling, in-home architectural review, housing improvement services to identify and modify any physical impediments in clients' homes, and social work consultations.

Determination of Level of Care. After the assessments are completed, the ACCESS case manager identifies what level of care is needed by the client, according to the five levels of care determined by the ACCESS program. The level of care reflects the type of long-term institutional care that may be needed as well as the equivalent and appropriate level of home care services.

After identifying which level of care is most appropriate, the case manager helps determine the most appropriate site for the client to receive care. For elderly clients who remain in their homes, the case manager helps with completion of forms and arranges for the provision of services in the client's home. For clients who need assistance but are not able to remain in the home, the case manager arranges for placement in a nursing home.

Service Plan Development. A service plan is created for all clients who remain in their homes. A client's service plan is developed by a community health nurse and documented on an alternate care plan (ACP) form. The ACP specifies the home care services recommended by the community health nurse, and the case manager often assists the community health nurse in developing a care plan.

Monitoring and Reassessment. Clients are monitored continually, to ensure that the services they are receiving are deemed medically necessary.[101]

In nursing homes, an admission review is completed within 5 days of a client's admission; continued-stay reviews are completed by utilization review staff at intervals of 30, 60, and 90 days, and every 90 days thereafter. The ACCESS supervisor is responsible for determining the appropriateness of nursing home admission and is responsible for evaluating continuing-stay reviews and certifying the medical necessity for the client's continued stay in the institution.

Clients receiving in-home care are monitored in several ways. First, continual communication is maintained among the case manager, the community health nurse, health care providers, and the client's family. Second, case managers telephone clients who are not receiving Medicaid-reimbursed services every 4 to 6 months. Third, a system of formal recertification of need is maintained for Medicaid beneficiaries every 120 days by the community health nurse through an abbreviated PAF form, called the Home Review Form.

Case managers visit clients in nursing homes or at home as needed, in order to provide additional quality assessments.

In addition to client monitoring, the ACCESS program uses two quality assurance mechanisms. First, a Case Management Systems Review Committee meets several times a year to review records and to evaluate the effectiveness of the case management functions. Second, quality of care in the ACCESS program is monitored by the Monroe County long-term care review team, which is supported by the Monroe County Department of Social Services.

(7) Funding and Financing

Case management costs for Monroe County Medicaid recipients are reimbursed through regular county Medicaid funds via a contract between Monroe County and ACCESS. This contract was developed because ACCESS performs functions that otherwise would be provided by the Monroe County Department of Social Services. The cost of services is paid through a 50 percent federal, 25 percent state, and 25 percent local match.

Case management costs for Medicare clients, as well as costs associated with their Medicare services, are covered through the Medicare Trust Fund. ACCESS approves all payment for services and then submits this information to Medicare and Medicaid to receive actual payment.

In addition to providing for expanded services, the waivers also have relaxed Medicaid financial eligibility requirements for the purpose of reimbursing assessment and case management services for non-Medicaid clients. This is done in order to deter either premature or inappropriate institutional admission.

(8)   ACCESS: Alzheimer's

Recently, ACCESS has added a new service—ACCESS: Alzheimer's—designed to serve 500 treatment clients and 500 control clients in eight counties. This demonstration project, funded by Medicare, marks the first time that Medicare has paid an amount beyond what is normally reimbursed for services for individuals (and their families) afflicted with Alzheimer's disease and related disorders. ACCESS is one of eight demonstration sites nationwide for this new program, which started in May 1991.

Clients who are eligible for the demonstration include Medicare beneficiaries who have Medicare Parts A and B or are enrolled in a Medicare HMO; reside in one of the eight counties covered by the service; live at home and not in a nursing home or adult care facility; and have a primary diagnosis of Alzheimer's disease or a related dementia.

Among the services for which these clients and their families are eligible are adult day care, skilled nursing, home health or personal care aides, housekeeping, general and specialized chore services (repairs and maintenance), companion services, transportation, adaptive and assistive equipment, consumable care goods, mental health services, family counseling and support, custodial home care, home safety equipment, educational sessions, support groups for family caregivers, case management, and medical assessments.

Because this is a demonstration project, half of those in the demonstration will be eligible for up to $250 per month for services not normally reimbursed by Medicare. The control group will remain eligible for services as provided and/or financed through the traditional Medicare system.

A physician satisfaction survey taken in 1991 indicated that 78 percent of the 128 respondents believed that the program had assisted the patient to more easily remain in the community; 67 percent said that the assistance with payment and arrangement of services had increased the patients' and caregivers' willingness to use needed services; and 81 percent believed that the Medicare Alzheimer's demonstration had been a worthwhile service for patients and caregivers.

This demonstration project will end in 1993 and will be fully evaluated at that time.

(h) CASE MANAGEMENT IN PROJECT OPEN

Project OPEN was a demonstration program designed to assess a co-ordinated hospital-based service delivery model in an urban setting. Project OPEN offered a cost-conscious approach to health care in which individual needs were assessed, appropriate community-based or home care services were provided, and independence was promoted.[102]

The specific objectives of Project OPEN were the following:

- To provide the necessary array of preventive and in-home support services, in order to reduce the use of acute care hospitals and skilled nursing facilities;
- To provide greater access to services;
- To maintain or improve the functioning levels of participants;
- To maintain or reduce total expenditures.

(1) History

Project OPEN was developed at Mount Zion Hospital and Medical Center in San Francisco. During 1975, Mount Zion participated in an adult day care demonstration project; in 1978, Project OPEN began, with the support of a long-term care research and development grant from the Health Care Financing Administration (HCFA). The first two years of Project OPEN were dedicated to planning and designing the project's consortium approach. From a pool of 18 providers, Project OPEN eventually selected two multiservice agencies, one hospital, and two senior centers to participate. Services provided by the consortium were designed to enable the frail elderly to function at an optimal level of independent living. In 1980, Project OPEN was awarded Medicare waivers by the Secretary of the

Department of Health and Human Services. The program was funded through September 1983.

(2) Clients

To be eligible for Project OPEN, individuals had to be age 65 or older, be covered by Medicare, reside within a certain geographic area of San Francisco, and have health or social needs that made it difficult to live or function independently.

Project OPEN had a total client population of 338 individuals: 220 demonstration participants and 118 control group participants. Approximately 55 percent of the clients were referred from various health and social service agencies, 17 percent were self-referrals, and the remaining 28 percent were referrals from family members, friends, or physicians.

The mean age of participants was 80; the youngest participant was 66 years old, and the oldest, 99 years old. Most of the clients were women (approximately 70 percent) and the group was ethnically diverse (68 percent White, 19 percent Japanese, 11 percent Black, and 2 percent other). Approximately 45 percent of the clients were widowed, 30 percent were married, 14 percent were single, and 11 percent were either separated or divorced. The clients generally belonged to the middle or the lower middle class.

(3) Services

Project OPEN services were provided through case management consisting of a needs assessment, care plan development, service coordination, and regular monitoring of each demonstration client.

Assessment.   A functional status assessment was administered to each client, in the home, by a service coordinator who was either a public health nurse or a social worker. The assessment, administered in an interview format, included:

Brief personal health history	Environmental satisfaction
Psychological status	Instrumental activities of
Mental status	daily living
Social support and activities	Physical status.
Activities of daily living	

Care Plan Development. The assessment information for each client was summarized and presented at an interdisciplinary case conference. The interdisciplinary team consisted of a nurse, a social worker, a physician, and other health professionals where appropriate (psychologist, physical therapist, occupational therapist, speech therapist). The interdisciplinary team developed an individually tailored 6-month plan of care for each participant. The care plan included: a priority list of needs; the appropriate services, providers, and locations; a start date; and the number of units of services recommended. Modifications and adjustments were made for the demonstration participants throughout the implementation of the care plan.

Service Coordination. Once the care plan was developed, the Project OPEN service coordinator contacted the designated service providers and arranged for service delivery—the beginning date and the total amount of service to be delivered. After the service delivery began, the service coordinator continually monitored the client's condition as well as the quantity and quality of services received. This process included consulting with the various providers to share information, to provide continuity, and to ensure appropriate, quality care.

Available Services. Project OPEN provided or arranged for comprehensive care, including the following services:

Adult day care	Medical social services
Adult social day care	Medications
Chore services	Mental health services
Dental services	Outpatient medical services
Escort services	Podiatric services
Financial services	Rehabilitative services
Home health services	Respite care
Homemaker services	Translation services (Japanese)
Meals (home delivered)	Transportation services
Medical appliances and supplies	Visual care services.

Additional services were available in the community. Those that were coordinated and arranged by Project OPEN but were not reimbursable by the Project included:

Acute care services

Companion Services

Counseling and referral

Housing services

Information

Legal aid

Meals (congregate)

Outreach services

Recreation

Senior center programs

Skilled nursing services

Telephone reassurance.

(4) Funding and Financing

Mount Zion Hospital and Medical Center acted as a Medicare fiscal channeling agent and authorized the reimbursement of services provided by the consortium of agencies. Certain limitations and requirements within Title XVIII of the Social Security Act (Medicare) were waived by the HCFA:

• Waiver of duration, amount, and scope of services;
• Waiver of level-of-care limitations, allowing payment for preventive care;
• Waiver of specific Medicare requirements, allowing Project OPEN to forgo coinsurance and deductibles as well as certain home care requirements.

Reimbursement for services provided under contract (i.e., by consortium members and other contracted services) was made on the basis of negotiated prospective rates. Other sources of funding included private insurance, Older Americans Act money, United Way and other philanthropic moneys, and individual client contributions. Even though Project OPEN was not able to pay for all services rendered to its participants, it did track the costs of all services rendered.

Project OPEN also used some cost containment measures. First, the service coordinator's actual functions—assessment, care plan development, and service authorization—all contributed to containing costs. As a broker, the service coordinator negotiated with the providers for the appropriate amount of services, and then monitored the cost and frequency of services used. In addition, the service coordinator acted as an advocate and educator in facilitating a heightened awareness among the clients regarding service costs, bills, and third-party statements.

(i) CASE MANAGEMENT IN THE CHANNELING DEMONSTRATION PROJECT

The Channeling project was a long-term care demonstration that tested the feasibility and cost effectiveness of using community-based long-term care services as a substitute for institutional care. Using a case management system, Channeling integrated health care and social services for the frail elderly. Specifically, Channeling tested whether case management for those at risk for nursing home placement could help control overall long-term costs while maintaining or improving the well-being of elderly clients. Case management included the following services: outreach, screening, and eligibility determination; comprehensive assessment of the individual's health and long-term needs; development of a care plan; service initiation; and monitoring and reassessment of the individual's needs and the adequacy of the care plan. Channeling started in 1980 and ended in 1985. Ten states participated in the Channeling demonstration, with each state engaging in a community project. The demonstration included a total of 6,327 participants.[103]

(1) History

Federal planning for the Channeling project began as early as 1978. The original plans for the project involved creating community agencies and assigning each of them to fulfill three specific functions: channeling all or part of the long-term care population; planning for the long-term care service system, to ensure that a sufficient supply of needed services and settings would be available; and coordinating, directly or indirectly, the provision of long-term care services.

The creators of Channeling originally anticipated that as much as $100 million annually would be allocated to the program, and the project was to include five organizational approaches to solving problems associated with long-term care delivery and financing. However, the Channeling project was not implemented on such an ambitious scale. In fiscal year 1980, Congress appropriated $20 million for the Channeling demonstration. Funding for the initiative came from the Health Care Financing Administration (HCFA) and the Administration on Aging (AoA). The responsibility for managing the initiative was given to the Office of the Assistant Secretary for Planning and Evaluation (ASPE). In 1980, the federal officials in charge of planning and organizing the Channeling project submitted a request for proposals from states that were interested in operating a Channeling project, and the participating states were selected in 1980. Although 12 states were originally selected for the project, Hawaii and Missouri were later dropped.

In the remaining 10 participating states, the Channeling project was implemented between 1980 and 1985 in four stages: demonstration planning, buildup, steady state, and closeout. The demonstration planning phase lasted from the time the Department of Health and Human Services (DHHS) signed contracts with the participating states in 1980 until the project became operational in 1982. The buildup phase consisted of intense outreach and screening efforts to build project caseloads, in order to achieve both the planned research sample size and the planned scale of operations at each site. This phase lasted until September 1983. The steady state phase began in October 1983, and lasted until June 1984. Projects were required to maintain a steady caseload, accepting new clients when participants died, left the program, or were institutionalized. In the closeout phase, community projects stopped accepting new clients to replace those who left the project, and implemented plans for terminating the Channeling program. This phase started in July 1984 and ended in March 1985, which was the end of the states' contracts with DHHS.

(2) Services and Financing

Two types of models were included in the Channeling demonstration project—the basic case management model and the financial control (or complex) case management model.

The *basic model* tested whether the major problems with the provision of long-term care services are caused mainly by lack of information, access, and coordination of services, rather than by lack of financial reserves. Under the basic model, case managers provided long-term care services to the program participants by coordinating already existing long-term services in the community. In other words, case managers acted as brokers arranging long-term care services for clients.

In providing case management under the basic model, case managers performed a variety of services—completing a comprehensive evaluation of participating clients; creating a care plan for each client; coordinating the services with providers in the community; monitoring patients to ensure that their care plans were appropriate; and periodically reassessing clients to identify any needed changes in care. Case managers operating under the basic model had limited financial authority of about $40 per month per client.

The *financial control model* tested whether the problems in providing long-term care services were the result of inadequate funding. The focus of this model was to determine need and to arrange and fund additional services. Under this model's increased financial control, the case manager had greater ability to access long-term care services. Still, the case managers' limit on average and individual service expenditures was equal to 60 percent and 85 percent, respectively, of nursing home costs,[104] and they had purchasing power of about $400 per month per patient. Case managers were given authorization to provide for a number of expanded services, some of which included:

Adaptive and assistive
  equipment

Adult foster care

Chore services

Companion service

Day health and rehabilitative
  care

Day maintenance care

Home-delivered meals

Home health aide services

Homemaker/personal care
  services

Housekeeping services

Housing assistance

Mental health services

Nonroutine consumable
  medical supplies

Occupational therapy

Physical therapy

Respite care

Skilled nursing

Speech therapy.

These services were paid for with funds made available through Medicare and Medicaid waivers. The case manager under the financial control model had more authority to determine the amount, duration, and scope of services paid for from the funding pool than did case managers under the basic model.

(3) Clients

Under a randomized experimental design, eligible applicants were randomly assigned to treatment group or control group status.

The clients served by Channeling were extremely frail, had low incomes, and reported many unmet needs. The average client age was 80 years, the average income was $542 a month, and 845 participants were restricted in their ability to perform activities of daily living (ADLs). The remainder, while having no ADL limitations, had multiple limitations to their instrumental activities of daily living (IADLs), such as grocery shopping, cleaning house, and check writing. About 70 percent of participants were women and about 31 percent were married.

(4) Staff

Each of the 10 Channeling agencies employed 4 to 10 case managers. Each case manager was responsible for conducting comprehensive assessments, completing formalized care plans, arranging both formal and informal services, and conducting ongoing case monitoring that included client reassessments.

Most of the case managers working under the basic and financial control models had bachelor's or master's degrees in social work, and the remainder had been trained in nursing or other related health or human service fields. Supervisory staff were either master's level social workers or public health nurses who had considerable experience in gerontology.[105]

(5) Intended Effects

Channeling expected the demonstration to have several outcomes including:

- Increased use of community services;
- Reduced use of nursing homes;
- Reduced use of hospitals;
- Reduced costs of long-term care;
- Maintenance of level of informal caregiving,
- Improved quality of life for clients and informal caregivers.

Overall, Channeling did not have the anticipated and desired effects. Ideally, Channeling should have reduced costs, lowered institutional rates, and improved client function. However, it was not successful in achieving any of these expected goals. The major benefit of Channeling was that it decreased clients' unmet needs and increased clients' (and especially caregivers') satisfaction and well-being.

NOTES

[1] Wright, M.C. "Case Management for the Aged: A Study of the Growth, Development and Implementation of Case Management Services in North Carolina." Unpublished paper, October 1986.

[2] Secord, L.J. *Private Case Management for Older Persons and Their Families: Practice, Policy, Potential.* Excelsior, MN: InterStudy, 1987.

[3] Dronska, H. "Focus: The Role of Case Management in Long-Term Home Health Care." *Pride Institute Journal of Long-Term Home Health Care* (Fall 1983), *2*(4): 19.

[4] Melemed, B.B. "Issues Related to Private Geriatric Case Management" (p. 9). Presentation at First Official Conference of Private Geriatric Case Managers, New York, October 5–6, 1985.

[5] American Hospital Association (AHA). *Hospital Statistics* (1986 Edition). Chicago: Author, 1986.

[6] Kemp, B.J. "The Case Management Model of Human Service Delivery." *Annual Review of Rehabilitation* (1981), *2:* 212–238.

[7] Weil, M., and Karls, J.M. *Case Management in Human Service Practice.* San Francisco: Jossey-Bass Publishers, 1985.

[8] Quinn, J. "Case Management: The Key to Integrating Long-Term Care Services." *Perspectives on Aging* (September–October 1986), *5:* 6–7, 18.

[9] National Council on Aging (NCOA). "Care Management Standards: Guidelines for Practice." Report prepared by National Institute on Community-Based Long-Term Care. Washington, DC: Author, 1988.

[10] *Ibid.*

[11] Wright, note 1.

[12] Weil and Karls, note 7.

[13] Austin, C.D., Low, J., Roberts, E.A., O'Connor, K., and Todd, M.R. *Case Management: A Critical Review.* Seattle: University of Washington, Institute on Aging, 1985.

[14] *Ibid.*

[15] Sterthous, L.M. *Case Management: Variations on a Theme.* Philadelphia: Temple University, Mid-Atlantic Long-Term Care Gerontology Center, 1984.

[16] Eggert, G.M., Zimmer, J.G., Hall, W.J., Brodows, B., Friedman, B., and Olcott, L. *Direct Assessment vs. Brokerage: A Comparison of Case Management Models.* Rochester, NY: Monroe County Long-Term Care Program, Inc., 1986.

[17] Sterthous, note 15.

[18] Office of Technology Assessment (OTA). *Confused Minds, Burdened Families: Finding Help for People with Alzheimer's and Other Dementias.* Washington, DC: Author, 1990.

[19] National Association of State Units on Aging (NASUA). *State Units on Aging: Understanding Their Roles and Responsibilities* (2nd ed). Washington, DC: Author, 1987.

[20] *Aging Network News,* March 1989, p. 2.

[21] NASUA, note 19.

[22] OTA, note 18.

[23] NASUA, note 19.

[24] Congressional Research Service (CRS), U.S. Congress. *Financing and Delivery of Long-Term Care Services for the Elderly.* Report issued May 25, 1988. Washington, DC: Government Printing Office, 1988.

[25] OTA, note 18.

[26] *Ibid.*

[27] CRS, note 24.

[28] NASUA, note 19.

[29] *Ibid.*

[30] *Id.*

[31] CRS, note 24.

[32] OTA, note 18.

[33] *Ibid.*

[34] *Id.*

[35] Parker, M., Polich, C.L., Fischer, L.R., Pastor, W., Krulewitch, H., Pitt, L., Olson, P., and Korn, K. *The Provision of Home Health Services Through Health Maintenance Organizations,* Excelsior, MN: InterStudy, 1988.

[36] Lerman, D. Manager, Home Care and Hospice Services, Division of Ambulatory Care and Health Promotion of the American Hospital Association (Chicago); Assistant Director, Society for Ambulatory Care Professionals. Personal communication, April 21, 1989.

[37] OTA, note 18.

[38] CRS, note 24.

[39] Cary, A.H., Project Director, Home Care Administration Program, The Catholic University of America, School of Nursing, Washington, DC. Personal communication, May 22, 1989.

[40] CRS, note 24.

[41] Mundinger, M.O. *Home Care Controversy: Too Little, Too Late, Too Costly.* Rockville, MD: Aspen Publications, 1983.

[42] Cary, note 39.

[43] CRS, note 24.

[44] Cary, note 39.

[45] Hobart, S. Director of Case Management, VNA Health Care Group Corporation, St. Louis, MO. Personal communication, April 17, 1989.

[46] *Ibid.*

[47] Webb, L.C. "Where Do We Start?" In Webb, L. C. (Ed.), *Planning and Managing Adult Day Care: Pathways to Success* (pp. 1–8). Owings Mills, MD: National Health Publishing (in cooperation with National Council on the Aging, Inc. and National Institute on Adult Daycare), 1989.

[48] National Institute on Adult Daycare (NIAD). *Standards for Adult Day Care.* Washington, DC: National Council on the Aging, 1984.

[49] Webb, note 47.

[50] NIAD, note 48.

[51] Von Behren, R. *Adult Day Care in America: Summary of a National Survey.* Washington, DC: National Council on the Aging, 1986.

[52] Webb, note 47.

[53] Ohnsorg, D., Coordinator, Adult Day Health Care, Veterans Administration Medical Center, Minneapolis, MN. Personal communication, April 20, 1989.

[54] Padula, H. *Developing Adult Day Care: An Approach to Maintaining Independence for Impaired Older Persons.* Washington, DC: National Council on the Aging, 1983.

[55] O'Brien, C.L. *Adult Day Care: A Practical Guide.* Monterey, CA: Jones-Bartlett Publishing Co., 1982.

[56] Kelly, W., and Webb, L.C. "The Development of Adult Day Care in America." In Webb, L.C. (Ed.), *Planning and Managing Adult Day Care: Pathways to Success* (pp. 9–17). Owings Mills, MD: National Health Publishing, 1989.

[57] U.S. Department of Health and Human Services (DHHS). *Health: United States, 1987.* DHHS Pub. No. 88-1232. Hyattsville, MD: Author, 1988.

[58] On Lok Senior Health Services. *Directory of Adult Day Care in America.* Washington, DC: National Council on the Aging, 1987.

[59] Von Behren, note 51.

[60] *Ibid.*

[61] Webb, note 47.

[62] OTA, note 18.

[63] Von Behren, note 51.

[64] Webb, note 47.

[65] Von Behren, note 51.

[66] Congressional Research Service (CRS), U.S. Congress. *Adult Day Care: Background, Funding, Cost-Effectiveness, Issues, and Recent Legislation.* Report issued June 11, 1986. Washington, DC: Government Printing Office, 1988.

[67] OTA, note 18.

[68] *Ibid.*

[69] Ohnsorg, note 53.

[70] Katz, K.S., and Maginn, P.D. "The Intake Assessment, Plan of Care, and Discharge Planning Process." In Webb. L.C. (Ed.), *Planning and Managing Adult Day Care: Pathways to Success* (pp. 145–158). Owings Mills, MD: National Health Publishing, 1989.

[71] Ohnsorg, note 53.

[72] *Ibid.*

[73] Iversen, L.H. *A Description and Analysis of State Pre-Admission Screening Programs.* Excelsior, MN: InterStudy, 1986.

[74] *Ibid.*

[75] *Id.*

[76] *Id.*

[77] Carnes, C., and Cook, A. "Nursing Home Preadmission Screening in Virginia." *Journal for Medicaid Management* (Winter, 1977), 2(1): 1–8.

[78] Garrick, M., Rubin, D., and Wilke, D. *Long-Term Care System Development Project: Final Report.* Olympia, WA: Washington Department of Social and Health Services, 1983.

[79] General Accounting Office. *The Elderly Should Benefit From Expanded Home Health Care But Increasing These Services Will Not Insure Cost Reductions.* Report

to the Chairman on Labor and Human Resources, U.S. Senate. Gaithersburg, MD: Author, 1982.

[80] Kemper, P., Applebaum, R., Brown, R., Carcargno, G., Christianson, J., Grannemann, T., Harrigan, M., Holden, N., Phillips, B., Schore, O., Thornton, C., and Wooldridge, J. *Channeling Effects for an Early Sample at 6-Month Follow-up: Executive Summary.* Report No. 85-05. Princeton, NJ: Mathematica Policy Research, Inc., 1985.

[81] Kramer, A., Pettigrew, M., Carter, D., Spencer, M., Trickler, A., Zahn, M., Foley, S., Caston, R., and Amos, R. *Colorado Medicaid Long-Term Care Program Level of Care Assessment.* Denver: University of Colorado Health Services Center, Center for Health Services Research, 1984.

[82] Polich, C. *The Pre-Admission Screening and Alternative Grant Programs: A Description and Analysis of Minnesota's Experience.* Minneapolis, MN: Health Futures Institute, 1984.

[83] Iversen, note 73.

[84] Secord, L.J. *Institution or Home Care? Predictors of Long-Term Care Placement Decisions.* Excelsior, MN: InterStudy, 1986.

[85] Sokoloff, S. and Auerbach, H. "Proprietary Case Management Services for the Elderly: An Overview." Providence, RI: New England Long Term Care Gerontology Center, August 1983. Unpublished article on survey results.

[86] Parker, M., and Secord, L.J. "Private Geriatric Case Management: Providers, Services and Fees." *Nursing Economic$* (July–August 1988) 6(4): 165–195.

[87] *Ibid.*

[88] Bartelstone, R. President, The National Association of Private Geriatric Care Managers. Personal communication, May 15, 1989.

[89] Parker and Secord, note 86.

[90] NAPGCM membership brochure, 1991.

[91] Bartelstone, R. President, The National Association of Private Geriatric Care Managers. Personal communication, December 1991.

[92] Metropolitan Council. *Reshaping Long-Term Care in the Metropolitan Area: Recommendations for Change.* St. Paul, MN: Author, May 1985.

[93] OTA, note 18.

[94] *Ibid.*

[95] Cantor, M., Rehr, H., and Trotz, V. "Case Management and Family Involvement." *The Mount Sinai Journal of Medicine* (November–December 1981), 48(6): 566–568.

[96] Kane, R.A. "Assessing Social Function in the Elderly." *Clinics in Geriatric Medicine* (February 1987), 3(1): 87–98.

[97] OTA, note 18.

[98] Seltzer, M.M., Ivry, J., and Litchfield, L.C. "Family Members as Case Managers: Partnership Between the Formal and Informal Support Networks." *The Gerontologist* (December 1987), 27(6): 722–728.

[99] Eggert, G.M., and Brodows, B.S. "Five Years of ACCESS: What Have We Learned?" In Zawadski, R.T. (Ed.), *Community-Based Systems of Long-Term Care* (pp. 27–48). New York: Haworth Press, 1984.

[100] Eggert, G.M., and Brodows, B.S. "The ACCESS Process: Assuring Quality in Long-Term Care." In *Quality Review Bulletin: The Journal of Quality Assurance* (February 1982), *8*(2): 10–15.

[101] Eggert and Brodows, note 99.

[102] Weiss, L.J., and Sklar, B.W. "Project OPEN: A Hospital-Based Long-Term Care Demonstration Program for the Chronically Ill Patient." In Zawadski, R.T. (Ed.), *Community-Based Systems of Long-Term Care* (pp. 127–145). New York: Haworth Press, 1984.

[103] Iversen, L.H. "Utilization Control: What's Appropriate for Long-Term Care?" In *InterStudy's Long-Term Care Expansion Program: Vol. II* (pp. 114–141). Excelsior, MN: InterStudy, 1988.

[104] Carcagno, G.J., and Kemper, P. "An Overview of the Channeling Demonstration and Its Evaluation." *Health Services Research* (April 1988), *23*(1): 1–22.

[105] Applebaum, R.A., and Wilson, N. "Training Needs for Providing Case Management for the Long-Term Care Client: Lessons from the National Channeling Demonstration." *The Gerontologist* (April 1988), *28*(2): 172–176.

Five

Acute Care Case Management

§ 5.1 INTRODUCTION

Case management in acute care settings has many of the same components as long-term care case management: screening/intake, assessment, care planning, service arrangement, monitoring/follow-up, and reassessment. The goal is also quite similar: to deliver quality, cost-effective care as efficiently as possible.

Acute care case management, however, is primarily focused on managing hospital costs and utilization, partly because hospital use comprises the single largest expense in health care. HMOs, insurers, and third-party utilization review companies manage other aspects of acute care (e.g., outpatient care and prescription drugs), but this management is not currently applied, to any significant degree, to the elderly.

§ 5.2 COMPONENTS OF ACUTE CARE CASE MANAGEMENT

This chapter examines some of the approaches to managing hospital care for the elderly. Although each approach is somewhat different, they all have similar components and attempt to manage similar issues: the appropriateness of the admission, the treatment plan to be performed in the hospital, the efficiency and timeliness of the treatment, and the discharge plan.

125

(a) APPROPRIATENESS OF THE ADMISSION

An increasing number of hospitals and payers use explicit criteria for determining the appropriateness of hospital admissions. These criteria are, or should be, reviewed by each of the individuals associated with a hospital stay. The patient, first and foremost, should feel comfortable that the hospitalization (and the procedure or treatment to be performed) is appropriate and necessary. The admission decision should be made after thorough discussions with the physician, and, possibly, after obtaining a second opinion. A second opinion may be particularly important when an individual is faced with a major surgical procedure; some payers require a second opinion before approving the admission. It is very important for the patient, the physician, and the hospital to know the requirements of the payer in this regard, because forgoing a required second opinion could impact whether the hospitalization is covered by the payer.

In addition to a second surgical opinion, some payers require preadmission certification for inpatient hospital care. The physician, the patient, or the hospital may be required to call for review and approval of the hospitalization prior to admission. This review may be performed by an HMO, an insurance company, or a third-party utilization review (UR) company. Typically, it is performed via telephone by trained nurses. The UR nurses use acute care criteria that are often computerized to make determinations of medical necessity. Physician advisers are also enlisted to review cases and discuss questionable admissions with the patient's physician.

Hospitals are increasingly performing preadmission certification as a risk management technique. Particularly with government payers, the hospitals may be at financial risk if an admission is retrospectively determined to be inappropriate: the payers may refuse to compensate the hospital for the care provided.

(b) TREATMENT PLAN TO BE PERFORMED IN THE HOSPITAL

After a patient is admitted to the hospital, the actual care provided to the patient can be monitored. This is a less prevalent approach to care management, because it is often perceived as interfering with the physician's practice of medicine. However, given the wide variations in practice patterns across the country (with little justification in terms of health status or outcomes), the actual care provided to patients is coming under increasing review.

This level of management is rarely provided for all patients in the hospital. Intensive care management is often coupled with a high-risk screening to identify those patients who would best benefit from care management. They might include patients who are clinically at high risk (with multiple conditions or complications), demographically or socially at high risk (the very old, for example), financially at high risk (uninsured or underinsured), or have a high-risk diagnosis. Patients who meet any of these criteria are identified and managed more intensively.

One approach to managing the treatment plan within the hospital is through use of "clinical care paths." This approach has typically been the responsibility of hospital nursing departments. Care paths provide information about what treatment should occur for specific diagnoses or procedures (lab tests, x-rays, medications, therapies), the expected course of recovery, and the activities of the various care partners. The care paths are, by definition, averages—the expected courses of treatment for average patients who have no complications. Variances from the care path are documented as part of the process. Whether there is further intervention regarding these variances depends on the nature and scope of the program. Many variances can be explained by unique patient characteristics—older, frailer, with complications. Occasional variances are typically disregarded. Patterns of variances for specific physicians, however, may be brought to the physician's attention, usually by the medical director or physician chair of the hospital's utilization review committee.

Increasingly, hospitals, HMOs, and utilization review companies rely on physician data to compare resource utilization and practice patterns. Physicians are then informed of how they compare with their peers. This information can be very powerful in changing variant practice patterns, but often needs to be accompanied by ongoing care management, to assist the physicians in determining how best to make use of the data. Although many physicians have been resistant to these approaches, dubbing them as "cookbook medicine," they are increasingly becoming part of medicine's mainstream.

(c)   EFFICIENCY AND TIMELINESS OF THE TREATMENT

When the treatment plan has been determined, care management contributes toward ensuring that the plan is carried out as efficiently as possible. A patient spends much of his or her time in the hospital waiting—for tests to be performed, for results to be delivered, for care to be provided. There are tremendous opportunities for savings by reducing the time it takes to perform the components of the treatment plan. The manager of care is charged with making sure that these time reductions occur, that nothing falls through the cracks. If the results of the lab test are not in the chart in time for the physician's rounds at the hospital, the care manager is responsible for finding them and making them available to the physician. If a patient is waiting to receive a test in the radiology department before a discharge order can be given, the care manager makes sure that the test is scheduled as quickly as possible. Length of stay, one of the key measures of the effectiveness of care management, can be reduced through monitoring and improving the efficiency of the treatment plan. Another prevalent approach to reducing length of stay is through discharge planning.

(d) DISCHARGE PLAN

Particularly for the elderly, the discharge plan is a very important component of care management and the hospital stay. Many elderly will require some type of care after they leave the hospital. Some may simply need education about medications and the recovery process, and arrangements for family support (help with meals and housekeeping) for the first few days following discharge. Others may require short-term care from a home health agency or skilled nursing facility. Some may require extensive rehabilitation in the home or nursing home; others may be facing a permanent move to a nursing home. All of these scenarios require assessment of need, planning, service arrangement, and social work.

The discharge plan may be performed by the hospital or by an HMO or insurer. For the elderly, it is largely the responsibility of the hospital, unless the patient is an HMO enrollee.

§ 5.3 CASE MANAGEMENT IN HOSPITALS

Political and demographic changes in the past decade have given hospitals strong incentives to manage the care provided to their elderly patients. One reason is that elderly persons are high users of hospital care and the number of older persons is growing rapidly. A second reason is Medicare's Prospective Payment System (PPS). PPS was implemented in 1983, in the hope that it would control the rate of growth in Medicare payments by giving hospitals strong incentives to deliver cost-effective care. PPS provides this incentive by capitating the rate paid to hospitals for each Medicare admission. This rate is based on a patient's primary diagnosis. Unlike the former cost-based payment system, hospitals must absorb any loss when the costs of caring for patients exceed the payment limit. Conversely, hospitals are entitled to retain any surplus when revenues exceed the costs of delivering care. Thus, hospitals have incentives to manage their costs to match the payments received. Doing so often requires a much more aggressive discharge planning/case management process than was used in the past.

Despite these incentives, few hospitals have developed comprehensive case management systems for older patients. A recent survey of over half of all U.S. community hospitals, for instance, found that only 2.8 percent have case management programs specifically directed toward the elderly.[1] However, most, if not all, hospitals have a discharge planning process that includes many aspects of the case management process. In a sense, discharge planning is a very limited type of case management.

The differences between discharge planning and case management are well articulated in the following excerpt from the "Model Case Management Program" developed by the Pittsburgh Program for Affordable Health Care (PPAHC):

> . . . hospital discharge planning and community or hospital-based case management are often perceived to be similar, or even the same, activities. Many similarities do exist between discharge planning and case management such as the one-on-one contacts with clients, evaluating the client, and planning for and coordinating community services. However, the discharge planner, unlike the case manager, is generally restricted to providing services from within the acute care hospital setting, and frequently under severe time constraints. As a result, the discharge planner has limited possibility for establishing more than a functionally supportive relationship with the patient and her/his support system, and little opportunity to accomplish more than the immediate task at hand: to assist the client and the informal support system (if available) to utilize the most appropriate postdischarge services that the community has to offer.[2]

(a) SCOPE OF SERVICES

The scope of services provided by hospital case managers and discharge planners varies widely by hospital. As noted above, individual client evaluation and immediate postdischarge care planning are standards of the hospital discharge planning/case management process. In discharge planning, the major goal is to arrange services that maintain or continue the rehabilitation of the client following discharge. A discharge planner may, for example, evaluate the client upon discharge and arrange for the client to receive in-home services or to be transferred to a nursing home. Discharge planning generally includes very limited follow-up that is conducted by telephone and continued only for a brief period of time.[3] The scope of services provided in a comprehensive case management program is much broader, primarily because client progress is monitored for a much longer period of time.

As the PPAHC has noted:

> Simply stated, discharge planners are responsible for the frequently intense activities surrounding discharge from an acute care setting while case managers handle the day-to-day activities involved in the continued maintenance of a client in the community. In other words, continued monitoring and responding to a patient's progress or deterioration in the community is not a standard function for discharge planners, but is for case managers.[4]

(b) STAFF

Case management and discharge planning are generally conducted by nurses and/or social workers, depending on the hospital's bias toward a medical, social, or integrated model of care planning and evaluation.

(c) CLIENTS

Older men and women comprise a large portion of hospital patients and have longer lengths of stay than younger persons. As of 1985, there were 5,732 community hospitals in the United States, with an average daily patient census of 649.[5] In 1987, there were approximately 34 million discharges from hospitals, with persons over 65 accounting for 31.2 percent of all those discharges. Elderly women accounted for more discharges than elderly men: in 1987, 4,677,000 discharges involved men over age 65 and 6,039,000 discharges involved women over age 65. The average older woman's length of stay was also longer (8.7 days compared to 8.2 days).[6]

Hospital discharge planning and case management clients include patients who have a wide variety of conditions and needs. As noted, because PPS has put hospitals under increased pressure to discharge patients as soon as possible, many patients are discharged to the home with a need for post-acute services that are medical (e.g., use of

IVs), therapeutic (e.g., physical therapy), and supportive (e.g., home-maker). According to the Prospective Payment Assessment Commission (ProPAC), the most common diagnoses among Medicare hospital patients are: heart failure and shock; angina pectoris; simple pneumonia and pleurisy (for persons over 70); esophagitis, gastroenteritis, and miscellaneous digestive disorders (for persons over 70); and specific cerebrovascular disorders, except ischemia attacks.[7]

Patients are often quite elderly. Persons aged 75 years and older, for instance, account for over one-fifth of all inpatient days in acute care hospitals.[8] As a result, hospital case management/discharge planning patients are frequently discharged to nursing homes. As noted by McIntosh in her excellent article on hospital case management, approximately one-third of all nursing home admissions are directly from acute care hospitals.[9]

(d) COST/REIMBURSEMENT

Case management in hospitals is typically funded as part of the hospital stay and included in the PPS payment for Medicare. However, like case management in community settings, it may also be funded by a variety of public and private sources. Public sources include Title III of the Older Americans Act, Title XX of the Social Security Act, state and local programs for the elderly, and Medicare and Medicaid research and demonstration projects.[10] A major source of private funding is large foundations. The Robert Wood Johnson Foundation, for example, is supporting 24 hospital-based case management programs across the country. As McIntosh explains:

> This project is one part of the larger "Program for Hospital Initiatives in Long-Term Care" that is sponsored by the AHA and National Governors' Association. The program's goal is to encourage hospitals to adopt the role of health centers that provide comprehensive social and health services for the elderly rather than acute medical care only. The fact that there were 500 initial applications for the Robert Wood Johnson Foundation grants, which are four-year grants of $650,000 each, indicates a widespread interest in hospital-based case management and geriatric programs. This represents the first major attempt to involve hospitals in long-term care of the elderly.[11]

(e) EVALUATION

As more and more case management programs are developed in hospitals, information regarding their effectiveness should become more available. At this point, it is believed that hospital-based case management and discharge planning can simultaneously assist patients and families in obtaining appropriate services and assist hospitals in managing costs. Cost management occurs if case management allows hospitals to increase control of patient flow, decrease lengths of stay, and decrease inappropriate resource use during the stay.

A perspective regarding the impact of hospital-based case management on a hospital's financial state may be gained from the following advice, offered by experts, to hospitals developing case management programs:

> Freestanding case management programs lacking third-party reimbursement are certain "money losers" and thus should be embedded within the context of revenue-providing programs in order to be effective.[12]

> The case management staff [should be financed] separately from the program itself [and] case management [should] be funded as an administrative cost. It is further recommended that hospitals contract with Medicaid or HMOs under a capitated financing program for funding for the remainder of the case management program.[13]

> Each hospital must design its own case management and geriatric program based on individual internal and external environments.[14] Just as no one general model of case management would fit every community setting,[15] the same holds true for hospital-based programs . . . .

(f) STRENGTHS AND WEAKNESSES

A major advantage of case management provided by hospitals is that "the hospital setting is an inexpensive and convenient means of case-finding because of immediate access to those who might require services."[16] Most hospitals also have an extensive knowledge of community resources available and a working relationship with home health agencies, nursing homes, and other providers. Further, hospitals may be viewed with trust by patients who are familiar with the hospital's staff and reputation. In rural areas, providing case management in a hospital setting may be an excellent choice if the hospital is the health care hub of the community and/or if other alternatives are not available.

On the other hand, providing case management in the hospital may be duplicative of efforts already being conducted by community agencies and nursing homes. This may make it unpopular with other case management and long-term care providers. Hospitals may be viewed with mistrust by patients who think the hospitals have strong incentives to control costs, and case management in hospitals may be limited by an acute care/medical bias in care planning and service implementation. This model may not adequately address the chronic, long-term needs of patients. Finally, case management in hospitals is limited by the fact that only those persons being discharged from the hospital receive the services. In reality, many other individuals with chronic conditions or acute conditions not requiring a hospital stay are in need of case management services.

§ 5.4   GERIATRIC ASSESSMENT UNITS

(a)   DEFINITION

Geriatric assessment is defined by Rubenstein as a "multidimensional—usually interdisciplinary—diagnostic process designed to quantify an elderly individual's medical, psychological, and functional capabilities and problems with the intention of arriving at a comprehensive plan for therapy and long-term follow-up."[17] Rubenstein goes on to say that geriatric assessment has become very important because of the increasing numbers of older persons, the complexity of caring for older persons with multiple chronic conditions, and the recently documented evidence that geriatric assessment can make a difference in the care outcomes of older patients.[18]

In another definition, developed at a National Institutes of Health consensus development conference in 1987, geriatric assessment is seen as "a multidisciplinary evaluation in which the multiple problems of older persons are uncovered, described, and explained, if possible, and in which the resources and strengths of the person are catalogued, need for services assessed, and a coordinated care plan developed to focus interventions on the person's problems."[19]

Geriatric assessment units can be found in many different settings. Among these are:

- Acute hospital inpatient units:
  - —Geriatric assessment/evaluation units;
  - —Geropsychiatric assessment units;
  - —Geriatric rehabilitation units;
- Chronic hospital inpatient assessment units;
- Inpatient geriatric consultation services;
- Hospital outpatient departments;

- Home visit assessment teams;
- Office settings or freestanding units.[20]

Geriatric assessment units (GAUs) serve multiple purposes. They provide the patient with a multidimensional diagnostic assessment and a plan of care; make available either limited or extensive treatment, depending on their mission, and arrange for rehabilitation services. GAUs help determine the best placement for the patient and facilitate both primary care and case management. They also optimize the use of health care resources and provide for geriatric education and research.[21]

GAUs are growing as a treatment setting for older persons in the United States because they "provide interdisciplinary assessment, treatment planning, case management, and often rehabilitation for frail elderly persons and are especially important for persons suspected of needing long-term institutional care."[22] Rubenstein attributes their development in the United States to a long, successful history in Great Britain and to their good record of producing results in helping families and providers serve the needs of the elderly. He credits GAUs with demonstrated effectiveness in better diagnostic accuracy, better care planning, more appropriate care decisions, a decrease in institutional placement for clients, and improved survival rates, well-being, and functional abilities for older persons.[23]

(b) HISTORY

Geriatric assessment began in Great Britain approximately 50 years ago when physicians became concerned with the large numbers of disabled elderly who were being institutionalized without having been evaluated either medically or psychosocially and with whom rehabilitation had never been attempted.[24] British physicians found that, with geriatric assessment, they were able to diagnose readily identifiable and treatable problems in the elderly and that patients often showed great progress with therapy and rehabilitation. Based on these early experiences, British geriatricians decided that many elderly patients would benefit from interdisciplinary geriatric assessments and that no elderly person should be institutionalized without a complete medical/psychosocial assessment and attempted rehabilitation.

Geriatric assessment units are credited with providing some crucial components of care not typically found in the usual hospital or outpatient care setting. As noted above, these include comprehensive, interdisciplinary assessments; treatment and rehabilitation; and placement determination based on the assessments and long-range follow-ups.[25]

Comprehensive geriatric assessment of older persons is important for several reasons. The assessment serves as the basis for developing the individual's rehabilitation program, establishes a baseline or benchmark for the individual, and helps providers see changes as they occur through time. In addition, the assessments of groups of people serve an important public health function: they aid in planning for future needs as demography changes and more elderly people live longer. Geriatric assessment also minimizes inappropriate institutionalization, which is very expensive, creates unnecessary dependency in the elderly, and reduces the likelihood that the older person will leave the institution and rejoin society.[26]

Hospital-based geriatric assessment units have become an important part of the national health care systems of Great Britain, Sweden, and Israel, and have been developing rather slowly in the United States for the past 10 to 15 years. Their slower growth here is in part linked to the fact that the United States has no national health plan to coordinate the development and financing of GAUs.[27] A 1987 survey of all hospitals, by the American Hospital Association, found that, of 6,821 hospitals, 1,407 provided comprehensive geriatric assessments and 874 hospitals had geriatric acute care units.[28]

GAUs are extremely varied in their settings and in the tools (either standardized or unique to each case) used to evaluate the elderly. Similarities among the units seem to center on the staffing mix and the groups of elderly targeted for service. The variety and heterogeneity of programs suggest that it will be difficult in the United States to make some overall judgments about the value of GAUs.[29] However, one extensive review of the impact of GAUs in many settings shows that outcomes can include improved diagnostic accuracy, placement location, functional status, and cognition; reduced use of prescribed medications; decreased nursing-home use; increased use of home health care services; reduced use of acute care hospitals; reduced medical care costs; and longer survival rates for the elderly.[30]

(c) SERVICES

When the target population has been identified, the major objectives of the geriatric assessment are:

- Improving diagnosis by multidimensional assessment (to screen for hidden diagnoses);
- Arranging for appropriate rehabilitation and care plans;

- Determining the optimum placement for the patient;
- Optimizing the use of limited health care resources (staff, finances, etc.);
- Facilitating long-term care plans and follow-up.[31]

In the process of assessment, the team reviews and individualizes the objectives and develops recommendations for the patient. This process may also involve some component of rehabilitative care. Most geriatric assessment programs use multi- or unidimensional instruments to gather data about patients. These instruments improve the reliability of data and the communication among team members (and between the team and the family), and are generally a more efficient way to gather the necessary information.[32]

(d) STAFFING

Geriatric assessment units almost always use multidisciplinary teams to assess and diagnose patients. The size and composition of the team may vary quite a bit, but the core team usually consists of a physician, a nurse, and a social worker. Other health care professionals—psychiatrists, psychologists, dieticians, public health nurses, pharmacists, occupational therapists, and physical therapists, to name a few—may also be part of the care team or may at least be available for consultation as needed.[33]

The importance of the multidisciplinary team in geriatric assessment cannot be overestimated. According to Campbell and Cole:

> In geriatric care, a form of teamwork is the recommended modality because of the complex biopsychosocial needs of the patient. The goal of geriatric assessment programs is to establish an intensive assessment of older adults which requires the competencies of several coordinated disciplines. Not only do teams have the capacity to assess patients in much greater depth, but also patients share different information with different providers. . . . The minimal level of team development would include establishing program goals, delineating professional responsibilities and roles, and implementing a system for exchanging and documenting information about patient plans.[34]

(e) CLIENTS

To be most effective and make the best use of scarce resources, geriatric assessment units must target their client populations carefully.

There must be standards as to who will be assessed and who will benefit most from the assessment. The targeting criteria usually include the following:

Age: 65 and older (often 75+).

Medical Diagnosis: Geriatric-specific problems, multiple medical or chronic problems.

Level of Care: Currently hospitalized, in rehabilitation, or about to enter a nursing home.

Functional Ability: Patients having difficulty with either the activities of daily living (ADLs, such as feeding, bathing, toileting), or the instrumental activities of daily living (IADLs, such as grocery shopping, cleaning house, check writing).

Social Support System: Patients who already have or potentially have a caregiver to help implement the care plan.[35]

Another view of the target population is presented by the Office of Technology Assessment (OTA) and by Rubenstein. According to the OTA, the target group should be those who are at risk for premature or inappropriate institutionalization and who have potentially curable medical and psychiatric problems.[36] Rubenstein is more specific:

> The individuals most likely to benefit from assessment are those who are on the verge of needing institutionalization, who are in the lower socioeconomic groups, who have inadequate primary medical care, and who have poor social support networks. These at-risk elderly people . . . appear to constitute between 5 and 10 percent of hospitalized elderly patients and a currently undetermined proportion (perhaps 2 to 5 percent) of unhospitalized elderly people.[37]

Most GAUs also use some exclusionary criteria. Patients excluded from geriatric assessment may include those who are terminally or acutely ill, have severe dementia, are disruptive, are already living in a nursing home, have no potential caregiver at home (i.e., no informal support system), have long-standing psychotic disorders, and are poor candidates for rehabilitation.[38]

(f) COST AND REIMBURSEMENT

The costs of providing geriatric assessments vary considerably, depending on the setting, the composition of the team doing the assessment, and the amount of time it takes. Medicare and Medicaid cover some costs, but many are borne by the patient and his or her family on a fee-for-service basis. The cost of the initial assessment can be approximately $300 to $450. If rehabilitation or inpatient care is recommended, costs increase. There are still no well-established reimbursement sources for geriatric assessments. Many programs are currently attached to large HMOs or Veterans Administration programs, or are recipients of research grants and moneys.[39]

In the United States, it is currently difficult and costly to start a GAU. To date, despite evidence that documents savings by reducing inpatient hospital and nursing home days for the elderly, third-party payers have been reluctant to pay for geriatric assessments.[40]

§ 5.5   LINKAGE

LinkAge is a geriatric care management system developed by United HealthCare Corporation (UHC) to manage high-cost, high-risk Medicare patients during hospitalization. LinkAge is applied within the hospital to reduce length of stay and resource use for the patients managed. The program is based on the premise that a relatively small proportion of Medicare patients account for the majority of problems because of excessive resource use and length of stay. These patients are prospectively identified. Focused care management techniques then reduce length of stay and costs.

LinkAge provides three broad categories of services:

- Identification of patients needing care management;
- Care management intervention;
- Performance evaluation.

(a)   IDENTIFICATION OF PATIENTS TO BE MANAGED

To appropriately target and identify patients needing focused geriatric care management, a diagnosis-related group (DRG) analysis is done. This analysis compares hospital data with normative data to identify the admitting diagnoses, the characteristics of patients, and the physicians who are associated with excessive lengths of stay and high costs. The purposes of the DRG analysis are to appropriately target LinkAge to the hospital's unique problem areas and to establish baseline data for performance evaluation. A report is provided to the hospital on the findings of the DRG analysis and the recommendations for appropriate adaptations and installation of LinkAge.

High-risk patient identification is a system that is integrated with the hospital's admission process to prospectively identify high-risk Medicare patients. Its purpose is to effectively target LinkAge to those patients who will most benefit from focused case management. The high-risk identification process is adapted for use at each hospital.

(b) CARE MANAGEMENT INTERVENTION

After they are identified, high-risk patients are assigned a geriatric care manager (GCM) who manages the patient's hospital stay. The required numbers of geriatric care managers are recruited and trained. The GCMs are registered nurses with experience in geriatrics, managed care, and care management. Their training includes two weeks of classroom training in the principles of geriatric medicine and the application of care management techniques to the elderly; two to three months of on-the-job training with a GCM coach—a seasoned, experienced GCM; ongoing support from the GCM coach; and biannual continuing education seminars. The goal is to provide the hospital with highly trained and effective care managers and ongoing supervision by experienced care management professionals.

The LinkAge information system, installed in the hospital for use by the GCMs, includes the data, forms, tools, and reports required by the GCMs to be effective in their role; the length of stay targets; and the practice guidelines for key diagnosis groups. The overall purpose is to improve the effectiveness of the GCMs in their role.

The work of the geriatric care managers is the centerpiece of LinkAge. Each GCM is assigned high-risk patients to manage throughout the hospital stay. The average daily caseload of the GCM is 10 to 15 patients. The LinkAge intervention varies substantially from patient to patient. In general, the GCM works to offset the three major reasons for high cost and long length of stay in the hospital: hospital operational/administrative inefficiencies; difficult discharge planning; and physician practice patterns related to geriatric patients. The goals of the LinkAge intervention are to reduce costs and length of stay associated with high-risk Medicare patients, thereby realizing significant cost savings for the hospital; to improve the quality of patient care; and to increase patient/family satisfaction with the hospital experience.

(c) PERFORMANCE EVALUATION

A critical component of LinkAge is the ongoing assessment of the effectiveness of the system within the hospital. On a quarterly basis, LinkAge provides the hospital with a customized performance report comparing the hospital's experience through use of LinkAge with the baseline data prepared for the DRG analysis and other normative data. The performance reports routinely provide such data as:

- Number of patients managed;
- DRGs of patients managed;
- Overall length of stay for managed patients;
- Length of stay by DRG for managed patients;
- Number of outliers;
- Number of readmissions;
- Available cost data on managed patients;
- Financial savings of LinkAge.

These reports also address, when appropriate, operational or administrative inefficiencies or problems that inhibit optimal performance by the GCMs, along with recommendations for correcting the identified problems.

Annually, the performance reports address such issues as:

- Outcomes of care for managed patients;
- Patient satisfaction with LinkAge;
- Physician and nurse satisfaction with system.

The results show that LinkAge has achieved significant savings in hospitals; the program's results are quantified in inpatient days saved. As of August, 1992, LinkAge saved an average of 1.2 days per case managed. The program has saved more than .8 day per case for Medicare patients with strokes (250 days saved for 318 patients managed); 1.7 days per case for patients with heart failure (742 days saved for 432 patients managed); and 1.6 days per case for patients with septicemia (298 days saved for 186 patients). LinkAge also saved 4.1 days for patients hospitalized with cholecystectomy or gallstone removal (209 days for 51 patients managed); 2.9 days for patients with vascular procedures (267 days saved for 93 patients); and 1.1 days per case for patients with respiratory problems (795 days saved for 748 patients). Importantly, the reduction in hospital days has not affected readmission or mortality rates.

Critical success factors for LinkAge include:

- Strong administrative support in the hospital;
- Early input from medical and nursing staff;
- Recruitment of experienced geriatric nurses;
- The hospital's ongoing commitment to the program and its goals;
- LinkAge's integration into the hospital's existing programs and its adaptation to the hospital's unique environment;
- the program's apparent success in larger hospitals (3,000+ Medicare admissions) with significant financial problems and with a Medicare average length of stay of 8 to 9+ days.

NOTES

[1] McIntosh, L. "Hospital-based Case Management." *Nursing Economic$* (September–October 1987), *5*(5): 232–236.

[2] Pittsburgh Program for Affordable Health Care (PPAHC). *Model Case Management Program.* Pittsburgh, PA: Author, 1989.

[3] *Ibid.*

[4] *Id.*

[5] American Hospital Association (AHA). *Hospital Statistics* (1986 Edition). Chicago: Author, 1986.

[6] Department of Health and Human Services (DHHS). *Health: United States, 1987.* DHHS Pub. No. 88-1232. Hyattsville, MD: Author, 1988.

[7] Prospective Payment Assessment Commission (ProPAC). Personal communication, May 1989.

[8] AHA, note 5.

[9] McIntosh, note 1.

[10] *Ibid.*

[11] *Id.*

[12] Jennings, M. "Financing Health-Care Services for the Elderly." In McIntosh, L. (Ed.), *The Hospital's Role in Caring for the Elderly: Leadership Issues* (pp. 84–87). Chicago: The Hospital Research and Educational Trust, 1982.

[13] Evashwick, C., Ney, J., and Siemon, J. *Case Management: Issues for Hospitals.* Chicago: The Hospital Research and Educational Trust, 1985.

[14] Gregory, D., Peters, S., and Reardon, T. "Role in the Hospital in Meeting the Health Care Needs of the Elderly." In McIntosh, L. (Ed.), *The Hospital's Role in*

Caring for the Elderly: Leadership Issues, (pp. 44–59). Chicago: The Hospital Research and Educational Trust, 1982.

[15] Steinberg, R.M. "Introduction." In Steinberg, R.M., and Jurkiewicz, V.C., *A National Directory of Case Coordination Programs for the Elderly: 1979–1980* (pp. 1–7). Los Angeles: Andrus Gerontology Center, University of Southern California, 1980.

[16] McIntosh, note 1.

[17] Rubenstein, L.Z. "Geriatric Assessment: An Overview of Its Impacts." *Clinics in Geriatric Medicine* (February 1987), 3(1): 1–15.

[18] *Ibid.*

[19] Office of Technology Assessment (OTA). *Confused Minds, Burdened Families: Finding Help for People with Alzheimer's and Other Dementias.* Washington, DC: Author, 1990.

[20] *Ibid.*

[21] *Ibid.*

[22] Rubenstein, note 17.

[23] *Ibid.*

[24] Von Sternberg, T., M.D., Riverside Medical Center, Group Health, Inc., Minneapolis, MN. Personal communication, May 3, 1989.

[25] Rubenstein, note 17.

[26] *Ibid.*

[27] OTA, note 19.

[28] *Ibid.*

[29] Branch, L.G., and Meyers, A.R. "Assessing Physical Function in the Elderly." *Clinics in Geriatric Medicine* (February 1987), 3(1): 29–51.

[30] Kane, R.L. "Contrasting the Models: Reflections on the Patterns of Geriatric Evaluation Unit Care." *Clinics in Geriatric Medicine* (February 1987), 3(1): 225–230.

[31] Rubenstein, note 17.

[32] Von Sternberg, note 24.

[33] *Ibid.*

[34] Campbell, L.J., and Cole, K.D. "Geriatric Assessment Teams." *Clinics in Geriatric Medicine,* (February 1987), 3(1): 99–110.

[35] Von Sternberg, note 24.

[36] OTA, note 19.

[37] Rubenstein, note 17.

[38] Von Sternberg, note 24.

[39] OTA, note 19.

[40] Rubenstein, note 17.

Six

Integration of Acute and Long-Term Care: Models

§ 6.1 INTRODUCTION

The creation of Medicare and Medicaid in 1965 cemented an already fragmented system of providing health and long-term care to the elderly population. Medicare was designed to provide for the acute medical needs of the elderly population. Medicaid, more by default than by design, became the primary funding source for long-term care (covering mostly nursing-home care). Unintentionally, the design of these programs exacerbated the social/medical dichotomy that has complicated efforts to provide a comprehensive continuum of care to the elderly. This dichotomy is reflected in the separate models of acute and long-term care case management that were described in previous chapters. Physicians, nurses, and hospitals provide and manage acute care financed by Medicare and related supplemental insurance. Social workers, counselors, aides, nursing homes, and home care agencies provide and manage long-term care financed by Medicaid, private payments, and a variety of community-based long-term care programs.

But what happens when the needs of the person (whether a "patient" or a "client") span the boundaries of what can be clearly defined as acute or chronic? In spite of those needs, the delivery systems remain steadfastly separate. They are separated by financing sources, program rules and regulations, provider discipline, and culture.

As the population ages and a higher proportion experience the frailty, chronic illness, and functional disability that often accompany extreme age, an integration of acute and long-term care will be essential to providing quality, appropriate care. Our "systems" fight against that integration. Fortunately, over the past 15 years, several programs have been launched to demonstrate the effectiveness of integrating acute and long-term care for both the frail and the healthy elderly. These programs, primarily through waivers of Medicare and Medicaid rules, have been successful in melding these disparate systems to the benefit of their participants. The bad news is that, with one exception, these programs have only been possible through the arduous waiver process. In addition, one of the programs discussed (Triage) had to cease operations when its demonstration status ended; without continued waivers, it could not survive. On Lok, another model of integration, has been successful only by obtaining "permanent waivers"—a very unusual accomplishment. The Social HMO demonstrations have received extensions of their waivers but live under uncertainty whether future waivers will be available. Only EverCare has operated outside of the waiver structure. It has been able to do so because it does not pay for the long-term care services of its enrollees; it only coordinates those services with acute care needs. The administrative costs associated with that coordination can be covered by acute care savings.

This chapter describes in detail these four models of integrating acute and long-term care.

§ 6.2   ON LOK

On Lok Senior Health Services is a consolidated, community-based long-term care program in which frail and elderly individuals are offered an alternative to nursing-home care and are provided with a full range of medical and social services. Program benefits are planned and coordinated by On Lok and directly provided by On Lok's multidisciplinary team and/or by authorized consultants. All services are integrated into one health program, which receives capitated payments from government programs (such as Medicare and Medicaid) as well as private funds for each participant. These payments form a large funding pool from which all services are paid.[1]

(a) HISTORY

On Lok Senior Health Services was begun in 1971 with the intent of providing quality long-term care services to frail elderly persons living in the local area of San Francisco's Chinatown—North Beach. Originally, the organizers of the program intended to build a nursing home; later, they decided to build an adult day-care facility instead. In 1972, with the help of a 3-year research and demonstration grant funded by the Administration on Aging (AoA), On Lok built a multipurpose day center. In 1974, On Lok received additional funds through a Medicaid demonstration project to develop an adult day health service. On Lok was the first program in the State of California to receive Medicaid reimbursement for adult day health services.

In 1975, On Lok received a 4-year AoA project grant to expand its day health center program and provide a continuum of community-based health and other services. At this time, On Lok added a social day-care center and expanded its in-home care, home-delivered meals, and housing assistance. In 1978, On Lok opened a second day health center in the Polk Gulch neighborhood of San Francisco. In the same year, On Lok received a 4-year federal grant to plan, implement, and study a comprehensive, consolidated model of long-term care for dependent adults in which On Lok formulated, coordinated, and provided all medical and social services. This program was called the Community Care Organization for Dependent Adults (CCODA). By 1979, On Lok's outpatient system, including primary medical care, was operational, with Medicare waivers covering all services; by 1980, acute inpatient components were added to complete the system. In 1980, On Lok opened On Lok House, with 54 apartments for the frail elderly, subsidized by the Department of Housing and Urban Development (HUD).

Initially, On Lok operated primarily as a Medicare demonstration project: services were paid for through Medicare waivers. In 1983, however, On Lok assumed full financial risk of providing all health care services and began receiving predetermined per-capita payments that were to cover all costs of providing care to its participants. At this time, federal legislation allowed On Lok to test a new financing system based on a fixed monthly per-person reimbursement from Medicare, Medicaid, and, when appropriate, private payments, to cover all medical and social services.

In 1986, On Lok successfully completed tests of its service delivery and capitated funding model, and was granted continuing waivers through federal legislation. Additional federal legislation provided waivers for 10 sites to replicate On Lok's service and funding throughout the country. In 1987, funding from the Robert Wood Johnson and Hartford Foundations allowed On Lok to provide technical assistance to 6 organizations, across the nation, that were interested in replicating the On Lok model. By 1988, On Lok's service and funding model was being replicated at 8 sites, from New York to Oregon. (This program, called PACE, is described below in greater detail.) In 1989, On Lok purchased and renovated a building in North Beach, California, to provide 35 units of low-income housing for the frail elderly, an adult day health center, and an intergenerational child-care center.

Today, On Lok continues to serve only the frail elderly—approximately 300 frail elderly men and women, over 55 years of age, who are state-certified as being eligible for nursing-home care. Participants must live in San Francisco's Chinatown, North Beach, or Polk Gulch communities, a 3.5 square-mile area.

(b) SERVICES

On Lok provides a variety of inpatient and outpatient services to its participants. The available services are listed in Table 6.1.

The majority of the services are provided in one of the three On Lok adult day-care centers, although some services are provided in participants' homes, nursing homes, and hospitals. Services are provided directly by On Lok staff, or by contract personnel under On Lok staff direction. In addition to these services, On Lok provides two forms of alternative housing for participants: the 54-unit house subsidized by HUD, and communal housing in private residences.

(c) STAFF

On Lok employs an array of employees who work in a variety of positions: physicians; nurse practitioners; registered nurses; nurse assistants; restorative therapists, including registered physical therapists (PTs), occupational therapists (OTs), and PT and OT aides; social workers; recreational staff; nutritional staff; licensed home health aides and home care attendants (both on-staff and contracted); drivers; center support; plant operations; program managers; and administrative personnel.

Table 6.1
Services Offered Through the CCODA Program

Provided By On Lok Staff	Hospice care
Primary physician services	Case management
Skilled nursing care, including medications	
	Provided By Part-time On Lok Staff
Physical, occupational, speech and recreational therapies (group and individual)	Primary physician (weekend, evening, and back-up services)
	Optometry
Social casework services (including financial management)	Audiology
	Dentistry (including dentures)
Nutritional counseling and education	Psychiatry
	Podiatry
Meals (both congregate and home-delivered, with special diets; Chinese and Western menus)	
	Provided By Contract
	Acute hospital care
Transportation (to and from centers and for other nonemergency services)	Skilled nursing care
	Pharmacy, prescription drugs
	Laboratory testing
Adult day health services	X-rays
Personal care appliances	Inpatient medical specialty
In-home attendant/homemaker services	Restorative and supportive aid
	Emergency medical transportation
Home health care	Cardiology
Discharge planning	Orthopedic care

In addition, several medical specialists, including an audiologist, dentist, and psychiatrist, visit each center weekly. On Lok also has medical specialty contracts with other physician consultants (including a cardiologist and orthopedist), and pharmacy, laboratory, and radiology services.

(d) CLIENTS

On Lok participants must be 55 years or older, be certified by the California Department of Health Services as being eligible for institutional care, and live within On Lok's 3.5-square-mile catchment area. This area, according to the 1990 census, contains approximately 18,500 people over the age of 65.

On Lok currently has approximately 300 participants. They are generally very frail and suffer from several chronic conditions and functional impairments. Participants are, on average, 81 years of age and have 5 serious medical conditions. Approximately 80 percent of the individuals enrolled in On Lok are Chinese; the remaining enrollees are of varied descent. About 58 percent of the participants are female.

Approximately 75 percent of On Lok's participants live alone, either in their own homes or in supportive housing such as On Lok House; the remaining 25 percent live with others in the community. The majority of participants require assistance with bathing, home care, cooking, and grooming and hygiene. Most On Lok participants have cognitive impairments, but fewer than half have a specific diagnosis of mental disorder.[2]

(e) COSTS AND FINANCING

Funding for On Lok services (other than housing) is provided by Medicare, Medicaid, and private payments. In order to provide the services it offers, On Lok has had to obtain several Medicare and Medicaid waivers. Each month, On Lok receives a fixed, capitated amount for each enrollee, from Medicare, Medicaid, and/or the participant, depending on the individual's eligibility. All the funds On Lok receives are pooled together into an unrestricted fund that covers all medical, therapeutic, social, and supportive services provided in either the inpatient or outpatient setting.

On Lok operates on a risk-based financing model, meaning that On Lok must provide all services with the reimbursements it receives from Medicare, Medicaid, and private payments. If On Lok spends more than it receives in capitated payments, the program suffers a financial loss. If the program spends less money than it receives in capitated amounts, On Lok retains the unspent funds. There is a strong incentive for On Lok to contain costs.

(f) CASE MANAGEMENT AND ON LOK

The primary goal of On Lok is to provide comprehensive services to program participants. Prior to being accepted into the On Lok program, each participant is screened by a social worker and receives an extensive evaluation of his or her medical, functional, and psychosocial status by a multidisciplinary team consisting of a physician, a nurse, a social worker, and a physical therapist/occupational therapist. Following the screening and assessment procedures, the state Medicaid representative determines whether the client is certifiable as needing either intermediate or skilled nursing-home care.

If the client is accepted into the On Lok program, a multidisciplinary team develops a care plan and provides medical, social, rehabilitative, and other services. The intake and assessment team function together as the "case manager"; services are authorized by the team based on the team members' assessment. Participants are reassessed regularly by the team, either at 3-month or 6-month intervals, depending on the participant's health and functional status.

The social worker who completes the initial client screening acts as the participant's counselor, case coordinator, and advocate, both within and outside the program.

On Lok has created a responsive, flexible service system. Case management in On Lok's consolidated model has three key characteristics:

1. A true multidisciplinary team of medical as well as nonmedical personnel who separately assess and then, as a group, plan with the client and/or the family the services to be given;
2. Use of the same team to assess needs and deliver services;
3. Access to a potentially unlimited array of services, with freedom to adapt or create needed services.[3]

(g) ON LOK'S PACE PROGRAM

The Program of All-inclusive Care for the Elderly (PACE) is On Lok's most recent endeavor to meet the long-term care needs of the very frail elderly. PACE is a nationwide effort to replicate the comprehensive service and financing model created by On Lok Senior Health Services. On Lok representatives describe PACE as the application of the managed care solutions developed by health maintenance organizations to long-term care.[4]

Each PACE demonstration site must be either a public or nonprofit organization. PACE is mandated to focus on the nursing-home-certified population; to maintain participants in the community for as long as it is medically, socially, and economically feasible; to provide comprehensive medical and supportive services through a multidisciplinary team; and to accept financial risk by accepting fixed capitation payments to cover all service needs.

Participants join PACE voluntarily and agree to receive all services from PACE while they are enrolled in the program. The average age of participants ranges from 77 to 83. Most enrollees have multiple acute and chronic medical problems such as heart disease, respiratory disease, and diabetes. Most also have some level of cognitive impairment and are severely impaired in the activities of daily living, such as dressing, walking, bathing, toileting, or eating.[5] (See Figure 6.1.)

PACE's all-inclusive care provides, in one organization, all medical, restorative, social, and supportive services. PACE's services far exceed traditional Medicare and Medicaid services, extending from hospital and nursing-home care to podiatry, dentistry, grooming, transportation, and home-delivered meals.

No matter how costly or complex a PACE participant's care becomes, continued coverage and care are guaranteed for the fixed monthly rate. In addition, services are provided as long as necessary; no artificial benefit limits are imposed and no additional co-payments or deductibles are required for any needed service. Like On Lok, most care for PACE participants is provided in adult day health centers and the enrollees' home settings, thereby preserving the participants' community residence, family relationships, and life-style.

The PACE multidisciplinary team—consisting of the primary care physician, geriatric nurse practitioner, nurse, social worker, rehabilitation specialists, recreation therapist, dietitian, health worker, and van driver—works together to diagnose each participant's full range

Figure 6.1

Percentage of Persons Ages 65 and Older in the United States Having Functional Limitations, Compared to PACE Participants

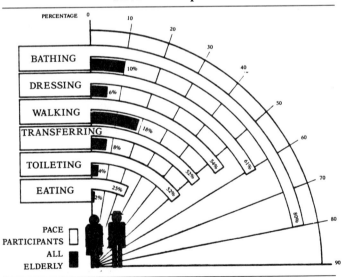

Source: Data PACE Reports, November 1990.

of social and medical problems. The team is responsible for formulating care plans; directly delivering most services (including primary care); managing the care given by contracted providers, such as medical specialists and acute care providers; observing treatment results continuously; and adjusting the care plan as needed.

Because the team members work closely with participants on a regular basis, they anticipate problems, use aggressive prevention measures, and work to avert health care crises before they occur. As a result, PACE participants use hospital and nursing-home services far less frequently than does the general elderly population. In spite of advanced age and functional disabilities, only 5 to 6 percent of PACE participants are placed in nursing homes. Hospital utilization is actually lower than that of the general elderly population. (See Figure 6.2.)

PACE is designed to cost less than services provided through traditional Medicare and Medicaid programs. Medicare achieves a 6 percent savings because PACE's capitation rate is 94 percent of the estimated Medicare costs for a comparable population in the fee-for-service system. Medicaid uses a rate-setting method similar to Medicare's. Depending on the state, this results in a 5 to 25 percent savings to

Figure 6.2
Hospital Days per Person per Year: PACE

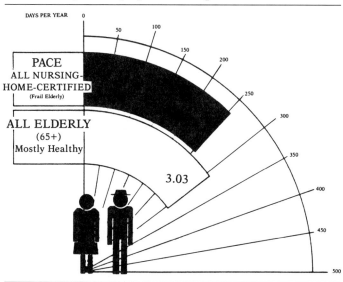

Source: PACE data for 1987.

Medicaid. Furthermore, participants eligible for Medicare and Medicaid pay nothing additional.

PACE is able to achieve these savings because service providers assume full financial risk, which sustains a strong incentive toward the efficient and effective use of resources. PACE's success depends, in large part, on very aggressive community-based preventive care, which helps maintain participants' health and averts the need for high-cost institutional care.

§ 6.3 TRIAGE

Triage was developed as a model project for the coordinated delivery of medical and social services to the elderly. Triage organized services around the needs of the client, stimulated the development of new services where needed, and ensured that all needed services were adequately monitored and reimbursed. Its purposes were to test the effectiveness and to measure the costs of this system of delivering care to the elderly.[6]

When Triage became operational in 1974, it resembled a health maintenance organization and focused on meeting the multiple needs of older adults. Triage was a freestanding agency that assumed an advocacy, coordination, and brokering role for both the elderly and service providers. The Triage project represented the first time that a full continuum of medical and nonmedical services for older people was provided under a unified program with a single funding source.

The single reimbursement system proved to be an effective mechanism for controlling costs, coordinating services, and ensuring quality of care. Thus, the Triage model proved to be an important influence in the evolution of later long-term care models around the country, despite the fact that the Triage organization itself was disbanded following the loss of federal funding.

The five primary objectives of Triage were:

1. To provide a single-entry mechanism to coordinate delivery of institutional, ambulatory, and in-home services on behalf of elderly clients;
2. To develop necessary preventive and supportive services;
3. To develop an integrated service delivery system at the local level;

4. To obtain public and private financial support for the full spectrum of services; and

5. To demonstrate the cost effectiveness of coordinated care, including:
   a. care to compensate for disability and to support independent living at home; and
   b. care deemed appropriate to need rather than dictated by third-party payers' service restrictions.

(a) HISTORY

The Triage project had its stimulus at the 1971 White House Conference on Aging, which had highlighted the deficiencies of the existing fragmented and poorly funded "nonsystem" of care. The desire to create a comprehensive, cost-effective, long-term care system in Connecticut resulted in the birth of the project.

Project Triage began in February 1974, with state funding and a start-up grant from the federal Administration on Aging. Triage's prime objectives were to increase the range and availability of services and to coordinate service delivery within a seven-town region in central Connecticut. The governing body of Project Triage was Triage, Inc., a private, voluntary, nonprofit organization that was a consortium of board members from provider agencies and elderly consumer representatives of the seven towns served by the project.

Joint state–federal efforts resulted in two subsequent phases of Triage. Between April 1, 1976, and March 31, 1979, federal funding was provided under a research grant to the Connecticut State Department of Aging from the National Center for Health Services Research, Public Health Service, and the U.S. Department of Health, Education, and Welfare. The State Department on Aging in turn contracted with Triage, Inc. for operations and with the University of Connecticut Health Center for evaluation. Between April 1, 1979, and September 30, 1981, the Health Care Financing Administration (HCFA) granted Triage continued funding for Phase II of project operations and evaluation ("Triage II").

(b) CLIENTS

During the 7½ years of Triage operation, a total of 2,628 people were enrolled in the program. A maximum of 1,750 were served at any one time prior to April 1979, but this number was reduced to 1,500 during Triage II.[7]

During Phase I of the program ("Triage I"), the only requirements for becoming a client were age (60 years or older), Medicare eligibility, and residence in the seven-town Triage area. For Triage II, staff determined that only those who were at high risk for institutionalization and who might benefit most from the Triage assessment and coordination would be accepted as new clients. To be considered high-risk, clients had to need the Triage assessment, coordination, and monitoring of medical and social services, and had to have a fragile or unstable informal support system at home. The new enrollees of Triage II had more complicated health problems and poorer functional status and were generally less able to obtain needed care from family and friends than clients who were enrolled during Triage I. Under Triage II, 495 persons were enrolled using the high-risk eligibility criteria. An additional 1,402 of those already enrolled in Triage I continued as clients during Triage II.

Clients enrolled under the Triage program consisted of a frail elderly group, predominantly widowed females, who lived alone and had less-than-adequate financial resources and limited educational attainment. At the end of the project's first grant period, 60.3 percent of the program's active client population was over age 75.

(c) SERVICES

The primary components of the Triage model were assessment of health and social needs; coordination of care; monitoring of services and client status; and client and family education about the health care system. The result was an individualized plan of care for each client that could be modified to meet changing health care needs.

(1) Assessment

Assessment consisted of a modified physical examination and an extensive health interview. The comprehensive assessment was completed during a home visit by a nurse-clinician or a nurse-clinician/social service coordinator team. The interview included a complete health history (i.e., physical and mental problems of an acute and chronic nature, prescription and nonprescription drugs taken); and information on the client's functional status, social background, nutritional status, physical environment, and living expenditures. Functional status was assessed using three standardized instruments:

- Activities of Daily Living (ADLs), a measure of the ability to perform the most basic functions, such as bathing, dressing, eating, and toileting;
- Instrumental Activities of Daily Living (IADLs), a measure of the ability to perform daily household and functional tasks, such as shopping, telephoning, cooking, taking medication, and handling money;
- Mental Status Questionnaire (MSQ), a measure of the client's cognitive functioning.

The assessment provided the basis for the problem-oriented client record, which was developed at the completion of the initial assessment.

(2) Coordination of Care

The Triage program offered a variety of services to its clients. Among them were:

Audiology	Nursing home care
Chore service	Nursing services
Companion service	Optometry
Dental care	Physical therapy
Financial counseling	Physician services
Home-delivered meals	Podiatry
Home health aide	Prescription drugs
Homemaker service	Psychological counseling
Hospital care	Transportation
Medical supplies and equipment	

Based on the initial assessment, the Triage team developed an appropriate care plan for meeting the needs of each client. The Triage team also selected the services and the service providers. Services were arranged by contacting the providers by telephone and establishing the type and the level of services to be rendered, the date for services to begin, and a reevaluation date for service continuation. This verbal arrangement was confirmed through a written service order, authorizing payment for services rendered. Bills were sent to Triage, not to the client, for reimbursement processing.

(3) Monitoring and Communication

The Triage team maintained frequent contact with the client to ensure that the quantity and quality of the services were meeting his or her current needs. Progress notes were made in the client's record on the basis of telephone calls and/or home visits. The Triage team also consulted with the service providers, who were required to submit reports that detailed the client's status, the services rendered, and the instructions given by the provider to the client.

(d) STAFF

Triage's staff consisted of a nurse-clinician or a nurse-clinician/social service coordinator team. These individuals were involved most directly with client assessment, care planning, and monitoring. Other providers played a more minimal role in the Triage process.

(e) PROGRAM FINANCING

In 1975, Triage received comprehensive waivers from the Secretary of the Department of Health, Education, and Welfare for the use of Medicare Trust funds. Waivers granted to the project included the following:

• Waiver of duration, amount, and scope of services—Triage was allowed to authorize payment for many ancillary and supportive services not traditionally covered by Medicare, such as prescription drugs, dental care, mental health services, homemaker services, eyeglasses, and hearing aids;
• Waiver of specific Medicare requirements—Triage was permitted to forgo deductibles and coinsurance, as well as several restrictions on home health care. For example, this waiver lifted the restrictions placed on an older adult's ability to receive home health care by eliminating the physician plan of care, the need for skilled nursing, and the Medicare requirement that the individual be homebound.

The federal fiscal intermediary (the agency that determines the reasonable costs of services and reimburses the providers) for Project Triage was the Office of Direct Reimbursement (ODR) of the Health Care Financing Administration (HCFA). Triage was responsible for verifying client eligibility and authorizing payment of providers by ODR. All bills for prescribed services were directed to the Triage office for review and approval and then forwarded to ODR, which issued payment to the provider. Reimbursement was limited to those services specifically authorized in writing by the Triage clinical teams.

Under Triage II, a new financial participation policy was adopted to encourage cost consciousness on the part of the client. Clients were asked for contributions to help defray the costs for waivered services that would otherwise have to be entirely self-paid. The amount of money requested from the Triage participants took into account individual income, the personal value to the client of the waivered service or set of services, and the cost of the service. The copayments ranged from 3 to 15 percent of the cost of the waivered services. Although client financial participation was encouraged, it was not mandatory for program eligibility. Between 1979 and 1981, Triage clients contributed about 10 percent of the cost of waivered services. All contributions were returned to the Medicare Trust Fund.

§ 6.4 EVERCARE

EverCare is a program designed to provide and manage comprehensive acute care services for nursing-home residents. In addition, EverCare coordinates those services with the long-term care provided to residents by nursing-home staff. It is essentially an HMO that specializes in the care of institutionalized frail elderly.[8]

(a) HISTORY

EverCare was first begun in Minnesota in 1987. The program, developed by a local HMO, was designed to reduce the costs of acute medical care for nursing-home residents (particularly costs associated with hospitalization); to improve coordination of care; and to improve the quality of health care. The HMO had a Medicare risk contract with a growing number of nursing-home residents. It became clear that, once an enrollee entered a nursing home, the HMO lost control over acute care utilization and costs. In addition, quality of care being provided to the nursing-home residents was not up to the standards expected. Because of the unique needs of this population, the HMO developed a program that would provide better, more cost-effective care. The program included:

- Developing a specialized provider network with expertise in geriatrics;
- Implementing strong and focused care management using geriatric nurse practitioners;
- Altering provider payment to encourage the use of more primary and preventive care and to prevent unnecessary hospitalization.

EverCare is made available to all nursing-home residents in the community. Enrollment in the program is completely voluntary. Growth in EverCare's first year (1987) was much slower than expected: 106 patients enrolled versus a projected 880. To stimulate growth in 1988, EverCare invested $150,000 in an advertising campaign. Unfortunately, the campaign's radio spots and direct mail did not prove effective in attracting enrollees. In 1989, EverCare hired a sales representative and developed a public relations program. This increased the enrollment to 244, but was still short of the 300-member enrollment needed to break even financially. Today, EverCare has over 500 enrollees in Minnesota.[9]

In 1991, EverCare started its second site in Chicago, in affiliation with Share Illinois. There were expected to be 50 enrollees by the end of its first year of operation.

(b) SERVICES

EverCare provides comprehensive acute care services, including hospital care, physician services, outpatient care, and skilled nursing. Specialty services brought directly to the nursing home by EverCare include dental care, optometry, intravenous (IV) therapies, laboratory and radiology services, dermatology, neurology, and mental health.

Although preventive care is not a new idea in health care, bringing it to the nursing home is one feature that makes EverCare unique. Emphasizing the importance of regular preventive care for nursing-home residents, EverCare seeks to reduce emergency room visits, outpatient and inpatient costs, and transportation costs.

EverCare provides enhanced personal health care to nursing-home residents by providing a physician/nurse practitioner team to regularly visit the member. EverCare also brings specific services directly to the nursing home. Encouraging more care to be provided within the nursing home has many advantages for the resident. It reduces transfers of the resident to the physician's office or hospital, which can be traumatic and disrupting. Preventive care is also encouraged.

(c) STAFF

Twenty-six physicians and 15 nurse practitioners (NPs) provide care for over 500 Twin Cities residents in over 80 nursing homes. These providers were selected for their expertise and interest in geriatrics.

The geriatric nurse practitioner provides nursing care with an emphasis on the psychosocial needs of the resident. EverCare nurse practitioners are registered nurses with advanced education in physical examination and the diagnosis and management of episodic and chronic illnesses. The nurse practitioner maintains close communication with both the family and the nursing home regarding the patient's physical, social, and psychological needs.

All EverCare physicians have taken geriatric fellowships or additional education in geriatric medicine and are specifically interested in caring for the frail elderly. Urgent care visits are made to nursing homes on nights and weekends, in addition to routine wellness visits. The physician provides expertise in the management of geriatric therapeutics and drug interactions, dementia-type debilitating diseases, chronic illnesses, and other specific geriatric conditions.

(d) CLIENTS

The direct clients of EverCare are the 500 nursing-home residents in Minnesota. The indirect clients are the residents' family members and the nursing homes. Residents benefit from EverCare's unique services in many ways. They receive enhanced medical care brought directly to them in the nursing home and integrated with their long-term care. Family members benefit from the regular communication that keeps them informed about their relative's condition and from the support systems gained through EverCare. The resident, family members, and nursing home all benefit from the time and cost savings that result from bringing these services directly to the nursing home. The resident is also spared the difficult and sometimes traumatic process of traveling to the physician's office or the hospital for care. The average age of EverCare clients is 88 years.

(e) COSTS AND FINANCING

EverCare is a primary care provider that contracts with an HMO to care for nursing-home residents. These residents and their families can choose EverCare as their provider option. Once a nursing-home resident becomes an EverCare member, the HMO pays EverCare a monthly capitated rate per member, to provide and manage all health care services that are part of the HMO's benefits package. In this way, EverCare is at full risk for the costs and utilization of health care services for its enrollees. Because EverCare is capitated for all health services, there is an incentive to be efficient in the provision of care and to be concerned about all aspects of the resident's health care—acute and long-term care, not just the hospital portion or the physician portion. There are no incentives to shift costs from one setting or payer to another.

EverCare has reduced the costs and utilization of acute care for the enrollees. Ambulatory costs average approximately $50 per member per month. EverCare enrollees have only 1,500 hospital days per 1,000 persons, compared to nearly 5,000 for nursing-home residents nationally. The average length of hospital stay for EverCare patients is less than 4.5 days, compared to over 9 for a comparable population.[10]

Using the physician/nurse practitioner teams improves efficiency and increases the amount of primary care and preventive care provided to nursing-home residents. However, EverCare further enhances the provision of primary care within the nursing home by giving the physician or nurse practitioner an incentive to visit the nursing home more often. Unlike Medicare, which provides nominal payment for one visit per month by a physician, EverCare pays its physicians and nurse practitioners on a fee-for-service basis for any and all visits to the nursing home, at significantly higher rates than Medicare. EverCare does not reimburse physicians or nurse practitioners when a nursing-home resident visits his or her office, unless preauthorized by EverCare. In addition, if any urgent visit is required, EverCare pays the physician or nurse practitioner a favorable fee to see the patient at the nursing home. The incentive to use the emergency room unnecessarily, in order to increase reimbursement for physician services, is lessened. This also reduces unnecessary, inappropriate hospital admissions and the resulting trauma and disorientation that often affect the older person adversely. EverCare pays the physician and nurse practitioner for comprehensive assessments and family conferences.

Furthermore, with the elimination of unneeded or duplicated prescriptions, the consumer saves on prescription drug costs and avoids complications due to overuse or improper use of drugs. Transportation costs are reduced because patients do not have to travel, unless needed, to a clinic or hospital for treatment.

(f) CASE MANAGEMENT AND EVERCARE

A major emphasis of the EverCare approach is care coordination and case management. Not only are costs controlled, but case management results in more closely monitored and better quality care. EverCare manages its patients' care and reduces health care costs by:

* Preventing duplication of services;
* Eliminating inappropriate and unnecessary services;
* Developing a network of cost-effective providers and facilities;
* Avoiding providers and facilities of questionable quality.

All new EverCare patients undergo extensive initial assessments by the physician/nurse practitioner team. The assessment includes a review of previous medical records, a comprehensive physical exam, preparation of a problem list, review of medications, review of routine laboratory and radiology tests, review of "do not resuscitate/do not intubate" (DNR/DNI) status, review of current therapies (physical, occupational, and speech), and an extensive meeting with family members.

EverCare assigns one physician/nurse practitioner team to each nursing home, and this team manages the care of all EverCare patients in the facility. This results in decreased travel time for the providers and establishes in-depth, ongoing relationships with the nursing homes. Because EverCare patients are concentrated in a few highly qualified nursing homes, providers can maximize their schedules to allow more time with patients and their families.

In addition, paying the team for family conferences increases involvement of the family and enhances family and resident satisfaction. Members of the EverCare team are available to answer questions or provide support to those who may feel they have nowhere else to turn. EverCare emphasizes ongoing communications; the family is kept continually apprised of both the patient's physical and psychological health.

§ 6.5 SOCIAL HMO DEMONSTRATION PROJECTS

One of the most important and innovative tests of integrating acute and long-term care in an HMO environment is the Social HMO demonstration. Conceived during the 1970s and designed during the early

1980s, four demonstration projects were implemented in 1985. These four sites are testing whether acute and long-term care benefits can economically be provided under one insurance and delivery system.

Social HMOs provide a comprehensive, integrated, prospectively financed and managed continuum of acute and long-term care. The goal is to achieve significant cost savings for both the government and individuals. In addition, the Social HMOs seek to demonstrate that improved primary care, case management, increased home care, and preventive health care can delay the dependencies and infirmities associated with aging and delay or prevent institutionalization.

The four Social HMOs are: Kaiser in Portland, Elderplan in New York, Seniors Plus in Minneapolis, and SCAN in Long Beach, California. Combined enrollment in the sites is approximately 18,000. Characteristics of each site are very briefly as follows:

- Kaiser/Portland is a large, established HMO that was an original site in the Medicare HMO demonstration project. Kaiser's size and the experience of the Kaiser Center for Health Research, which manages the Social HMO, were factors in its decision to develop the long-term care services needed for this new Social HMO project— Medicare Plus II—on its own, without taking on a formal partner.
- Metropolitan Jewish Geriatric Center (MJGC) (Elderplan) owns two large nursing homes and operates a variety of community-based programs. It saw the Social HMO as a way to extend and consolidate its services to the elderly. For medical services, MJGC created a new geriatric medical group with Cornell University Medical College. Hospital services are purchased from two community hospitals, and long-term care is provided through MJGC. MJGC also formed Elderplan, Inc., a nonprofit HMO, to operate the Social HMO.
- Seniors Plus, Minneapolis, Minnesota, was a joint venture between the Ebenezer Society and Group Health, Inc. The Ebenezer Society is comprehensive long-term care provider with a range of services similar to MJGC's. Rather than starting its own HMO, however, Ebenezer chose to affiliate with Group Health, Inc., the largest and oldest staff-model HMO in the Twin Cities area. This partnership provided all the required services for the Seniors Plus plan.
- Senior Care Action Network (SCAN), Long Beach, California, is a brokerage-model case management agency that provides no direct services on its own. Instead, it relies on an extensive network of referral relationships with existing community providers, in both

acute and chronic care. Like MJGC, SCAN established and closely
controls a new HMO, the SCAN Health Plan, Inc. (SHP). SHP uses
St. Mary's Hospital and an Independent Practice Association (IPA)
based at that hospital, paying them on a capitation basis with
strong risk incentives.

(a) SERVICES

Social HMO benefits include comprehensive Medicare services, as well
as the extended benefits typically offered by Medigap supplements or
Medicare HMOs (such as extended hospitalizations and preventive
care). In addition, Social HMOs offer chronic care or long-term care
benefits. Although varying in detail (e.g., benefits range between $6,500
to $12,000 per benefit or calendar year, with varying levels of cost
sharing, depending on site), long-term care benefits include both home-
and community-based care and institutional nursing-home services.[11]

For example, long-term care benefits include homemaker and home
health aides, medical transportation, home nursing, adult day care,
respite care, and institutional care. For Medicaid enrollees, the benefit
package contains those services to which the beneficiary is entitled
under Medicaid. All Social HMO sites also offer prescription drugs,
eyeglasses, hearing aids, and nonemergency transportation.

(b) CLIENTS

Unlike earlier demonstrations, designed to target services to the impaired elderly only, the Social HMO demonstrations seek to serve a
cross-section of the elderly, including both the functionally impaired
and the nonimpaired elderly. All four sites have been successful in
enrolling a balanced mix of impaired and well elderly in each local
community.

At enrollment and annually thereafter, all Social HMO members fill
out a Health Status Form (HSF), which provides information on general demography as well as data on members' use of long-term care
services, mobility, and the activities of daily living. Those who are functionally impaired or who are becoming increasingly impaired, speak
with site case management staff by telephone. These specially trained
case managers collect more information about the enrollees and record
the information on the Comprehensive Assessment Form (CAF). In all
four sites, those enrollees selected to fill out the CAF tend to be older,
female, widowed, living alone, with lower incomes, and with more ADL,

IADL, and mobility deficits. At the time of the interview, these impaired enrollees are usually receiving one or more health treatments and using one or more community services and one or more pieces of adaptive equipment (durable medical goods). They self-identify as having increasingly poor health (a very accurate measure of one's future health status); have entered the hospital within the past year; and indicate that their health interferes with their activities.

Harrington and Newcomer, for the year 1989, compared the number of enrollees, the percent who were nursing-home-certified, and the percent receiving chronic care at year-end, for Elderplan, Medicare Plus II, Scan Health Plan, and Seniors Plus (see Table 6.2). For the same year and the same plans, they reported on hospital days per 1,000 members per year, average length of stay (ALOS), and admissions per 1,000 members per year (see Table 6.3). In terms of utilization of chronic care services per 1,000 members per year, for 1989, Harrington and Newcomer's research revealed some extreme variations. For example, Elderplan had 1,636 chronic care skilled nursing facility/intensive care facility (SNF/ICF) days, compared to Seniors Plus's 458 days. For the same year, Elderplan experienced zero chronic care home health visits and Seniors Plus had 377. Elderplan provided 40,277 chronic care respite/homemaker/home aide/chore hours; SCAN provided 4,520. Elderplan provided 15 adult day-care center days compared to Seniors Plus's 1,009.[12] (See Table 6.4 for the detailed comparative data.)

(c) COSTS AND FINANCING

The Social HMO demonstration projects were designed in 1980 by Brandeis University and funded by the Health Care Financing Administration (HCFA) with waivers from the Medicare and Medicaid

Table 6.2
Social HMO Enrollment and Chronic Care Utilization, 1989

	Number of Enrollees	Percent Nursing-Home-Certified	Percent Receiving Chronic Care
Elderplan	5,082	5.4%	7.7%
Medicare Plus II	5,412	11.4	7.7
Scan	2,824	7.9	8.5
Seniors Plus	3,256	8.5	13.7

Source: C. Harrington and R. Newcomer, "Social Health Maintenance Organizations' Service Use and Costs, 1985–89." *Health Care Financing Review* (Spring 1991), *12*(3): 37–52.

Table 6.3
Social HMO Hospital Utilization, 1989

	Hospital Days Per 1,000	ALOS	Admissions Per 1,000
Elderplan	2,271	9.3%	245
Medicare Plus II	1,779	5.8	308
Scan	2,135	6.8	308
Seniors Plus	2,060	10.0	207

Source: C. Harrington and R. Newcomer, "Social Health Maintenance Organizations' Service Use and Costs, 1985–89." *Health Care Financing Review* (Spring 1991), *12*(3): 37–52.

programs. Costs of all services in the Social HMO demonstrations are covered by premiums paid into a prepaid capitated pool of funds by Medicare, Medicaid, and by the members themselves through supplemental premiums, copayments, and deductibles. The Social HMOs assumed full financial risk for all service costs at the end of the first 30 months of the demonstration.

One of the most important goals of the Social HMO demonstration project was to control enrollees' service utilization/costs and to develop a fiscally sound organization that would be able to sustain itself after the demonstration period ended. This goal, with variable success from site to site, has been achieved.

During 1989, the total average expenditures varied site to site but ranged from $331 to $404 per member per month. Total chronic care expenditures per member per month ranged from $19 to $44.[13]

Table 6.4
Social HMO Chronic Care Utilization, 1989

	Chronic Care Services Per 1,000	Chronic Care Home Health Visits Per 1,000	Homemaker/ Chore Hours	Adult Day-Care Days
Elderplan	1,636	0	40,277	15
Medicare Plus II	1,050	38	16,090	880
Scan	831	0	4,520	279
Seniors Plus	458	377	8,907	1,009

Source: C. Harrington and R. Newcomer, "Social Health Maintenance Organizations' Service Use and Costs, 1985–89." *Health Care Financing Review* (Spring 1991), *12*(3): 37–52.

(d) CASE MANAGEMENT IN DEMONSTRATION SITES

All Social HMOs provide comprehensive case management, including such components as screening and assessment, monitoring, and some utilization review and discharge planning. A summary of the primary case management roles in the various Social HMOs is found in Table 6.5.

According to the interim report to Congress on Social HMOs in 1987, the key components of care planning, while not identical, were similar across Social HMOs. They included:

1. Developing problem-oriented care plans with specific objectives, scope, and duration of services;
2. Exploring care options with the client and the family;
3. Explaining service costs and copayments to the client and family;
4. Reinforcing and supporting family caregiving;

Table 6.5
Primary Case Management Roles

Roles	Medicare Plus II	Seniors Elderplan	SCAN Plus	Health Plan
Screening/Assessment	Yes	Yes	Yes	Yes
Care planning and service arrangement	Yes	Yes	Yes	Yes
Monitoring chronic care services and resource allocation	Yes	Yes	Yes	Yes
Utilization review				
Hospital	Monitor only	Yes	Monitor only	Limited
Nursing home	Monitor only	Yes	Monitor only	Yes
Discharge planning				
Hospital	No	Yes	No	Limited
Nursing home	No	Yes	No	Yes
Record keeping/ Developing MIS	Yes	Yes	Yes	Yes
Other membership services	Yes	Yes	Yes	Yes

Source: Cathleen L. Yordi, "Case Management in the S/HMO Demonstration," In *Interim Report to Congress: Evaluation of The Social HMO Demonstration,* chap. 6. Berkeley, CA: Berkeley Planning Associates in conjunction with the Institute for Health and Aging, 1987.

5. Developing the most cost-effective mix of services within the constraints of the benefit package.

In general, the Social HMOs allocate 4 to 10 full-time equivalent (FTE) positions to perform case management functions. Interestingly, the proportion of time devoted to various case management functions (e.g., administrative matters and client case management) vary considerably by site. Table 6.6 shows the variation and average caseload for the fourth quarter of 1986.

Table 6.6
Allocation of Case Management Staff Time by Functions

Social HMO	FTE	Average Caseload, 4th Quarter, 1986[a]
Medicare Plus II		
Administrative matters	1.55	N/A[b]
Client case management	4.50	70
Utilization review/Discharge planning	0.00	N/A
Total FTE	6.05	N/A
Elderplan		
Administrative matters	3.00	N/A
Client case management	3.00	45
Utilization review/Discharge planning	1.00	N/A
Total FTE	7.00	N/A
Seniors Plus		
Administrative matters	2.00	N/A
Client case management	2.50	100
Utilization review/Discharge planning	0.00	N/A
Total FTE	4.50	N/A
SCAN Health Plan		
Administrative matters	3.75	N/A
Client case management	5.20	80
Utilization review/Discharge planning	0.50	N/A
Therapist	0.50	N/A
Total FTE	9.95	N/A

[a] Average caseload per full-time equivalent case manager.
[b] N/A indicates information was not available.

Source: Cathleen L. Yordi, "Case Management in the S/HMO Demonstration," In *Interim Report to Congress: Evaluation of The Social HMO Demonstration*, chap. 6. Berkeley, CA: Berkeley Planning Associates in conjunction with the Institute for Health and Aging, 1987.

NOTES

[1] Ansak, M.L., and Zawadski, R.T. "On Lok CCODA: A Consolidated Model." In Zawadski, R.T. (Ed.), *Community-Based Systems of Long-Term Care* (pp. 147–170). New York: Haworth Press, 1984.

[2] On Lok, forthcoming publication.

[3] Zawadski, R.T., and Ansak, M.L. "Consolidating Community-Based Long-Term Care: Early Returns from the On Lok Demonstration." *The Gerontologist* (August 1983) *25*(4): 364–369.

[4] *PACE: The National Replication of On Lok's Long-Term Care Model*, pamphlet, n.d., p. 5. (Available from On Lok.)

[5] *Data PACE Reports* (November 1990). San Francisco: On Lok, Inc.

[6] Quinn, J.L., and Hodgson, J.H. "Triage: A Long-Term Care Study." In Zawadski, R.T. (Ed.), *Community-Based Systems of Long Term Care* (pp. 171–191). New York: Haworth Press, 1984.

[7] *Ibid.*

[8] Bayard, J., Jacobson, R., Polich, C., and Parker, M. "A Nurse-Run Business to Improve Health Care for Nursing Home Residents." *Nursing Economic$* (March/April 1990), *8*(2): 96–101.

[9] Jacobson, R. Vice President of Operations, EverCare. Personal communication, November 1991.

[10] *Ibid.*

[11] Harrington, C., and Newcomer, R. "Social Health Maintenance Organizations' Service Use and Costs, 1985–89." *Health Care Financing Review* (Spring 1991), *12*(3): 37–52.

[12] *Ibid.*

[13] *Id.*

Seven

Managing the Costs of Postretirement Health Benefits

§ 7.1 BACKGROUND

Postretirement health benefit (PRHB) plans provide health care coverage to a population of former employees who are currently retired. These programs do not comprise a large portion of health care revenue for the elderly, but they are generating increasing interest and controversy.

Employers that fund coverage through PRHB plans are facing escalating costs associated with the plans. The cost increases have resulted from cutbacks in Medicare benefits and a growing and aging retiree population. Possibly even more important, the financial implications of reporting future PRHB obligations have caused many employers to seriously reconsider their retiree health plans. From their perspective, providing a PRHB plan is, at best, a necessary evil and, at worst, a legal obligation that prevents their organization from maintaining a competitive advantage.

169

From the perspective of the retiree, a well-designed postretirement health benefit plan can make a significant difference in the individual's financial position by providing a combination of premium sharing and more attractive group rates. In addition to the potential financial advantage afforded through PRHB plans, group coverage provides the additional security of knowing that premium increases will reflect the shared risks of the group instead of the actual experience of a covered individual.

For current employees, the existence of PRHB plans may be incorporated into planning for future retirement. For employees who are confident that these benefits will be available when they retire, this future benefit is significant. Caution is advised, however, for people who work for employers that are not legally obligated to maintain their PRHB plans. It is very likely that these benefits will be changing or have recently changed to limit the employers' potential financial exposure.

(a)   WHO RECEIVES BENEFITS?

According to 1988 Employee Benefit Research Institute (EBRI) data,[1] 43 percent of individuals ages 40 and over had some form of post-retirement health benefit coverage available through their own or their spouse's current or former employer. Approximately 39 million people are potentially covered through both private and public employer-sponsored plans. Although these individuals may actually receive benefits under these plans when they retire, there are usually eligibility requirements that restrict coverage. Some plans incorporate eligibility features that mirror the pension plan coverage—years of service, or eligibility for early retirement. In addition, PRHB plans are not generally portable, and no benefits will be paid if the employee leaves without completing the required eligibility standards.

In 1987, estimates of retirees from the National Medical Expenditure Survey included 8.6 million individuals receiving postretirement health benefits and another 2.2 million covered under these plans as dependents.[2] This survey, conducted by the National Center for Health Services Research, included retirees ages 55 and older (22 million people). The number of people currently receiving benefits under PRHB plans will grow in the future because of the aging of the population and the increasing numbers of potentially eligible persons.

There is a strong likelihood that the proportions of men and women receiving benefits under PRHB plans will shift in the future as well. In 1988, although 54 percent of persons ages 40 and over were women, only 39.4 percent of women were covered by their own or their spouse's employer plan for PRHB. In contrast, 46.9 percent of men received PRHB under a plan sponsored by their own or their spouse's employer.[3]

In addition to gender variations, the likelihood of receiving PRHBs varies with family income. The percentage of individuals with retiree health coverage increases steadily as the income level increases. For example, 90.7 percent of persons over age 40 with annual family income of under $5,000 have no retiree health coverage. For persons 65 and over with annual family income of under $5,000, 93.1 percent have no coverage. At the other end of the spectrum (annual incomes of $50,000 and over), 37.6 percent of persons 40 and over and 55.6 percent of those 65 and over have no coverage.[4]

Another factor related to an individual's probability of being covered by a PRHB plan is the size and type of industry of the past employer. In 1988, EBRI reported that, of retirees receiving health coverage from their employer, 3.7 percent had been employed by companies with fewer than 20 employees. In contrast, 61.8 percent had been employed by companies with 1,000 or more employees. Although these data may suggest that smaller firms do not offer PRHB plans, this is not the case. Jonathan C. Dopkeen has disputed the myth that "few smaller firms offer PRHBs" by analyzing a variety of surveys. His data indicate that 42 percent of small firms (50 to 99 employees), 46 percent of small to medium firms (100 to 499 employees), 62 percent of medium firms (500 to 999 employees), and 86 percent of large firms (1,000 or more employees) offer PRHBs.[5] He has also disputed the myth that PRHBs "are provided mostly by the older smokestack industries which are heavily unionized."[6] Table 7.1 reveals a broad array of industries offering PRHBs.

Table 7.1
Percentages Providing PRHBs—Major Industries

Industry	Percentage
Finance/Banking/Insurance/Trust	82.8%
Communication/Transportation/Utilities	82.7
Sales (retail & wholesale)	58.3
Industrials	77.3
Services	47.8
Sample average prevalence	71.4

Source: J. C. Dopkeen, "Post-Retirement Health Benefits," *Health Services Reprint* (February 1987), *21*, 6: 812.

(b) TYPES OF BENEFITS PROVIDED

In structuring the benefits provided under PRHB plans, employers will consider the relationship of their benefits to Medicare benefits and to the health benefit plan offered to their employed population. Coordination of benefit design with Medicare is a critical factor because Medicare will be the primary payer and the employer health plan the secondary payer. Employers have generally elected to utilize six different plan designs, each coordinating benefits with Medicare in a different fashion. In a survey conducted in 1988 by Johns Hopkins University and the Health Insurance Association of America, 1,665 firms reported on the design options they utilized. This information is summarized in Table 7.2.[7]

The most popular PRHB plan design is the "Medicare carve-out" plan. Typically, this type of plan looks like the active employees' benefit plan; however, when a claim is filed, the amount paid by the employer is reduced by the Medicare benefit amount. This has the effect of leaving the retiree with the responsibility for the full deductible and any copayments, including those required by Medicare. Because of the sharing of the deductibles and copayments, carve-out plans tend to be the least expensive to the employer.[8]

The second most popular design is a coordination of benefits plan. In this design, the plan sponsor applies the Medicare benefit first against the plan copayments and deductibles, reducing the retiree's

Table 7.2
Relationship Between Firm's Retiree Health
Benefit Plan and Medicare Coverage

Plan Relationship to Medicare	Percentage of Firms
Firm pays Medicare supplement	13%
Firm pays Medicare Part B	11
Firm pays for Medigap coverage	8
Firm offers "Medicare carve-out" plan	52
Firm offers "coordination of benefits" plan	27
Firm offers "Medicare exclusion" plan	14

Note: The percentages do not add to 100% because some firms offered multiple plans.

Source: "Changes in Retiree Health Benefits: Results of a National Survey," *Inquiry* (Fall 1990), *27*, (3): 291.

potential liability to little or nothing. This design is an attractive option to retirees because it has the appearance of a continuation of the regular health benefit plan for active employees. However, coordination of benefit plans are a costly design option for employers.

Under the Medicare exclusion design, the Medicare portion of a claim reduces the total claim before any deductibles or copayments are calculated. The beneficiary shares in the deductibles and copayments, but not to the full extent of the Medicare amounts.

With a Medicare supplement (or wraparound) plan, the employer provides only coverage for benefits not covered under Medicare, such as prescription drugs. In this plan design, the retiree is still responsible for all Medicare deductibles and copayments, plus any deductibles and copayments on the supplemental coverage.

To provide ease of administration, 11 percent of employers utilize a Medicare Part B plan. With this option, the employer pays the Part B premium for its retirees. The retiree, however, remains responsible for all Medicare (Parts A and B) deductibles and copayments.

The least popular design option, although still utilized by 8 percent of employers, is Medigap coverage, which pays for all retiree deductibles and copayments under Medicare.

§ 7.2   EMPLOYER PERSPECTIVES

Employers began offering postretirement health benefit plans in the early 1940s when the Internal Revenue Code was changed to recognize employee benefits as a business expense. Some minimal growth of this benefit continued during the post-World War II era and the 1950s; business was booming, and the numbers of retirees in comparison to active employees were low. When Medicare enacted health coverage for the elderly in 1965, more public attention was focused on health care coverage for the population 65 and over, including retirees. Corporations responded to the need to supplement the gaps left by Medicare, and retiree health plans rapidly expanded in number.

In 1960, there were approximately 17 million people ages 65 and over in the United States, or 9 percent of the total population. By the year 2000, that number is expected to grow to close to 35 million. Adding more difficulty to the anticipated growth in the aged population is a rate of inflation for medical care that has far exceeded the overall rate of inflation in the past 10 years. This is illustrated in part by the increases for out-of-pocket health care expenses experienced by seniors. From 1977 to 1986, annual average senior out-of-pocket health expenditures rose from $712 to $1,850.

In addition to the growing pressures exerted by the changing demographics of an aging society and rising health care costs, employers now face the impact of a change in financial reporting of their future obligation for postretirement health benefits.

(a) IMPACT OF FAS 106

The Financial Accounting Standards Board (FASB) is the primary body for the determination of standards for generally accepted accounting principles (GAAP). By determining standard ways of reporting financial information across all businesses, one goal of the FASB is to allow readers of financial reports to rely on the comparability of reporting of types of accounts and transactions.

The FASB first began exploring how to account for postretirement benefits in the mid-1980s, when it became clear that many organizations were recording the costs on a pay-as-you-go basis. This method of cost recognition is not consistent with accrual accounting, where expenses are recorded as known, and matched with related revenues. This treatment is also not consistent with the accounting for pensions that was established by Financial Accounting Standards (FAS) 87 and 88. In December 1990, the FASB issued FASB Statement No. 106, "Employers' Accounting for Post-retirement Benefits Other Than Pensions" (FAS 106). In contrast to the pay-as-you-go practice frequently used by employers, FAS 106 requires an estimate of the future obligation for postretirement health and other benefits to be included as a liability on the financial statements, a treatment that is consistent with the reporting of the liability for pension expenses.

Although the effective date of FAS 106 requires implementation for fiscal years beginning after December 15, 1992, most employers have already assessed the impact of this change in financial reporting. A Securities and Exchange Commission Staff Accounting Bulletin requires that public companies must disclose, as known, any material effects of changes to future financial statements.

Some large employers have already announced the estimated impact of FAS 106 on their organizations. The "Big Three" U.S. automakers, for example, collectively have a liability of up to $39 billion. The announcement of the automakers did not specify whether this liability would be a one-time charge against earnings or would be recognized evenly over the greater of plan participants' average remaining years of service, or 20 years. However the corporations choose to record it, the magnitude of these potential liabilities is staggering. Table 7.3 illustrates these liabilities for some of the nation's largest companies.

In 1988, the EBRI estimated the present value of private employers' liabilities for current retiree health benefits at $241 billion. The General Accounting Office (GAO) took the process one step further: in addition to an estimate of $217 billion for current liabilities, the GAO calculated the additional liability to be incurred in the future by current employees—a $175 billion item!

These two estimates illustrate the problems employers and their benefit consultants will encounter in making an estimate for a liability that requires a sophisticated actuarial calculation. This calculation must incorporate assumptions regarding changes in health care costs, which could be affected by health care inflation; changes in projected utilization and delivery; technological advances; changes in health status of the plan participants; and the discount rate on future costs.[9]

Because organizations have only recently begun to report their estimates of the FAS 106 liability, it is not yet clear how large the impact on financial markets will be. An estimate by Integrated Administrative Services predicted net income decreases of 30 to 60 percent for some companies. If true, this could seriously reduce the stock market values of these organizations' securities. However, some analysts believe that the companies that will be affected most have already seen a market adjustment for the potential liability. One thing is clear: FAS 106 has resulted in all employers with postretirement health benefits evaluating the pros and cons of providing this coverage.

(b) EMPLOYERS' RESPONSES

Table 7.4 describes the results of a survey of 1,665 employers conducted in 1988 by Johns Hopkins University and the Health Insurance Association of America. This survey showed clearly that large numbers of employers are planning or considering specific changes in their retiree health benefits. Although a good portion reported that the changes considered were linked to FAS 106, a larger percentage were considering changes for other reasons. The most popular alternative for change—increasing employee cost sharing—was favored by nearly half the respondents. Other alternatives included in the survey were: tightening eligibility for retiree health benefits, limiting health plan coverage or benefits, and expanding use of managed care health plans to control costs.

Table 7.3
Effect of FAS 106—Major Corporations

Accounting Rule's Fallout

Here are estimates of how some companies' equity and profits could be affected by the new rule, which requires accrual of costs of retirees' future medical benefits

Company	One-Time Charge (in millions of dollars)	Charge as Percent of Equity	Annual Continuing Charge (in millions of dollars)	Percentage Reduction in Pretax Profits
COMPANIES THAT HAVE ALREADY ADOPTED RULE				
Bell Atlantic	$1,550	17%	$183	0%*
Equifax	49	13	10	6
General Electric	1,799	8	279	0*
General Mills	70	11	12	1
Georgia-Pacific	119	4	23	3
IBM	2,263	5	394	8
Int'l Paper	215	4	37	3
Pennzoil	49	4	12	8
Philip Morris	921	8	216	2
Woolworth	115	5	14	1
COMPANIES THAT HAVE DISCLOSED RULE'S IMPACT BUT NOT ADOPTED IT				
Alcoa	$ 1,200	24%	$ 150	11%
American Brands	175	4	35	2
American Express	120–180	2	42–76	4–9
AT&T	5,500–7,500	34–46	558–725	0–4*
Chrysler	2,400–6,000	35–88	358	41
Deere	1,200–1,700	42–60	178	64
Du Pont	3,000–4,000	18–24	500–750	6–12
Ford Motor	5,000–9,000	22–39	915	22
General Motors	16,000–24,000	59–88	2,023–2,356	22–33
Sears, Roebuck	1,750–2,500	14–19	250–415	9–28
USX	1,200–1,800	20–31	317–483	14–27

*Zero means earnings are unaffected because company was already "pre-funding" to cover retirees' future medical costs.

Note: Figures are estimates, based on recent financial results.

Source: Lee Berton and Robert J. Brennan, "New Medical-Benefits Accounting Rule Seen Wounding Profits, Hurting Shares," *The Wall Street Journal,* April 22, 1992, p. B-1. Reprinted by permission of *The Wall Street Journal,* © 1992 by Dow-Jones & Co., Inc. All Rights Reserved Worldwide.

Table 7.4
**Proportion of Firms Planning or Considering
Specific Changes in Retiree Health Benefits**

Considered Alternatives	Percentage of Early Retirees		Percentage of Regular Retirees	
Tighten eligibility for retiree				
health benefits	32%	(44/139)[a]	28%	(43/154)[a]
Change due to FAS 106	43		40	
Change for other reasons	57		60	
Increase employee cost sharing	39	(53/136)[a,b]	37	(56/152)[a,b]
Change due to FAS 106	25		27	
Change for other reasons	75		73	
Limit health plan coverage				
or benefits	12	(17/138)[a]	14	(21/155)[a]
Change due to FAS 106	24		38	
Change for other reasons	76		62	
Expand use of managed care				
health plans (PPOs, HMOs)	38	(41/107)[a,c]	35	(37/106)[a,c]
Change due to FAS 106	13		28	
Change for other reasons	87		72	

[a]Denominator represents the number of firms responding to this item; numerator is the number of affirmative responses.

[b]Firms where the employee paid the full cost of health benefits excluded from the denominator.

[c]Firms offering only an HMO or PPO benefit excluded from the denominator.

Source: G. deLissovoy, J. D. Kasper, S. DiCarlo, and J. Gabel, "Research Notes and Data Trends: Changes in Retiree Health Benefits: Results of a National Survey." *Inquiry* (Fall 1990), 27:289–293. (See p. 292.)

The approaches described in the survey still leave the employer with some level of risk for costs of PRHBs. By shifting to a defined-contribution plan, an employer can shift the risks to the plan beneficiary. As with a defined-contribution pension plan, an employer would allocate to each employee's account a specific contribution amount that could be used in the future to purchase retiree health benefits. By prefunding only specified amounts, the risk of whether these amounts will be adequate to provide future health coverage is shifted to the beneficiary.

Another approach that shifts future risks to the employee is the defined dollar benefit. By establishing a maximum annual dollar amount to be used to purchase health benefits after retirement, employers limit their liability. This is the approach taken by International Business Machines (IBM). IBM is capping the amount paid for premiums on retiree health benefits to $7,000 for retirees under age 65 and $3,000 for those who are 65 and over (Medicare-eligible).

Both of these options would require the funding of an account designated for postretirement health benefits. In other words, to limit liability using these designs, an employer must also give the beneficiary control over the investment decision of accumulated benefits. Although funding of pension accounts is required by federal law, there are currently no laws or pronouncements requiring PRHB funding.

(c) VEHICLES FOR FUNDING

Imitating the concept found in a pension plan, many employers are providing options for advance funding of the liability for postretirement health benefits. Unlike pension plan prefunding, which is required under the Employee Retirement Income Security Act of 1974 (ERISA) and receives tax-preferred treatment, PRHB prefunding is not mandatory and prefunding investment vehicles vary in tax treatment.

One example of a currently used prefunding vehicle is a trust established under Internal Revenue Code ("the Code") Section 501(c)(9). Commonly known as a VEBA (Voluntary Employee Beneficiary Association), a "501(c)(9) trust" allows the employer to make tax-deductible contributions up to certain limits. These limits include not allowing contributions to reflect an assumption for future expected health inflation or increased utilization. In addition, investment earnings in VEBAs are only tax-exempt for plans established under collective bargaining agreements. These plans impose strict antidiscrimination rules that were legislated in the Deficit Reduction Act of 1984 (DEFRA).

In spite of the restrictions imposed on VEBAs, some employers have chosen to utilize this vehicle for prefunding PRHBs. Since April 1990, current employees at American Airlines contribute $10 each month into one of two 501(c)(9) trusts, one for union (collective bargaining) and one for nonunion employees. Employees who began work after the effective date pay a monthly rate ranging from $12.00 to $91.50, which is actuarially age-based.[10]

Another option used for prefunding PRHBs is a "401(h) plan," named for the Code Section that dictates its use. This vehicle establishes a separate account for PRHBs within a defined-benefit pension plan. Medical benefits are explicitly limited and become subordinate to the pension benefits. This clause is interpreted to mean that the health benefit contributions cannot exceed 25 percent of the annual total contributions to all retiree benefits (pensions included).[11] For many employers, particularly those without rich pension plans, this limitation restricts funding of PRHBs.

A "401(k)" plan is most commonly identified by employees as a vehicle for funding retirement income needs. This type of plan can also be used to pay for retiree health benefits, although the success of communicating this to employees will rest with the employer. Like the other vehicles, there are limitations to the 401(k) plan. Annual contributions of both the employer and employee cannot exceed $30,000 (or 25 percent of the plan dollar limit, if greater) or 25 percent of the employee's compensation. The 401(k) contributions can be made on a pretax basis by the employee and are tax-deductible to the employer. Fund investment earnings are also accumulated without annual taxation. In retirement, however, fund distributions to the retiree are taxed and would be available to pay for retiree health benefit premiums with after-tax dollars only.

Corporate-owned life insurance (COLI) is another vehicle in use by some employers for prefunding PRHBs. By purchasing life insurance on employees and/or retirees, the employer can create a potential future cash flow of funds to be used for paying for PRHBs. This cash flow is created through nontaxable death benefits or loans on accumulated cash surrender value. COLI can offer some significant tax advantages over a period of time, but, during the initial years of funding COLI (when there is a cash drain), there are minimal advantages. In addition, the ability to prove an insurable interest by the employer is a challenge, depending on location. Some states are silent on how an insurable interest is defined in an employee–employer relationship, but others have limited this definition to key employees only. Because of these disadvantages, COLI may not be a viable prefunding choice for all employers.

Using an employee stock ownership plan (ESOP) as a prefunding vehicle for PRHBs is similar in concept to the use of a 401(k) plan. By educating its employees that an existing ESOP should be used for funding future health benefits, the employer shifts the responsibility of prefunding to the employee. This may be an attractive option to the employer, but employees would prefer health insurance benefits after retirement. In an EBRI/Gallup poll, 69 percent of people 18 and over reported a preference for employer-paid PRHBs in lieu of a share in the ownership of the company that could be cashed out at retirement.[12]

Many employers are crafting approaches for providing PRHB plans that incorporate a combination of changes to existing benefit designs with prefunding vehicles. An example of this approach is the Libbey-Owens Ford Company plan, made effective in 1989.

The main features of this plan include funding retiree health care benefits with a portion of active employees' cost-of-living increases, using managed care arrangements, and freezing the company's defined-benefit pension plan while changing to a defined-contribution approach with a 401(k) plan.[13]

An approach utilizing a combination of funding vehicles is being employed by Procter and Gamble. Incorporating an ESOP with a 401(h) plan, this plan, referred to as an HSOP, allows the assets to grow tax-free and provides an asset to offset the employer's liability under FAS 106.[14]

(d)   LEGAL ISSUES ASSOCIATED WITH MODIFYING OR ELIMINATING PLANS

As employers struggle with the financial obligations of PRHB plans, they may be forced to ask: "What will be the legal consequences of eliminating or modifying the PRHB plan?"

Answering this question is a difficult task. Some authorities maintain that retiree health benefits plan documents stating that the employer has the right to make plan changes will protect the employer from a legal liability. This position was supported in a 6th U.S. Circuit Court of Appeals ruling that allowed American General Corporation to alter its PRHB plan for a recently acquired subsidiary.[15] Other cases, such as *Moore v. Metropolitan Life Insurance Company*, also established the right to change benefits based on plan language explicitly providing that right.[16]

Being able to withstand a legal challenge to changing PRHBs does not mean that the decision to modify or eliminate plans is an easy one. Other factors that an employer will need to consider include the impact on employee morale, the ability to offer competitive benefits to attract the best work force, and the ethical dilemma of keeping promises of future benefits made in prior years.

§ 7.3   EMPLOYEE AND RETIREE PERSPECTIVES

Employers are clearly struggling to meet their obligations under PRHB plans. Some of the same forces that cause employers to struggle are having a significant impact on employees and retirees as well. For most employees and retirees, the high rate of medical care inflation increases their out-of-pocket costs every year. This is equally true for coverage provided under Medicare. In addition to facing increased costs, many health plans have incorporated more restrictions on obtaining different treatments or utilizing certain providers, in an attempt to manage the escalating costs more closely.

(a) RETIREES' PERSPECTIVES

A survey exploring retirees' perspectives on health benefits was sponsored by the American Association of Retired Persons (AARP) and conducted by Brandeis University researchers from the Policy Center on Aging. The survey results indicated that (1) coverage under a PRHB plan dramatically reduced the purchase of supplemental health insurance by retirees, and (2) many retirees purchase more coverage than is necessary, primarily because supplemental plans are not designed to coordinate with PRHB plans.

Retirees' greatest worries (in order of priority) were: (1) out-of-pocket costs will increase, (2) benefits under Medicare will be cut, (3) they won't be covered for long-term care, (4) Medicare costs will increase, (5) private insurance costs will increase, and (6) their own health or their spouses' health will deteriorate.[17] Many of these worries are realities of health care benefits in the 1990s.

(b) EMPLOYEES' PERSPECTIVES

A 1991 survey conducted by Northwestern National Life explored employees' perspectives on retiree health benefits. The results indicated that, although 90 percent of employees were either very confident or somewhat confident that their major health care costs will be taken care of while they are employed, this number dropped to 60 percent regarding postretirement costs. Only 42 percent reported feeling knowledgeable about Medicare and the cost of health care for retired people.[18] Employers need to build strong educational programs around their retiree benefit plans. This education should be given to both current employees and retirees, and should encompass all aspects of planning for retirement.

§ 7.4 PUBLIC POLICY ISSUES SURROUNDING PLANS

Employers currently receive tax deductions for providing retiree and employee health benefits. Is this an appropriate incentive for private industry to provide coverage to its employees? This is one of many public policy issues that surface relating to the tax treatment of retiree and employee health benefits. A related issue is whether benefits paid for by employer health plans should be taxable income to the individual. Current law does not tax the individual for company-provided health benefits (employee or retiree plans). Does this provide an inequitable benefit to those working for employers that offer rich benefit packages? Would it make sense to legislate that the value of such benefits is only nontaxable up to certain defined dollar limits?

Should PRHB plans be subject to mandated minimum benefit levels? This would provide a sound protection for retirement planning, but the cost to employers of mandating benefits would be substantial. Such legislation may result in employers eliminating PRHB plans that currently provide less than the mandated benefits. These plans may not provide adequate coverage currently, but many employers provide no PRHBs.

Should prefunding of PRHB plans be required? This would help ensure employees that funds will be available to provide future benefits. With the implementation of FAS 106, prefunding will become more common on a voluntary basis. With a phased-in schedule for establishing the funds necessary to provide for PRHBs, legislated prefunding could provide an important protection for employee and retiree interests.

§ 7.5   MANAGING RETIREE HEALTH CARE: COST CONTROL

As described in earlier chapters, applying managed care techniques to the aged has both rewards and challenges.

One of the challenges encountered in applying managed care to the retiree population is geographic diversity. Many regular employees are concentrated in particular geographic locations, but retirees frequently resettle and tend to be a mobile population, particularly in their early retirement years. Geographic diversity makes it more difficult to utilize networks of preferred providers and hands-on case management.

Another significant challenge in managing health care for retirees is that Medicare is typically the primary payer, with the employer plan as secondary payer. Coordinating and managing benefits with Medicare is a complicated task. In addition, successful managed care techniques incorporate a strong hospital utilization review program. As the secondary payer, the employer-sponsor may not sufficiently benefit from the dollars saved with strong hospital utilization review.

(a) TEFRA RISK HMOS

One option for applying managed care to a retiree population would be enrollment in health maintenance organizations (HMOs) with risk contracts to provide Medicare services under the Tax Equity and Fiscal Responsibility Act of 1982 (TEFRA). HMO plans generally provide better coverage than Medicare and may significantly reduce the employer's retiree liability. Because HMOs receive a fixed monthly payment from the government to provide all Medicare benefits, these plans typically incorporate strong managed care techniques. With the HMO as the central financing source for all services, the retiree and employer will experience reduced administration and paperwork.

Although Medicare HMOs provide some significant benefits, there are some potential disadvantages in servicing a retiree population through them. The prime disadvantage is that the program is not designed to provide the nationwide coverage that an employer may require. Medicare HMOs contract to service specific contiguous counties; very few contracts have large geographic concentrations. Because PRHB plans tend to vary significantly in benefit design, additional riders to the Medicare HMO benefit package may be required to mirror the existing retiree plan.

These types of benefit riders have not been commonly available through the HMO, although more plans are now providing greater flexibility in design options. Another disadvantage to many employers is that Medicare HMOs generally require the member to use the participating provider network, and open access in Medicare risk plans is not common. To many retirees, this could mean having to change physicians to become a member of the Medicare HMO.

In spite of the disadvantages described, the potential benefits to both employers and retirees of the Medicare HMO program deserve consideration.

(b) OTHER WAYS TO MANAGE CARE OF RETIREE POPULATION

For many employers, a Medicare HMO will not be a viable option, but these employers do not have to rule out managed care as an option for controlling retiree costs. The techniques that allow a Medicare HMO to cost effectively manage the care of the elderly can be applied in other settings. For example, a retiree benefit plan may benefit from telephonic case management, particularly if applied to catastrophic or costly benefits. For example, assigning a case manager to all inpatient stays that exceed 10 days may result in significant reductions in the use of drugs, outpatient services, and other benefits covered only up to certain maximums under Medicare.

Another effective managed care technique that can be applied to a retiree population is to create preferred provider networks that specialize in certain services. An example is a network that contracts with centers of excellence to provide transplants on a fixed-price basis. Because of the significant costs of these services, the savings generated through such a network can be significant.

In a somewhat similar vein, programs that focus on managing a specialized health care need of the elderly can be effective managed care applications. These programs could focus on such things as controlling the use of services for mental health or prescription drugs.

A recent additional managed care alternative for employers is the Medicare Insured Groups (MIGs) demonstration project. Under this project, employers would receive a fixed monthly amount to provide all Medicare and retiree health benefits. The rate they receive would be based on the employer's individual experience for a retiree health plan. The employer would be at risk for delivering the services within that fixed amount, but there would be significant advantage to folding the financing and administration of retiree health benefits into Medicare. In spite of the appeal of this concept, the government has not been overwhelmed by interested employers, and no MIGs are currently operating.

§ 7.6 CONCLUSION

Postretirement health benefit plans provide valuable benefits to retirees. Although these benefits are expensive to maintain, employers are able to attract and maintain employees by offering them. In spite of the perceived value for both employees and employers, the future existence of PRHB plans is being jeopardized by escalating health care costs, Medicare benefit cutbacks, the impact of implementing FAS 106, and the changing demographics of an aging society.

To date, managed care techniques have not been applied to the elderly population in great numbers. Applying managed care to the health care needs of the elderly, such as retirees, would help the continually limited funds to be utilized in more cost-effective ways.

NOTES

[1] Employee Benefits Research Institute (EBRI). "Retiree Health Benefits: Issues of Structure, Financing and Coverage." *Issue Brief,* March 1991, No. 112.

[2] Congressional Research Service (CRS). "Health Benefits for Retirees: An Uncertain Future." *Issue Brief.* Update written by B.C. Fuchs, Education and Public Welfare Division. Order code 1B88004. Washington, DC: Author, June 5, 1991.

[3] EBRI, note 1.

[4] *Ibid.*

[5] Dopkeen, J.C. *"Post-retirement Health Benefits."* Health Services Research *Reprints* (February 1987), *21*(6).

[6] *Ibid.*

[7] de Lissovoy, G., Kasper, J.D., Di Carlo, S., and Gabel, J. "Changes in Retiree Health Benefits: Results of a National Survey." *Inquiry* (Fall 1990), *27:* 289–293.

[8] Dopkeen, note 5.

[9] EBRI, note 1.

[10] "American Airlines Employees Prefund Postretirement Health Care Benefits." *Employee Benefit Plan Review* (September 1990), *45*(3): 17–20.

[11] CRS, note 2.

[12] EBRI, note 1.

[13] Greenwald, J. "Libbey-Owens Overhauls Retiree Plans." *Business Insurance, 22,* December 12, 1988, pp. 1, 10–11.

[14] EBRI, note 1.

[15] Geisel, J. "Court Says Firm Can Alter Retiree Health Plan Benefits." *Business Insurance, 23,* January 2, 1989, pp. 2, 7.

[16] EBRI, note 1.

[17] American Association of Retired Persons (AARP). *Health Benefits: Retiree Experiences and Attitudes.* AARP Worker Equity Series, undated monograph PW4049 (1287) D10349.

[18] Northwestern National Life Insurance Company. *Retirement at Risk: The Growing Threat of Health Costs.* Presentation at forum for public policymakers, November 14, 1991, Washington, DC.

Eight

Employer-Sponsored Long-Term Care Services

§ 8.1 EMPLOYEES AS CAREGIVERS

As described in Chapter 7, the aging of our population is having a significant impact on employers. In addition to addressing health care needs for workers who are retiring, employers are facing increasing numbers of active employees who are caring for disabled elderly parents or spouses. It is estimated that 13.3 million Americans, including over 7 million full-time workers, have a disabled elderly parent or spouse.[1]

Not all of these workers are the primary caregivers, but the issues facing family members of disabled elderly are not limited only to this group. Many stresses emerge in balancing the needs of a disabled elderly relative with regular work and other family pressures. This group of employees is often referred to as the "sandwich generation," caught between the demands of aging parents and young children.

Employers are now realizing that the need to balance these stresses may have a negative impact on a worker's on-the-job performance. The problems often associated with these pressures include lost time and lost productivity. Sixty percent of respondents to a survey of corporate executives reported being aware of specific work-related problems associated with elder caregiving, including employee stress, unscheduled days off, late arrivals and early departures, above-average use of the telephone, and absenteeism.[2]

According to one estimate, 25 percent of the work force has responsibility for the care of an aging relative. They lose an average of 9.3 hours of work each month.[3] Another estimate places the value of lost productivity for each caregiving employee at $2,500 per year.[4] Although not quantified in the research, there may be an additional financial burden of helping an elderly relative pay for the ongoing long-term care services that they need.

Employers are beginning to recognize the high cost of lost time and lost productivity associated with caring for an elderly relative. In response, some employers are now offering a variety of employee programs to address these concerns. These programs include: (1) personnel policies designed to support families, (2) direct or indirect support for social service and other agencies that deliver long-term care services, (3) consultation, information, and referral services focusing on eldercare issues, and (4) employer-sponsored long-term care insurance offered to employees and their immediate relatives. This chapter examines these employer responses in detail.

§ 8.2 PERSONNEL POLICIES

The most important aspect of establishing personnel policies that support caregivers of the elderly is to create flexibility. By incorporating such features as flexible hours, job sharing, and unpaid family leave, employers can create a work environment that is supportive of the individual needs of the family, whether they relate to caring for children or the elderly. By accommodating the changing family needs through personnel policies, employers can retain valuable employees and avoid turnover and retraining expenses. In a recent employer survey, 56 percent of respondents reported allowing for an extended leave of absence, 58 percent provided part-time work options, and 30 percent offered flextime options.[5]

Flexibility can also be incorporated in employer benefit plans. Establishing a dependent care spending account provides employees a tax-preferred vehicle for funding expenses related to both child care and elderly dependents. The account provides up to $5,000 of annual contributions, to be made without taxation, when utilized to provide allowable dependent care expenses.

§ 8.3   SUPPORT TO SOCIAL SERVICE OR OTHER AGENCIES

Employers can also help their employees address the problems associated with caring for an elderly relative by establishing relationships with community or social service agencies. This step may include selecting one or more service organizations in the employer's community for direct or indirect funding. Employees can then access these agencies for help in their caregiving responsibilities. In a recent employer survey, 18 percent of the respondents reported making contributions to community agencies that provide services to the elderly.[6]

§ 8.4   CONSULTATION, INFORMATION, AND REFERRAL SERVICES

An increasing number of employers are providing or contracting for specialized consultation, information, and referral services focusing on eldercare issues. These services, made available to all employees and retirees, are generally accessed telephonically and include some or all of the following components.

(a)   TRAINED COUNSELING

Trained counseling to address a variety of questions and concerns relating to the care of an elderly relative is an important feature. The counseling helps families to cope with and relieve the stresses of informal caregiving. It may also include emotional support to people facing the burden of evaluating care options.

(b)   INFORMATION ABOUT CARE OPTIONS

The information service component, delivered via telephone, provides the caller with publications or other resources that offer education on the specific issues that he or she may be facing. Frequently, this information provides help in guiding the person through the complex and ever changing eligibility requirements for public programs providing long-term care services. This information may also relate to dealing with a chronic medical condition, evaluating long-term care service providers, selecting a private case manager, applying for available public programs, or even selecting and purchasing supplemental health care or long-term care insurance. To deliver high-quality service, a trained counselor would make a follow-up call to individuals receiving information, to ensure that their needs have been addressed.

(c)   REFERRAL TO SERVICE PROVIDERS

Because the long-term care service delivery system is very fragmented, many people have difficulty negotiating it effectively. For this reason, referral to specific long-term care service providers is linked closely with the information service. In some current services, this referral may be based on such criteria as location, state licensure, and availability of services. The next generation of eldercare referral services will include establishing a network of preferred long-term care providers that deliver services in accordance with quality standards. Although consultation, information, and referral services for eldercare are growing, they are still relatively new employee benefits. As yet, no data are available on the number of people served by the outcomes of these programs.

Another setting for eldercare consultation, information, and referral programs is in employer-sponsored long-term care insurance programs. In this setting, the service provides assistance in securing the informal long-term care services not generally provided through insurance.

§ 8.5   EMPLOYER-SPONSORED LONG-TERM CARE INSURANCE

An increasing number of employers have begun to offer group long-term care (LTC) insurance as an employee benefit. Although this benefit offering is relatively new, the number of employers instituting group LTC programs is growing rapidly. For example, the number of employers offering group LTC insurance increased from 2 in 1987 to 81 by the end of 1990.[7] At least 51 other companies reported plans to begin such offerings in 1991, according to the Health Insurance Association of America.[8]

In spite of the rapid growth in employer-sponsored offerings of LTC insurance, a relatively small number of people are covered by these plans. By the end of 1990, just over 130,000 employees, retirees, and relatives of employees had purchased coverage through these plans.[9] The answer to why more people are not covered under employer-sponsored LTC insurance lies in a lack of understanding about the features and pricing of the products offered.

(a) FINANCING GROUP LTC INSURANCE

Most employer-sponsored group LTC insurance is offered to employees as an optional benefit, with the cost of the insurance paid for by the individual. One exception to this is found in the group LTC coverage provided by International Business Machines Corporation (IBM). IBM provides 20 percent of the cost of the LTC insurance to its employees, an amount believed to approximate the portion of the premium representing medical expenses, a tax-deductible contribution.[10]

Some employers have linked their provision of subsidies for purchasing group LTC insurance to making changes in postretirement benefit plans. An example of this type of trade-off is found in Security Pacific Corporation's plan, which subsidizes the LTC insurance costs for employees who retired before January 1, 1991, and elected to move from the company's traditional retiree medical plan into a new, flexible benefits plan.[11]

The employers cited above subsidize the employees' cost of group LTC insurance; however, most employers are not able to provide this help. To the individual employee, the cost of such products is not insignificant. Table 8.1 illustrates the range of average annual premiums for various ages.[12] Because group LTC insurance premiums are level funded and based on issue age, the premium should remain the same over the life of the policy. The cost of purchasing LTC insurance is therefore directly related to the age of the purchaser. For this reason, it may make sense for employees to purchase LTC insurance when they are young and coverage is relatively inexpensive.

(b) PRODUCT FEATURES OF EMPLOYER-SPONSORED GROUP LTC INSURANCE

There is not a standard for LTC insurance products. Because the products are relatively new, there has been a rapid evolution in product features over the past 5 years. For this reason, it is impossible to describe all the possible combinations and choices currently offered under employer-sponsored group LTC insurance. Instead, this section discusses desirable product features that are available in some policies.

Table 8.1
Average Annual Premium at Selected
Ages for Employer-Sponsored
Long-Term Care Plans[a]

Age	Annual Premium[b]
30	$ 125
40	176
50	328
65	1,108
79 to 80	4,438

[a]Generally, for a plan providing $80 per day for nursing-home care, a 90-day deductible period, and 5 years of nursing-home coverage.

[b]Includes data from six insurers for ages 30 and 40 and seven insurers for ages 50, 65, and 79 to 80. Premium data were not available for two of the insurers surveyed. Premiums are level (i.e., they remain at the level shown, over the course of the insured's lifetime).

Source: Health Insurance Association of America, *Long-Term Care Insurance: A Market Update.* Washington, DC: Health Insurance Association of America, 1991.

LTC insurance will provide coverage for costs (skilled or custodial) incurred during a stay in a nursing home. This coverage is generally based on reimbursing 100 percent of actual expenses, up to a daily benefit maximum. The insured generally may choose a daily benefit maximum ranging from $40 to $150.

In addition to providing nursing-home coverage, a good LTC policy will provide coverage for home health care services. This coverage is typically reimbursed at 50 percent of the daily benefit maximum selected for nursing-home coverage. Home health care covered services tend to be limited to services provided through licensed home health care agencies for nursing services; physical, occupational, or respiratory therapy; or assistance by a home health aide. Most policies do not provide home health care benefits for alternative types of services and service settings. Although not standard features, it is desirable to include coverage for respite care and adult day care in a group LTC insurance offering. If a respite care benefit is available, it will provide a way for an informal caregiver to temporarily place the disabled person in an alternative care setting. An example would be a situation where a daughter cares for her mother in her own home on a regular basis. Her mother has Parkinson's disease and is unable to dress, bathe, or feed herself. By placing her mother in a nursing home for two weeks, the daughter is able to take a vacation from her caregiving duties. The insurance coverage for the respite care provides financial support for this service, which helps keep the impaired person from residing in a nursing home permanently. An adult day-care benefit also provides an informal caregiver the much needed relief that helps keep an impaired person in a home setting.

In addition to daily benefit maximums, LTC policies generally provide the insured the option of limiting total benefits to a selected maximum or choosing an unlimited lifetime maximum. An unlimited lifetime maximum provides the best coverage for catastrophic care, but this feature makes the product very expensive, particularly when purchased at younger ages. Research suggests that the likelihood of spending 5 years or more in a nursing home is only 9 percent.[13] Consequently, it may make better sense to utilize premium dollars for other optional features.

Generally offered as a policy rider, and not a standard policy feature, is an inflation option. An inflation rider will automatically increase the daily benefit maximum and total benefit maximum at a rate specified in the contract. A common selection for inflation coverage is 5 percent compounded annually. This protection does not guarantee that the costs of long-term care will increase at the same rate. For this reason, some insurance companies prefer to offer the insured the option to periodically purchase additional coverage in lieu of inflation riders.

Another policy feature with several options open to the insured is the elimination (sometimes referred to as the deductible) period. This period is the time frame for which covered services will not be reimbursed. A new elimination period will begin each time there has been a break in meeting the eligibility requirements for services. Standard elimination periods that are commonly selected are 10, 20, or 90 days. The longer the elimination period selected, the lower the related premiums will be.

A policy feature that is gaining attention recently is the provision of nonforfeiture benefits. Because design features in LTC insurance have been rapidly evolving in recent years, the rate of policy lapses has been high. Regulators and employer-sponsors have been concerned that the insured is not adequately protected in a policy that does not provide nonforfeiture benefits. A nonforfeiture benefit is designed to return a certain portion of the level funded premium to the insureds if they lapse the policy. Because insurance industry pricing reflects an estimated lapse rate, carriers legitimately argue that nonforfeiture benefits will increase the cost of LTC insurance. As a result, some policies do contain nonforfeiture benefits, but these policies are more costly.

Determining eligibility for benefits under LTC insurance policies is an area that has evolved in recent years. Initially, many policies only provided nursing-home benefits following 3 days' hospitalization, the Medicare skilled care criterion. Most current policies have moved to determining eligibility for benefits based on limitations in activities of daily living (ADLs). An individual who requires assistance with two of five or three of six ADLs is generally eligible for the nursing-home benefit. Better policies will also pay benefits for impairments in cognitive functioning.

The selection of the best policy features for a particular individual's need may be based on a variety of factors—age, affordability, goals in purchasing the product, and costs of services in the area. Employers will need to weigh the costs of providing many design options against the benefits of individualizing coverage to meet the employees' needs. A significant service that an employer can provide in offering LTC insurance is to educate employees on how to select features that will best meet their own unique situations.

Employers provide a valuable service by making certain that the insurance carrier they select to offer coverage is a reputable and financially sound organization. They must also make certain that the policies offered to their employees will be portable if an employee leaves the organization.

Large employers who offer LTC insurance have significant influence over the insurance carrier in determining policy features, terms of the offering, and, sometimes, price. It is not uncommon for large employers to offer group coverage on a guaranteed issue basis. With guaranteed issue, active employees must be insured regardless of the individual's health. This is in contrast to the individual underwriting, including health and cognitive screening, that is common in individual policies.

Many refer to group LTC insurance as the "employee benefit of the '90s." Although recent growth in the number of employees insured under these products is positive, the increasing number of employers offering these products is even more compelling evidence of a bright future.

(c) PROMOTING GROWTH IN EMPLOYER-SPONSORED LTC INSURANCE

Currently, the only clear tax-preferred treatment of long-term care services is provided through the dependent care tax credit and expenses paid from a dependent care spending account.[14] Although some interpret the Internal Revenue Code definition of medical care to include long-term care, there is no definitive Internal Revenue Service ruling to support this position. Congress has considered legislation to provide tax incentives to employers and employees for purchasing long-term care insurance. In addition, many bills were introduced in the 102nd Congress that would provide the same tax treatment for LTC insurance as for accident and health insurance. Although no bill has yet passed into law, this legislation seems inevitable because of the government's need to encourage a private-sector solution to the growing Medicaid expenditures for long-term care.

Another hope for stimulating future growth in LTC insurance is found through managed care. By creating an innovative managed care insurance product for LTC, the needs of a greater number of people can be met.

Managed care in LTC insurance can include such features as:

1. Providing an initial care plan that addresses the insured's needs and potential service settings to meet those needs;
2. Providing ongoing care management services to insureds receiving benefits;
3. Providing alternative benefits and service settings to insureds receiving benefits with the assistance of a care manager;
4. Providing consultation, information, and referral on a wide variety of informal and formal long-term care services to insureds;
5. Providing the convenience of paperless claims;
6. Creating and incorporating networks of long-term care providers who provide quality services, preferred access, and discounted fees.

The long-term goal of incorporating managed care with LTC insurance is to bring together a continuum of care for acute and long-term care services. By integrating acute and long-term care service delivery, customers will receive seamless service that will best meet their needs. This level of service will also provide employers with a vehicle that will accommodate their desire to be responsive to the needs of their employees in meeting their caregiving obligations.

NOTES

[1] Stone, R.I., and Kemper, P. "Spouses and Children of Disabled Elders: How Large a Constituency for Long-Term Care Reform?" *The Milbank Quarterly* (1989) *67*(3–4): 490.

[2] Fortune Magazine and John Hancock Financial Services. "Corporate and Employee Response to Caring for the Elderly: A National Survey of U.S. Companies and the Workforce" (1989), p. 6.

[3] Glickman, L.L., Birchander, E.L., and Greenberg, J.N. "Helping Companies Solve Elder Care Problems." *Compensation and Benefits Management* (Spring 1989), *5*: 197–201.

[4] Scharlach, A.E. "Four Ways to Avoid Problems in Corporate Elder Care." *The Aging Connection* (June/July 1990), *11*(3): 13.

[5] Sullivan, S.E., and Gilmore, B.J. "Employers Begin to Accept Eldercare as Business Issue." *Personnel* (July 1991), *68*: 3–4.

[6] *Ibid.*

[7] "Sales of Long-Term Care Policies Soaring: Report." *AHA News*, September 2, 1991, p. 3.

[8] *Ibid.*

[9] Health Insurance Association of America. "Who Buys Long-Term Care Insurance?" (1992), p. 51.

[10] Shalowitz, D. "Some Employers Starting to Pay LTC Costs." *Business Insurance*, April 1, 1991, p. 26.

[11] *Ibid.*

[12] Employee Benefit Research Institute. "Long Term Care Financing and the Private Insurance Market." *Issue Brief*, August 1991, No. 117, p. 11.

[13] Kemper, P., and Murtaugh, C.M. "Lifetime Use of Nursing Home Care." *New England Journal of Medicine*, February 28, 1991, pp. 595–600.

[14] Employee Benefit Research Institute. "Long Term Care Financing and the Private Insurance Market." Issue Brief, August 1991, No. 117, p. 8.

Nine

Comparative Analysis: Reform Proposals on Health and Long-Term Care

§ 9.1 INTRODUCTION

Over the past several years, public policymakers and private community organizations have developed proposals geared to reform the nation's health and long-term care system. This chapter examines several of the prominent proposals. All are designed to expand access, control costs, and improve quality of care delivered, although they vary in intensity, scope, and method. Specific proposals covered in this chapter are:

- The Pepper Commission's acute and long-term care proposals;[1]
- Senator George Mitchell's medical care bill entitled "HealthAmerica: Affordable Health Care for All Americans Act";[2]
- Senator John H. Chafee's medical care bill entitled "The Health Equity and Access Improvement Act of 1991";[3]

197

- Senator Robert Packwood's long-term care bill entitled "Secure Choice";[4]
- The long-term care proposal of the Physicians for a National Health Program.[5]

This chapter provides summaries of the proposals, a comparative analysis of recommendations, a discussion of how and whether these recommendations meet the health and long-term care needs of the elderly, as identified earlier in this book, and a look at what changes health care providers may expect in the future. As of this writing, none of the proposals has been passed into law.

§ 9.2 HEALTH CARE REFORM PROPOSALS

(a) THE PEPPER COMMISSION'S PROPOSAL

In 1989, Congress mandated the U.S. Bipartisan Commission on Comprehensive Health Care, known as the Pepper Commission (after Congressman Claude Pepper, a long-term advocate of health care reform), to recommend legislation that would ensure all Americans coverage for health and long-term care. In 1990, the Commission, chaired by Senator John D. Rockefeller IV (D—West Virginia), released its recommendations.

For medical care, the recommendations are designed to guarantee coverage for those currently uninsured and to ensure adequate coverage for those who have some insurance but not enough to cover catastrophic costs associated with a major illness. The plan would be phased in over 5 years; when fully implemented, the plan's total annual federal costs are projected at $24 billion (see Table 9.1).

(1) Basic Coverage

Under the proposal, all workers would be entitled to a minimum level of health coverage through their own jobs. The Commission recommended that all firms with more than 100 employees should be required to provide coverage to all their workers (and nonworking family members) by purchasing private insurance or by contributing to a newly established federal plan. Contributions to the public plan would be set at a fixed percentage of the employer's payroll.

Table 9.1
Impact of Commission Plan on Federal Expenditures

	Billions
Nonworkers covered under public plan	$11.0
Federal contribution to the public plan for workers (7.0% cap on employer costs)	5.3
Tax expenditure*	5.6
Payment of premiums and cost sharing for workers below 200% poverty	4.1
Augmented Medicaid physician and hospital payments	4.0
Savings to Medicare, CHAMPUS,† Medicaid	(6.0)
Total	$24.0

*Tax expenditure = a loss of tax revenue.
† Civilian Health and Medical Program to the Uniformed Services.
Source: The Pepper Commission, *A Call for Action: The Pepper Commission, U.S. Bipartisan Commission on Comprehensive Health Care.* Washington, DC: U.S. Government Printing Office, 1990, p. 69.

For employers with 100 or fewer employees, insurance market reforms and tax credits/subsidies were recommended as a way of encouraging greater purchase of private insurance for employees. Nonworkers, including those covered by Medicaid, and the self-employed would be covered through a new federal plan. All individuals would be required to obtain coverage either through their employers or from the federal plan.

(2)   Private Insurance Reform

The Commission recommended four changes to reform the small group health insurance market. Geared toward expanding access and increasing affordability for small businesses, these changes were:

- Prohibit preexisting condition exclusions;
- Guarantee acceptance of all small groups wishing to purchase health insurance;
- Set premiums on the same terms for all groups within specified areas;
- Prohibit selectively increasing rates for a particular group of policyholders.

Insurers would be allowed to require minimum enrollment periods so that they could spread out the costs of advertising and of forming a new group. Insurers in the small group market would be required to include small groups in managed care systems if they offer managed care options to larger employers in the area.

(3) Federal Public Program

A federal program would replace the federal/state Medicaid program and would guarantee all persons similar protection, no matter where they live. The federal program would pay providers Medicare rates and/or rates determined according to Medicare rules.

(4) Minimum Benefit Package

A federally specified standard benefit package would supersede current laws and would apply to everyone, regardless of enrollment in a public or private, traditional or managed care plan. Benefits would include: hospital care, surgical and other inpatient physicians' services, physician office visits, diagnostic tests, and limited mental health services. In addition, certain preventive services would be provided, including prenatal care, well-child care, mammograms, pap smears, colorectal and prostate cancer screening procedures, and other preventive services that evidence shows are cost-effective.

(5) Cost Sharing

Whether covered by the private or public plan, employees would pay a maximum of 20 percent of premium charges, and employers would be required to pay at least 80 percent. Those not covered through employment would pay the full costs of coverage in the public plan, based on their ability to pay.

Cost sharing for basic services would include a deductible of $250 for an individual and $500 for a family. For all services except mental health, outpatient services, and preventive care services, individuals would pay 20 percent coinsurance. Outpatient mental health services would be subject to 50 percent coinsurance, and there would be no deductibles or coinsurance for preventive services. Cost sharing would be capped at $3,000 for individuals and families.

Premiums and cost-sharing requirements would be subsidized for low-income people. Those with incomes below 100 percent of the federal poverty level would pay no premiums or coinsurance. Premiums and cost sharing would also be subsidized on a sliding scale for people with incomes up to at least 200 percent of the federal poverty level. For this population, premiums could not exceed 3 percent of income.

(6) Impact on Private Insurance Market

The Commission predicted that the job-based private insurance market would expand under its recommendations. The cap on payroll taxes for firms choosing the public plan would be set at a rate high enough—7 percent—to encourage as much participation in the private sector as possible. At this level, the Commission estimated that the number of workers brought into the public plan would be approximately equal to the number covered under job-based private insurance (24 million and 26 million, respectively). The total number of Americans covered by job-based private plans is expected to reach 171 million.

(7) Impact on Service Use

The Commission predicted that its proposal would increase total health care spending by $12 billion a year. Of this total, $5.3 billion would go toward inpatient hospital care and $3.5 billion to physician services. (See Table 9.2.)

(8) Strengthening the Health Care System

Along with expanding access, the proposal included recommendations for strengthening America's health care system. The Commission recommended developing a national system for quality assurance, public and private initiatives to contain health care costs, specific interventions to ensure availability of care to underserved people and areas, and support for programs of health promotion and disease prevention.

(9) Quality Assurance and Malpractice Reform

The Commission recommended that the federal government develop and implement a comprehensive national system of quality assurance that included five components:

1. Development and implementation of national practice guidelines and standards of care, which the Commission believed would

Table 9.2

**Impact of the Pepper Commission Plan on
Health Care Expenditures, by Type of
Service for Noninstitutionalized People***

Type of Service	Billions	
	Expenditures	Utilization
Hospital inpatient	$181.4	$5.3
Hospital outpatient	38.7	1.4
Physicians	146.6	3.5
Dentists	49.7	0.3
Other professionals	17.9	0.3
Prescription drugs	33.2	0.9
Eyeglasses and appliances	12.4	0.0
Other health	13.4	0.3

*Assumes Commission's plan fully implemented in 1990.

Source: The Pepper Commission, *A Call for Action: The Pepper Commission, U.S. Bipartisan Commission on Comprehensive Health Care.* Washington, DC: U.S. Government Printing Office, 1990, p. 71.

reduce unnecessary, inappropriate, and ineffective care. The Commission estimated that $1.5 billion to $22 billion could be saved annually from changes in practice patterns.

2. Development and implementation of a uniform data system that would cover all health care encounters, regardless of payment source or setting. This system would be designed to provide a common foundation for all payers' quality assessment activities and for examining the effectiveness of medical care. It would also be designed to help identify health policy and research concerns.

3. Development and testing of new, more effective methods of quality assurance and assessment.

4. Development and oversight of local review organizations that have skills in data integration and analysis, quality assessment, and quality assurance. This recommendation was designed to enhance the performance of a quality assurance program while making reviewers more accountable for their performance.

5. Demonstration projects related to medical malpractice reform that would lead to recommendations for federal action, Congressional hearings on malpractice issues, and professional liability reform incorporated in access legislation.

(10) Cost Containment

The Commission believed that the cost sharing included in the recommended minimum benefit package would make consumers sensitive to price and more prudent in the medical services they choose.

In addition, the Commission believed that its recommended insurance reform would lead insurers to compete around efficient service delivery rather than for good risks. The requirements that insurers accept all group applicants and use comparable rating systems for all covered groups would, it was believed, ensure that the greatest rewards no longer go to the insurers who are most adept at attracting low-risk clients.

Efficient service delivery would be encouraged by extending managed care to small employers and including managed care as a means to provide the minimum benefit package to private insurance and the public plan. The Commission stated that extending Medicare payment rules to the public program would expand these effective payment controls and serve as a model for private insurance. In addition, adoption of comprehensive quality assurance strategy, including malpractice reform, would ensure greater value in the delivery of health care services.

(11) Reduction of Cost Inequities Among Groups

The following provisions were designed to reduce the health care costs for groups that now bear a disproportionate share of the health care financing burden:

- The current cost shifting from the uninsured to the insured population would be reduced. This would reduce costs for the employers and insurers currently paying indirectly for uncompensated care.
- The current cost shifting from employers that do not cover workers to employers that do would be reduced. This would reduce costs for employers already providing coverage.
- Small business insurance reforms would make insurance more affordable for small businesses.

(12) Preventive Health

The Commission recommended federal support for programs of health promotion, disease prevention, risk reduction, and health education. This program would be geared toward reducing excess morbidity and mortality and increasing healthy life-styles. The Commission recommended an additional $1 billion of federal funds for this effort.

(13)　Improving Protection for Those Ages 65 and Over

The Commission included a separate set of recommendations for the elderly, focused largely on addressing the gaps in Medicare coverage. Recommendations, which the Commission stated would serve 30 million elderly and would cost an additional $2.8 billion in federal spending, included the following:

- Medicare, or the public plan that would replace Medicaid at the federal level, would provide assistance with the Medicare premium, deductibles, and cost sharing to all elderly people with incomes below 200 percent of the federal poverty level. Elderly persons with income between 100 and 200 percent of the poverty level would receive assistance on an income-based sliding scale; those with incomes below the poverty line would receive full assistance. This program would undergo strong outreach efforts to ensure participation.
- Medicare would be expanded to provide selected preventive services, including mammography and colorectal and prostate screening services. Other services would be added when they are established as being cost-effective.
- To guard against Medigap abuse, the Commission recommended federal action to ensure the nonpoor elderly access to adequate coverage through insurance reforms similar to the insurance reforms recommended by the Commission for the nonelderly. In addition, legislation would be enacted to fund state or local programs that would advise Medigap purchasers on the quality, price, and benefits of Medigap policies.

(b)　THE "HEALTHAMERICA" BILL

In June 1991, Senator George Mitchell (D—Maine) introduced the Senate Democratic leadership bill, entitled "HealthAmerica: Affordable Health Care for All Americans." This proposed legislation would ensure that every American has basic health care coverage. The coverage would be provided either through a private plan offered by an employer or through a public federal/state insurance program, referred to as "AmeriCare." AmeriCare would replace Medicaid except for long-term care services. Many of the provisions in the bill are similar to the

Pepper Commission's recommendations for health care reform. The plan would be phased in over 5 years and, when fully implemented, would cost $18 billion annually.

(1) Employment-Based Coverage

For employees and their families, businesses would have the choice of providing coverage that meets minimum standards or making a contribution to the public plan. The contribution would be set as a percentage of payroll, at a rate that would encourage employers to offer private coverage. Employers with a high percentage of low-wage or part-time workers would receive a substantial subsidy.

Employees would be required to accept coverage for themselves and their families if offered by their employers, and they would be required to pay a share of the premium as well as copayments and deductibles. If an employer provides private coverage rather than making a contribution to the public plan, all workers working at least 17.5 hours a week must be covered for themselves and their families.

(2) Basic Benefit Package

Plans must cover hospital services, physician services, diagnostic tests, limited mental health, and the following preventive health services: prenatal, well-baby, and well-child care; mammograms; and pap smears.

Employees would pay a maximum of 20 percent of the premium, deductibles of $250 per individual and $500 per family, and copayments of 20 percent. Out-of-pocket payments for catastrophic care would be capped at $3,000. For low-income workers, out-of-pocket payments would be subsidized by the public plan.

(3) Consumer Protection

No limits on coverage could be imposed based on preexisting conditions. A set of legal protections would be established for insured individuals, including the right to full information on plan provisions and the right to appeal coverage decisions.

(4) Public Plan

Except for long-term care services, Medicaid would be replaced by a new federal/state program called "AmeriCare." The program would be administered by the states subject to national standards for eligibility, reimbursement, and coverage. Benefits under AmeriCare would be the same as for employment-based coverage, except that AmeriCare would provide for early and periodic screening, diagnosis, and treatment.

Individuals below the federal poverty line would have access to optional services that each state could choose to provide. Those who are below the poverty line and are covered by an employer-based plan would have the option of receiving such services through the public plan.

Those below the poverty line would pay no premium, and other low-income individuals would pay on a sliding scale. The public plan would also subsidize low-income workers covered through the private plan.

States would be encouraged to establish purchasing consortia to reduce the overall inflation rate of health care costs. States would also be encouraged to set up and enroll beneficiaries in managed care systems. Providers would be reimbursed at levels at least equivalent to the levels that would be provided by the use of Medicare reimbursement rules.

(5) Financing

The public program would be financed by state and federal contributions. States would receive an enhanced federal match for coverage of newly eligible persons and other new costs in the public program. This enhanced match would be a specified percentage of increase over a state's current matching rate for the Medicaid program.

(6) Expanding Access

Over a 5-year period, approximately $1.3 billion in additional funding would go toward the creation of community health centers, to provide primary care services to underserved areas. Authors of the bill estimated that such additional funding would increase service capacity from 5.8 million to 15 million persons each year.

(7) Controlling Costs

The bill's authors believed that providing universal health care coverage would in itself reduce the cost of health insurance coverage. They would take the following additional steps to reduce costs.

Reduce Unnecessary or Ineffective Care. Legislation would raise the authorization level for the Agency for Health Care Policy and Research (AHCPAR) by $50 million, to enable it to conduct additional outcomes research and develop practice guidelines for more procedures.

Government programs would be required to use practice guidelines in utilization review activities. Additional measures would be adopted to ensure dissemination of guidelines (once developed) to providers and payers. Research on technology assessment at AHCPAR would also be expanded.

Steps would be taken to encourage managed care. State legislative barriers to managed care would be preempted. Small businesses would be given guaranteed access to managed care through small business insurance reform. The public program would include managed care options.

Eliminate Unnecessary Administrative Costs.   Four programs would be established in an effort to reduce excessive administrative costs:

- Claims forms would be standardized;
- Small insurance companies would be required to form an insurance consortia for the purpose of paying providers, thus reducing the number of payment entities with which providers must deal;
- New agencies would be established in each state to work with providers on a program of continuous quality improvement and implementation of cost-effective methods of delivering care, including practice guidelines;
- Small business reform would be implemented.

Ensure Provider Price and Volume Restraint.   A Federal Health Expenditure Board would be established to set national expenditure goals, overall and by sectors of the health care industry. Advisory goals would also be established for states and regions. The Board would convene providers and purchasers to conduct negotiations on rates and on methods of achieving the expenditure goals. If the negotiators agree, then these rates would be mandatory and enforceable. If the negotiators do not agree, the Board would issue mandatory rates.

States would be required to establish insurance/purchasing consortia, which would require insurance companies with small market shares to participate for the purpose of reducing administrative costs. The consortia would make all direct payments to providers on behalf of insurance companies with small market shares and would work with providers to establish other administrative efficiencies, such as paperless processing. The states would have the option of allowing larger insurers to join the consortia. The consortia would be allowed to carry out such functions as price negotiations, volume negotiations, capital allocation, rational distribution of providers, data collection, consumer protection, and promotion of managed care/competition.

Develop and Disseminate Cost and Quality Data on Individual Providers. The Federal Health Expenditure Board would collect, analyze, and disseminate data that would assist consumers and purchasers of care in evaluating the efficiency and quality of individual providers. This is intended to assist in developing managed care networks, identifying quality providers for patients, and encouraging providers to improve their performance.

(8) Special Programs for Small Businesses

The legislation would reduce the cost of insurance for businesses that employ predominantly low-wage or part-time workers by offering these businesses the opportunity to make a contribution based on a percentage of payroll instead of providing coverage directly.

Federal standards for health insurance sold in the small group market would be designed to accomplish the following: remove barriers to group health insurance by eliminating preexisting condition exclusions and denials of coverage on the basis of health status; promote equity in insurance premiums by moving toward a community-rated system; and improve the affordability of coverage for small employers by preempting state benefit laws and ensuring access to managed care.

Small businesses not profitable enough to provide health insurance coverage to their workers without difficulty would receive a tax credit to cover up to 25 percent of the cost. This credit would be in addition to the deduction currently available (at the time the bill was written) for the cost of such insurance. Self-employed owner-operators would be able to deduct 100 percent of the cost of health plan insurance premiums.

(9) State Single-Payer Option

States would be allowed to adopt a single-payer, tax-supported system rather than following the combination of employer- and public-based model established in the bill.

(c) THE CHAFEE PROPOSAL

In November 1991, Senator John H. Chafee (R—Rhode Island) introduced the Republican Congressional leadership's health care reform bill, entitled "Health Equity and Access Improvement Act of 1991." The basic principle of the bill is that the current system has definite strengths and they should be built on, not replaced. The proposal attempts to expand the advantages of the current system while adding some reforms designed to expand access and control costs.

(1) Standardized Benefits

The National Association of Insurance Commissioners would develop a model health care benefit plan containing standard benefits and coverage that health insurers would have to meet. Standard benefits would include basic hospital, medical, and surgical services, including preventive care services "determined appropriate by the Secretary of Health and Human Services." Standard cost sharing, copayments, and deductibles would also be outlined. In addition, a managed care advisory committee would be formed to develop standards that insurers offering managed care plans would have to meet with respect to benefits, coverage, and services provided under such plans.

(2) Cost Containment

Aimed at slowing the trend of increasing medical costs, the proposal encourages the development and utilization of managed care techniques. Businesses that begin to offer a managed care plan would receive a tax credit for the first 5 years they offer the plan. State anti-managed-care laws would be preempted for approved managed care plans. States would receive a 3 percent enhanced match for each low-income participant in the public program who is enrolled in a managed care setting.

(3) Expanded Access

Tax credits would be available for individuals with family incomes below $32,000 or individual incomes below $16,000. Credits would be $1,200 for a family and $600 for an individual. The credit could be used to purchase health insurance and health care services.

Tax credits would be provided to small businesses that begin to provide health insurance to employees, as well as to those that extend coverage to include dependents. Employers that join a purchasing group (as defined in the bill) would receive a tax credit.

To encourage the purchase of insurance, tax deductions would be available for those without employer-provided insurance and for those who are self-employed.

A tax credit would be available for preventive services such as cancer screening tests, childhood immunization, and well-child care.

The proposal would increase authorization levels by $2.9 billion over the next 5 years, for community health centers. Authorization would also be expanded for the National Health Service Corps. A grant program would be established under the Public Health Service Act. States would allocate funds to health care providers that propose to expand services in medically underserved areas or health professional shortage areas. The Centers for Disease Control would receive a $50 million increase to expand the childhood immunization program.

(4) Public Program

States would be permitted to establish a new program to provide basic health coverage for low-income, uninsured individuals who are not eligible for Medicaid. States would set eligibility requirements for the new program, with two restrictions. First, individuals would have to live in families with incomes below 200 percent of the federal poverty level. States would be allowed to charge premiums, deductibles, and/or copayments for those with incomes between 100 and 200 percent of the poverty level. Premiums could not exceed 5 percent of adjusted gross income. Second, individuals would not qualify for Medicaid as currently covered by the state. States could target eligibility to specific age groups, locations, income levels, or employment groups.

States would set benefit packages and reimbursement levels. However, federal financial participation would not be available for long-term care residential settings, including nursing homes and group housing.

(5) Assistance to Small Businesses

Small business purchasing groups could be established by small businesses in an area. The groups would be nonprofit, membership corporations with full-time staff and a board of directors comprised of participating businesses. Start-up grants would be available through the Secretary of Health and Human Services for approved groups certified by the state. Small employers who purchase insurance through an approved group would receive a small tax credit if more than 60 percent of their work force elects coverage.

(6)   Expanded Access in Rural Areas

The bill includes several provisions to expand access to health care in rural areas that are currently underserved. Recommendations include: reallocating funding under the Health Professionals Training Act and Nurse Education Act, to increase the number of health professionals in medically underserved areas; and providing demonstration grants to improve the quality and availability of health care in rural areas by encouraging the sharing of resources, developing managed care cooperatives, and establishing mental health outreach programs.

(7)   Demonstration Projects

The bill's authors recommended establishment of a Waiver Board made up of the Secretaries of Health and Human Services, Treasury, and Labor, with authority to waive requirements of federal programs such as Medicare, Medicaid, Public Health Service Grants, ERISA, and other programs, for the purpose of allowing states to implement statewide demonstration programs.

(8)   Medical Liability Reform

The cost of medical liability is estimated at $15 billion annually. As part of overall cost control mechanisms, the proposal attempts to reform the liability system by encouraging the development of alternative dispute resolution systems designed to reduce court costs and backlogs and to increase access to the liability system for those with small claims. Other recommendations include: encouraging early claims settlements whenever possible; preempting state tort laws in certain areas; sending punitive damage awards to consumer protection agencies and state disciplinary boards; and strengthening the ability of states to ensure that the quality of care provided by physicians and other health care professionals remains high.

§ 9.3   LONG-TERM CARE PROPOSALS

(a)   THE PEPPER COMMISSION'S PROPOSAL

The basic principles of the Commission's long-term care proposal are: (1) long-term care should be treated as an insurable event whose risk can be spread through private and/or public coverage; (2) people in nursing homes should be guaranteed an ample floor of protection, ensuring that no one will become impoverished; and (3) all but the poorest should contribute to the costs of care. The Commission recommended a program of federal "social insurance" for home- and community-based care and extended nursing-home coverage. The plan would be designed to ensure access, control costs, and promote research on preventing and reducing disabilities. It would be phased in over a period of 4 years at a total additional cost of $42.8 billion for the 4-year period, $31.8 billion of which would be for the elderly.

(1) Public Program

The proposal includes a public program, a role for private insurance, and a research agenda. In terms of the public program, there would be a single point of entry for all beneficiaries, a single set of eligibility rules for all services, a standardized assessment to determine eligibility, and a mechanism for managing the care process across settings. The program would be designed to allow individuals the opportunity to choose care settings and types of care and to help ensure efficient administration and service coordination.

Under the public program, an individual would qualify for long-term care benefits at home or in a nursing home if he or she meets one of the following disability criteria:

- Need for hands-on or supervisory assistance with three out of five activities of daily living (ADLs were not defined in the Commission's proposal);
- Need for constant supervision because of cognitive impairment that impedes ability to function;
- Need for constant supervision because of behaviors that are dangerous, disruptive, or difficult to manage.

The program would encourage the expansion of home care services and would include minimum federal standards for managing care and ensuring quality. The Commission believed these efforts would expand and improve services for the entire long-term care population, not just the severely disabled. Availability of services would increase, and, even for those who do not receive benefits under the public program, services would be better and more accessible.

(2) Home- and Community-Based Care

The Commission "considers financing home- and community-based care a top priority." Benefits for the severely disabled would be intended to complement support that families provide and to help disabled people continue functioning at the highest possible level of independence. The Commission recommended that public program benefits include the following:

- A broad range of personal care services, including feeding, transferring, and tasks related to personal hygiene;
- Homemaker/chore services;
- Medication management;
- Day-care services for those who are unable to leave their homes.

Respite services and support counseling would be provided to family caregivers, as well as training on how to deliver home-based care more effectively. The Commission also recommended that skilled nursing care and physical, occupational, speech, and other appropriate therapy services be covered.

(3) Cost Sharing

Beneficiaries would be required to contribute 20 percent of the actual costs of care or 20 percent of the national average cost of home- and community-based care, whichever is lower. Full federal subsidies for the poor, and partial subsidies for those who have income up to 200 percent of the poverty line, would be granted.

(4) Case Management

Home care services would not be designed to replace family caregiving. They would be designed to supplement family care, and case managers would be the cornerstone for organizing this cooperative effort. Case managers would develop and oversee individual care plans, helping to integrate care and service delivery for multiple problems.

The case manager would operate within a budget set by the federal government. This budget would be based on a per-capita amount set according to the service needs of individuals with different levels of disability. Working within the budget, the case manager would develop a plan of care tailored to the needs of the individual. The case manager would also be responsible for monitoring implementation of the care plan and conducting periodic reassessments to determine whether changes in the amount or type of services are needed. Case managers would be audited periodically by an assessment agency. The Commission recommended that a federally certified state or local government or nonprofit assessment agency determine people's eligibility for the public program and that a standardized assessment criterion be used.

(5) Nursing-Home Care

Along with community- and home-based care, the Commission's proposed social insurance program would cover short-term nursing-home stays. Those who are declared to be eligible for nursing-home care by the federally certified assessment agency would be covered for the first 3 months of institutional care, with each 3-month period of coverage considered an episode of care. Individuals would be required to contribute 20 percent of the actual costs of care, or 20 percent of the national average cost of nursing home care, whichever is lower. Federal subsidies for the poor and near-poor would be similar to those for community- and home-based coverage.

For those with nursing-home stays of more than 3 months, the Commission would establish a floor of asset protection and more generous income protection than is available under current law, to ensure that no individual or noninstitutionalized spouse faces impoverishment. For the poor who are severely disabled, this program would replace Medicaid.

The Commission's plan would prevent impoverishment from long-term nursing-home stays. Individuals would be allowed to keep $30,000 and couples $60,000 in nonhousing assets. Individuals would be required to contribute toward the costs of nursing-home care after this portion of their income was protected. In addition, single individuals would be allowed to keep 30 percent of their monthly income for the first year of stay, to enable them to maintain their homes in the community. Married persons would be eligible for this housing allowance as long as the community spouse is alive. The program would also provide a personal needs allowance of $100 per month for nursing-home residents (compared to the $30 per month allowed now for Medicaid recipients).

(6) Financing the Public Plan

The federal government would be responsible for financing the social insurance components of the public plan. Federal and state governments would share the financial responsibility for the part of the program that covers longer nursing-home stays.

(7) Administering the Public Plan

The federal government would contract with states to administer the public plan and would be responsible for setting guidelines and adequate standards for this administration. Guidelines would be established for quality assurance and for certifying case managers, to ensure adequate training and the capacity to undertake the assessment, service allocation, and monitoring functions.

Provider payment rates for both home- and community-based care and for nursing-home care would be determined at the federal level. The states would administer the public plan and certify the providers who participate in the public plan, in accordance with federal guidelines. The state would also develop a review and appeals process with respect to benefit termination and denial, subject to federal guidelines.

(8) Ensuring Quality and Controlling Costs

The case manager (who is most likely to develop a personal relationship with the client and family) would monitor the quality of services being provided formally and informally in the home. The auditing function of the federally certified assessment agency over the case manager would provide an additional quality check.

(9) Integration with Existing Federal Long-Term Care Programs

Medicare benefits would be expanded to cover nursing-home care, and Medicare would become the first payer for nursing-home users who qualify. Through the social insurance program, Medicare coverage would be extended to cover up to a total of 3 months of care.

For those who meet the definition of severely disabled, the social insurance program would replace all Medicaid programs that currently fund home health and home care services. Medicaid would remain intact for the less severely disabled who meet the current financial standards. The new program would not replace Medicare's role in covering skilled home health care.

For the chronically mentally ill and developmentally disabled, services would continue under the veterans' health system, Title III of the Older Americans Act, the Social Services Block Grant, and other programs. The case manager would be responsible for coordinating services across programs.

(10) The Role of Private Long-Term Care Insurance

Private insurance would be designed to supplement coverage provided by the public program. Insurance could be purchased to cover cost sharing and to protect additional income and assets in case of long-term nursing-home stays. The Commission recommended the following measures to promote and regulate private long-term care insurance:

- Clarification of the Internal Revenue Code so that long-term care is explicitly defined as appropriate for preferential treatment;
- Treatment of long-term care insurance premiums paid and benefits received in the same manner as health insurance, which would enable employers to pay for long-term care insurance without obligating the employee to include premiums or benefits as taxable income;
- An allowance for employers to include long-term care insurance in employee cafeteria plans.

These provisions would give long-term care insurance the same tax preferences as health insurance, pensions, and other employee benefits.

(11) Research Agenda

The Commission recommended research on ways to prevent the need for long-term care, on the kinds of services most likely to enhance people's capacity to function, and on program management tools and delivery systems that promote efficient delivery of quality care. The Commission recommended total funding of $1 billion annually.

(12) Beneficiaries and Costs of Recommendations

The Commission believed its recommendations will make home- and community-based care, now limited in most communities and virtually nonexistent in many, both available and affordable. The choice between care in the home or in an institution would depend on need and preference rather than on resources.

For the severely disabled elderly, new federal spending would be split almost evenly between home care ($15 billion) and nursing-home care ($16.8 billion). (See Table 9.3.) For nursing-home care, the floor of protection against impoverishment would cost an estimated $11.3 billion, and expanded coverage for short stays would cost an additional $5.5 billion.

Under the new program, the Commission projected that 2 million severely disabled elderly people at home would use care—double the number who now use paid care. For the 1 million who would have purchased their own care in the absence of the public program, out-of-pocket savings are estimated to reach $900 million, or about $1,000 per user.

(b) THE "SECURE CHOICE" PROPOSAL

In July 1991, Senator Robert Packwood (D—Oregon) introduced a long-term care bill entitled "Secure Choice," which is designed to make long-term care services for the elderly more affordable and available. The bill

Table 9.3
Beneficiaries and Net Federal Costs of
Commission Long-Term Care Recommendations,
by Age Group and Type of Service

	Home Care	Nursing Home Care	Total
Total beneficiaries (in millions)			
Elderly	2.0	1.2	3.2
Nonelderly	1.0	0.2	1.2
Total	3.0	1.4	4.4
New federal costs (in billions, 1990)			
Elderly	$15.0	$16.8	$31.8
Nonelderly	9.0	2.0	11.0
Total	$24.0	$18.8	$42.8

Source: The Pepper Commission, *A Call for Action: The Pepper Commission, U.S. Bipartisan Commission on Comprehensive Health Care.* Washington, DC: U.S. Government Printing Office, 1990, p. 130.

would provide services to the poor elderly, set up a public–private partnership to make insurance more affordable for low-income elderly, and remove existing tax barriers in order to provide incentives for the elderly to purchase long-term care insurance. The bill would also expand coverage for home- and community-based care.

(1)   Federal/State Program

The bill would establish a new federal program to provide long-term care services to low-income elderly who are below the federal poverty line, under a new Title (XXI) of the Social Security Act. Long-term care services now provided to the elderly through Medicaid would be moved to this new Title XXI. Eligibility would be changed so that it is based on age, income, assets, and impairment. (Impairment is defined as limited ability to carry out three of five activities of daily living (toileting, eating, transferring, bathing/dressing, and mobility).)

(2)   Benefits

Covered services would include nursing-home care and a mix of home- and community-based services. Community- and home-based services would include homemaker/home health aide services; personal care services performed by a qualified nonfamily member; home health care; adult day care; nursing services provided by or under the supervision of a registered nurse; physical therapy and related services; and respite care. Other covered benefits would include prescription drugs, case management services, and respiratory care services.

(3)   Case Management

Anyone participating in the state plan would receive case management. The case manager would design a plan of care to maximize functioning, coordinate long-term care services, identify the mix of formal and informal services available, and contain costs by choosing the appropriate services based on available resources and service needs. The case manager would not be permitted to provide care.

(4)   Eligibility

States would be required to cover eligible individuals with incomes up to 100 percent of the federal poverty level, and they would have the option of covering individuals up to 240 percent of the poverty level. Individuals qualifying for benefits could not exceed income or resource levels of $2,000 to receive nursing-home care coverage, or $5,000 to receive home- or community-based coverage. No cost sharing would be required if the beneficiary meets these requirements.

Under the federal/state plan, the minimum monthly personal needs allowance for nursing-home residents would be $35 for individuals and $70 for a couple. States would have the option of increasing this allowance.

(5) Relationship with Medicaid

Medicaid would retain its current structure, except for provisions related to long-term care services for functionally impaired elderly persons. Nursing facility services, home health services, and other services would remain covered under Medicaid; however, states would limit these services to 45 days for the functionally and cognitively impaired elderly. A stay of longer than 45 days would indicate a chronic condition requiring long-term care services covered under Title XXI.

States would be able to purchase home- and community-based care services more easily than they currently can under Medicaid because the need to obtain Medicaid waivers for these services would be eliminated.

(6) Standards

A single state agency would administer or supervise the administration of the plan. This entity would determine eligibility for long-term care assistance, establish and maintain standards for private and public providers, and ensure that all qualifying individuals have the same services available. Standard rates for nursing home services would be established, and states would have to file uniform cost reports from nursing facilities.

(7) Public–Private Partnership

The bill would give states the option of participating in a public–private partnership. Individuals who had purchased qualified long-term care insurance policies would be eligible to have part of their coverage subsidized once they became functionally or cognitively impaired, were over age 55, and had an income between 240 and 400 percent of the federal poverty level. The state and federal governments would subsidize the costs of coverage on a sliding scale. Subsidies would be established by the Standards and Performance Organization (see below). A maximum benefit subsidy would be equal to 75 percent of the costs of services provided under the policy minus the amount to be paid by the qualified insurer. Individuals who purchase qualified policies would be allowed to protect assets above the Title XXI levels, up to $20,000.

States choosing to participate in the insurance option would be required to expand their Title XXI programs to cover functionally and cognitively impaired elderly individuals with income up to 240 percent of the federal poverty level, to eliminate gaps in coverage between Title XXI and the insurance option.

(8) Benefits and Coverage

Qualified insurers would be required to offer case management, nursing-home facility services, and home- and community-based services similar to those offered under the public plan.

For nursing-home facility services, the maximum daily benefit required under a long-term care insurance policy would be 80 percent of the per diem rate. For community- and home-based services, the maximum daily benefit would be 60 percent of the maximum daily benefit for nursing-home facility services.

The maximum lifetime benefit offered by qualified insurance policies would equal $80 per day (for FY 1991; the amount would increase by 5 percent each succeeding year), multiplied by 730 days. In other words, the maximum lifetime benefit would be equal to 2 years of the price of nursing-home care. This maximum benefit could be used for any combination of nursing-home and home- and community-based care or services.

(9) Increased Accessibility to Private Insurance

Qualified insurance policies would have to guarantee renewability, adjust benefits for inflation, have no more than a (cumulative) 30-day elimination period, and limit the waiting period for preexisting conditions.

(10) Standards

A Standards and Performance Organization would be required in each participating state, to ensure that plans meet license, certifying, and other standards. The Organization would assess the quality and appropriateness of case management services, ensure that plans comply with standards and cover appropriate services, determine whether qualified insurers are using appropriate managed care techniques, ensure that long-term care services meet developed standards, and monitor the income of participants.

(11) Tax Incentives

The bill would clarify the tax laws relating to long-term care expenses and insurance so that they are treated the same as medical expenses and medical insurance. The following provisions would become effective:

- Out-of-pocket long-term care expenses and the cost of qualified long-term care insurance would be tax-deductible (above 7.5 percent of adjusted gross income);
- Payments for insured long-term care services under qualified long-term care policies would not be taxable;
- Employer-paid long-term care services and qualified long-term care insurance would be tax-free employee benefits;
- Insurance company reserves set aside to pay benefits under qualified long-term care insurance policies would be tax-deductible;
- Death benefits paid under a life insurance policy to terminally ill individuals would be tax-free.

(c) THE PROPOSAL OF PHYSICIANS FOR A NATIONAL HEALTH PROGRAM

Physicians for a National Health Program (PNHP) published their recommendations for a national long-term care program in the December 4, 1991, issue of the *Journal of the American Medical Association.* The goals of their proposal are to achieve the following: make long-term care coverage universal, with access to services based on need rather than age, cause of disability, or income; provide a continuum of social and medical services aimed at maximizing functional independence; coordinate medically and socially oriented long-term care with acute inpatient and ambulatory care; spread financial risk across the entire population, using a progressive financing system rather than having payment for long-term care fall disproportionately on the severely disabled; and provide support for long-term care that assists rather than supplants informal caregivers.

(1) Coverage

Everyone would be covered for all medically and socially necessary services under a single public plan. Long-term care services would be intended to supplement and be integrated with acute care services. (As of this writing, PNHP is in the process of developing its recommendations for medical care reform.) Covered services would include:

- Home- and community-based benefits, including nursing, therapy services, case management, meals, information and referral, in-home support, respite, transportation services, adult day health, social day care, psychiatric day care, hospice, community mental health, and "other related services";
- Residential services, including foster care, board and care, assisted living, and residential care facilities;
- Institutional care, including nursing homes, chronic care hospitals, and rehabilitation facilities;
- Drug and alcohol treatment, outpatient rehabilitation, and independent living programs;
- Preventive services (specific services are not listed).

(2) Administrative Structure and Eligibility for Care

Under federal mandate, each state would set up a long-term care system with a state Long-Term Care Planning and Payment Board and a network of local, public, long-term care agencies. These local agencies would employ panels of providers to assess individuals' long-term care needs, develop a plan of service, coordinate care, conduct provider certification, and sometimes provide services. An agency would serve as the entry point for local long-term care use, certify eligibility for specific services, and assign a case manager "when appropriate."

The Long-Term Care Planning and Payment Board and local long-term care agencies in each state would pay for the full continuum of covered long-term care services. Each state's long-term care operating budget would be allocated to the local long-term care agencies based on population, the number of elderly and disabled, the economic status of the population, case mix, and cost of living. Each long-term care agency would allocate funds from the available budget to cover the operating costs of approved providers in its community. The actual payment structure would be centralized in the state's Board.

Each institutional provider could negotiate a global operating budget with the local long-term care agencies. PNHP suggested another option in which the provider could contract to provide comprehensive long-term care services or integrated long-term care and acute care services on a capitated basis. Physicians could be paid on a fee-for-service basis or receive salaries from institutional providers.

Coverage would extend to anyone needing assistance with one or more activities of daily living (defined as bathing, dressing, going to the toilet, getting outside, walking, transferring from bed to chair, or eating) or instrumental activities of daily living (defined as cooking, cleaning, shopping, taking medication, doing laundry, making telephone calls, or managing money). High-risk patients who did not specifically meet these criteria would be eligible for services needed to prevent worsening disability and possible future institutional care. Local panels would have the flexibility, within their defined budgets, to authorize a wide range of services, taking into account such social factors as the availability of informal care.

PNHP stated that "not all those needing long-term care require case management." Therefore, when case management or care coordination is needed, the local agencies would conduct or delegate this service to capitated providers who offer comprehensive services.

(3)   Utilization and Cost Controls

PNHP predicted that their proposal could result in a 20 percent increase in nursing-home utilization and a 50 to 100 percent increase in community- and home-based care utilization. They predicted this increase would continue for about 3 years.

(4)   Financing

The program would be completely financed by tax revenues, without premiums, deductibles, copayments, or coinsurance. People permanently living in residential care would use part of their Social Security or Supplemental Security Income to contribute to living costs.

(5)   Cost Controls

The proposal relies on enforceable overall budgetary ceilings to contain costs. With a defined fixed budget, local long-term care agencies would allocate finite resources to those in need. PNHP argued that local agencies would therefore have strong incentives to support more cost-effective informal providers and community-based services, in an effort to forestall costly institutionalization. Funding for ongoing evaluation was recommended, to quickly disclose problems and allow rapid correction.

(6) Quality of Care

Each long-term care provider would be required to meet uniform national quality standards in order to be paid by the public plan. These standards would include structural measures, process measures, and outcome measures.

Each long-term care organization and agency would be required to establish a quality assurance program meeting national standards and a quality assurance committee with representatives of each category of service provider—clients, family members and other caregivers, and community representatives. The committee would review the quality of care provided and resolve problems and disputes.

Unresolved issues would be reported to a public regulatory system, defined as a body consisting of all existing regulatory entities, such as peer review organizations and certification agencies.

Funding would be provided for training and in-service education of long-term care professionals, paraprofessionals, and informal caregivers. Formal providers would be required to meet minimum training and competency standards. The program would be geared toward the special needs of the frail elderly, the disabled, and the mentally impaired, and would be designed to work with multidisciplinary teams, in order to develop community services.

(7) Cost and Financing

Public expenditures would cover the $52 billion PNHP said is spent each year (in 1990 dollars) in total long-term care costs. PNHP estimated that the increased utilization resulting from expanded access would add $21.5 billion in home health care costs and $16 billion in nursing-home costs each year. Quality improvement measures would cost an additional $2 billion per year.

PNHP estimated that a total of $70 billion to $75.5 billion in new tax revenues would be needed to finance the program. They suggested that revenues could be raised from several sources, including the Social Security system, general taxes, and estate taxes.

§ 9.4 COMPARATIVE ANALYSIS

All the proposals are similar in their goals of increasing access, containing costs, and centralizing and streamlining the health and/or long-term care delivery system. However, they differ in their approach to these goals and in the extent to which they would change the current system. Tables 9.4 and 9.5 provide comparisons of the various provisions of these proposals. The following describes their similarities and differences.

(a) IMPROVING ACCESS TO SERVICES

All the proposals include measures to improve access to health care services, and all attempt to base access to services more on need than on ability to pay. But they differ on who would receive government-supported services and on the level of service that would be provided.

Both the Pepper Commission's and Senator Mitchell's proposals for medical care would guarantee all Americans health insurance coverage, either through private, job-based insurance or through entry into a public plan. Both would mandate a minimum benefit package focused largely on physician and hospital services, with minimal preventive services. Both include insurance reforms designed to make the purchase of private insurance easier for businesses, particularly small businesses.

Table 9.4
Provisions of Health Care Reform Proposals

	Pepper	Mitchell	Chafee
Those covered	All firms with over 100 employees required to provide coverage for employees by purchasing private insurance or contributing to a public plan; all workers required to obtain coverage; those not working buy into public plan.	All employers are required to provide coverage for employees by purchasing private insurance or contributing to a public plan; all workers are required to obtain coverage; those not working buy into public plan.	Provides tax credits to help low-income individuals and families purchase insurance; states allowed to establish public program for those with incomes below 200% of the federal poverty level; program would include deductibles, premiums, and copayments.

Table 9.4 *(Continued)*

	Pepper	Mitchell	Chafee
Benefits	Hospital care, surgical and other inpatient physicians' services, physician office visits, diagnostic tests, limited mental health, prenatal care, mammograms, pap smears, colorectal and prostate cancer screening.	Hospital care, physician care, diagnostic tests, limited mental health, prenatal care, well-baby care, well-child care, mammograms, and pap smears.	Hospital, medical and surgical services; preventive services to be determined by Secretary of Health and Human Services; tax credit for cancer screening, child immunization, and well-child care.
Cost sharing	Employees pay 20% and employers pay 80% of premiums; cost sharing capped at $3,000; deductibles are $250 for individuals and $500 for families.	Employees pay 20% and employers pay 80% of premiums; cost sharing is capped at $3,000 for catastrophic care; deductibles are $250 for individuals and $500 for families.	Intended, but amount not specified.
Assistance for low-income people	Copayments subsidized for those living at up to 200% of federal poverty level.	Subsidies provided for low-income people.	Tax credits only for low-income people—families with incomes below $32,000 and individuals with incomes below $16,000.
Quality assurance/ cost containment	Develop and implement national practice guidelines and standards, uniform data system, demonstration programs related to malpractice reform; encouragement of managed care; extension of Medicare payment rates to public program.	Establish national expenditure goals, outcomes research, and development of practice guidelines which government programs would be required to use in utilization review activities; encouragement of managed care; efforts to reduce administrative costs.	Malpractice reform to encourage development and implementation of managed care techniques; incentives provided to encourage enrollment in managed care.

Table 9.5
Provisions of Long-Term Care Proposals

	Pepper	Packwood	PNHP
Benefit qualifications	All individuals impaired in 3/5 ADLs or cognitively or behaviorally impaired.	For elderly below federal poverty line who are impaired in 3/5 ADLs; option of covering those up to 240% of poverty line.	Anyone with one or more impairments in ADLs.
Home- and community-based benefits	Personal care services, homemaker/chore services; medication management; day care; respite care.	Homemaker/home health aide services, personal care, home health care, adult day care, nursing services, physical therapy and related services, respite care, prescription drugs, respiratory care.	Nursing, therapy, case management, meals, information and referrals, in-home support, transportation, adult day health, social day care, psychiatric day care, hospice, community mental health.
Cost sharing	Beneficiaries pay 20% of costs of care.	None.	None.
Special assistance for low-income individuals	Subsidies for those up to 200% of poverty level.	Benefits are for low-income elderly only.	All benefits the same for all income levels.
Case management	For all; develop plan of care, monitor and assess care.	For all in program; design a plan of care, coordinate long-term care services, contain costs.	Only when deemed appropriate by local assessment agency.
Institutional benefits	Covers short-term nursing-home stays up to 3 months; individual contribution is 20% of cost of care; for longer stay, floor of asset protection and income protection are extended; individuals keep $30,000 and couples $60,000		

Table 9.5 *(Continued)*

	Pepper	Packwood	PNHP
Institutional benefits *(continued)*	in nonhousing assets; single individuals keep 30% of monthly income for first year of stay, and personal needs allowance for residents would be $100 per month; individuals contribute to cost of nursing home care beyond these provisions.	Income or resource level could not exceed $2,000; minimum monthly allowance of $35 for individuals and $70 for couples.	Includes nursing home, chronic care hospitals, and rehabilitation facilities.
Quality improvements/ Cost controls	Case manager monitors quality.	Standards developed for providers; standard rates developed for nursing-home providers.	Providers required to meet uniform national quality standards; training for providers to help improve care; development of overall budgetary ceilings; ongoing evaluation to quickly disclose and correct problems.
Role of private insurance	Could be purchased to cover cost sharing and to protect additional income and assets.	For those 240 to 400% of poverty line, states have option of private–public partnership to subsidize purchase of private insurance on sliding scale; private insurers would have to offer case management, nursing-home services, and home- and community-based services similar to the public plan.	None.

Senator Chafee's proposal does not guarantee coverage for everyone; rather, it is designed to make coverage more affordable by giving tax credits to middle- and low-income people to use to buy insurance and/or services. States would have the option of providing basic coverage to those who have incomes below 200 percent of the federal poverty line, but nursing-home and other residential long-term care would not be included. Tax credits would also be provided for small businesses that offer insurance to employees.

Both the Chafee and Mitchell proposals include provisions to expand services specifically for the underserved. Mitchell would create community health centers to provide primary care to underserved areas, and Chafee would allow more funds for Public Health Service programs that help address health professional shortages in certain underserved areas. Chafee would also increase funding for the Centers for Disease Control's childhood immunization program. The Pepper Commission would focus on expanding access to the underserved by guaranteeing them health insurance coverage.

These different approaches raise the issue of whether the primary obstacle in reaching the underserved involves a lack of financing or a lack of accessible service providers.

The long-term care proposals also focus on expanding access to care. Both the Pepper Commission and the Physicians for a National Health Program (PNHP) would base eligibility for long-term care benefits on need—specifically, level of impairment—and not on financial status. Both would provide a range of benefits that includes social supports and other nonmedical services, and both would be designed to supplement, not replace, informal care. Both would also improve access by extending government support for nursing-home care to those who are not impoverished.

The PNHP proposal seems the most flexible in terms of benefit eligibility. The proposal allows patients who do not specifically meet the eligibility criteria to qualify for services, if these services would prevent worsening of a disability. The Pepper Commission claims its plan would "indirectly benefit" those who need long-term care but do not qualify for the public program, because home-based care and other services would be expanded and improved as a result of the public program.

(b)   DEFINING IMPAIRMENT

The three long-term care proposals differ in their definitions of the level of impairment necessary to qualify for benefits. PNHP would only require beneficiaries to need assistance in carrying out one ADL or one IADL. The Pepper Commission offers benefits to those who require assistance with three out of five ADLs, who have cognitive impairment, or who have behavioral dysfunction.

In Senator Packwood's bill, qualifying for government aid would still be based on income, although the bill would raise the qualifying floor substantially. Support for community- and home-based care would be greatly increased, and qualifying for any assistance would be based on level of cognitive and functional impairment.

The three proposals differ in what they define as ADLs. This is important because identifying which ADLs are used as a measure of qualification for benefits affects the scope of eligibility. The Katz Index of ADLs, developed over 25 years ago by Dr. Sydney Katz, has become the standard in objective evaluation of chronically ill and elderly populations. The Katz Index includes bathing, dressing, toileting, transferring, continence, and feeding.[6] However, none of the proposals discussed in this chapter includes continence as an ADL, and eligibility for benefits will be affected by its exclusion.

The Pepper Commission and Packwood proposals include only five ADLs in their definitions. The Long Term Care Group, Inc., which develops long-term care products and is an expert in the field of long-term care, points out that having five instead of six ADLs can have a significant impact on a person's eligibility for benefits.[7] As Figure 9.1 shows, if bathing and dressing are combined into one ADL, as is done in the Packwood proposal, ability to qualify for care may not be measured the same as if dressing and bathing were separate categories. The Pepper Commission mentions only five ADLs as well, and, although these are not identified, it can be assumed that the same problem would occur.

The Long Term Care Group also states that needs differ for those who have two versus three ADL impairments. Both will require assistance, but the intensity of service and needed training of providers will differ.[8] PNHP only requires impairment in one ADL to qualify for benefits. Such a benefit package would have to take into account that, once a person becomes impaired in three ADLs, care and training needs would intensify. The lower the number of ADLs needed to qualify for benefits, the more people become eligible, which will lead to higher government expenditures.

(c) RESPONSIBILITY FOR CHOOSING MEDICAL INSURANCE

The Pepper Commission's medical care proposal and Senator Mitchell's bill place the responsibility of obtaining health insurance with the

Figure 9.1
Impact of Five versus Six Basic ADLs in
Qualification for Benefit Eligibility.

Benefit Eligibility for Home Care

PLAN A	PLAN B
Requires 2/6 ADLs	Requires 2/5 ADLs
BATHING *dependent*	*Bathing loss not counted*
DRESSING *dependent*	DRESSING *dependent*
TOILETING	TOILETING *dependent*
TRANSFERRING	TRANSFERRING
CONTINENCE	CONTINENCE
EATING	EATING
Total ADL Loss based on 6 standard ADLs: 2	3

Benefit Eligibility for Nursing-Home Care

PLAN A	PLAN B
Requires 3/6 ADLs	Requires 3/5 ADLs
BATHING *dependent*	*Bathing loss not counted*
DRESSING *dependent*	DRESSING *dependent*
TOILETING *dependent*	TOILETING *dependent*
TRANSFERRING	TRANSFERRING *dependent*
CONTINENCE	CONTINENCE
EATING	EATING
Total ADL Loss based on 6 standard ADLs: 3	4

Source: Long Term Care Group, Inc. *Issues in Understanding Activities of Daily Living (ADLs) and Implications for the Design of Long-Term Care Insurance Products.* Unpublished report.

employer. The employer can choose whether to buy private insurance for employees or to buy into a public plan, but some form of coverage must be provided. In Senator Chafee's proposal, the employee is responsible for choosing insurance, and no one is required to obtain or provide coverage. Middle- to low-income people are given a tax credit, and they choose how to spend it.

In terms of long-term care, the Pepper Commission and PNHP proposals provide long-term care coverage for all the impaired elderly (i.e., no choice); Senator Packwood's bill would provide coverage to all those below the poverty line and then encourage others to purchase private coverage through subsidies and tax incentives.

(d) POINT OF ENTRY FOR LONG-TERM CARE

The Pepper Commission and PNHP long-term care proposals attempt to centralize long-term care services by having one entity serve as the point of entry for all persons seeking long-term care services. Such a system would address the problem of multiple delivery systems, multiple payers, and uncoordinated providers by allowing all consumers and all services to be administered under one umbrella.

The proposals differ, however, in who should serve as the point of entry. The Pepper Commission's proposal would have a case manager serve as the point of entry, and this manager would develop and oversee all individual care plans. All service and eligibility decisions would be made through the case manager. Therefore, every person seeking service would work with a case manager. In effect, the case managers would also serve as the point of entry for all those qualifying for public assistance under Senator Packwood's proposal. The case manager would determine eligibility, coordinate service delivery, and monitor appropriateness and quality. However, those insurers and beneficiaries not involved in the public program would not be required to use case management, and coordination of care would not necessarily occur across the entire elderly population.

PNHP recommends that a local or state government or nonprofit agency serve as the assessment vehicle to determine people's eligibility and service needs. This agency would be responsible for determining, locating, coordinating, and sometimes providing services. PNHP would provide case management only when the agency determined it was necessary. PNHP believes that "not all those needing long-term care require case management." When case management or care coordination is needed, the local agencies would conduct or delegate this service to capitated providers who offer comprehensive services.

(e) UTILIZATION OF SERVICES BASED ON NEED

Each of the proposals strives to base utilization of services on need rather than on ability to pay, as often occurs under the present system.

Both of the Pepper Commission's proposals and the Mitchell and PNHP proposals expand coverage so that everyone would be guaranteed financial coverage for the same services. Senator Chafee's bill increases the income available to families and individuals that is specifically geared toward the purchase of health care services or insurance, and Senator Packwood's bill expands the availability of public assistance to a greater population.

The Pepper Commission's and PNHP's long-term care proposals state that their goal is to support, not supplant, informal caregivers, and utilization of services is to reflect this goal. Respite care, training, and counseling would be provided to support informal caregivers under both proposals. Respite care and coordination of formal and informal services are recommended in Senator Packwood's bill, but there is no language or control mechanism to gear services toward enhancing, not taking the place of, informal care.

Each of the proposals in some way increases the role of public financing and increases equity in private financing. By providing everyone with some type of coverage, the Pepper Commission and Mitchell proposals spread the risk of health care financing across the population. By mandating copayments for employees/beneficiaries and by capping these payments per service (20 percent) and for overall total out-of-pocket payments ($3,000 for individuals and families), risk is further spread more evenly, instead of making those who are the most ill pay for such a disproportionate cost of care.

Equity is also increased by reducing the cost of shifting from the uninsured to the insured, which has resulted in employers and insurers paying indirectly for uncompensated care. Small business reform, included in Senator Chafee's proposal, would make insurance more affordable and thus further increase equity of payments for coverage across groups. However, because Senator Chafee's bill does not guarantee health insurance for all and because the tax credits would not, in most states, cover the cost of insurance, Senator Chafee's proposal leaves inequities in the system by not allowing the same financial access to services for everyone.

The Pepper Commission and Mitchell proposals would greatly increase the public-sector role in providing health care coverage; Senator Chafee's proposal would keep the system primarily financed by the private sector. Tax credits would be available for middle-income and low-income individuals and families; however, actual public insurance coverage would only be extended to those below 200 percent of the federal poverty line. There are also no caps on total allowable spending by individuals or families. Therefore, risk would still be based on severity of individual cases of illness and would not be spread as much among the total population.

In terms of long-term care, the Pepper Commission and PNHP proposals would guarantee coverage for all the severely disabled. The Pepper Commission would require copayments similar to those recommended for medical care. PNHP, however, would have the public system pay for all care, with no premiums, deductibles, copayments, or coinsurance. With money for this extensive public program to be raised from tax revenues, PNHP's proposal would put everyone at the same risk for the cost of care, and no one would be limited in choice of services because of income or assets.

The Packwood proposal would increase public financing on a sliding scale, to cover those living at up to 400 percent of the poverty level. Unique to this proposal is its cap on the total amount of coverage under the private–public plan—the equivalent of 2 years of nursing-home care. (This money could be used for nursing home, community-based, or home-based care.) The Packwood proposal does not include an estimate of how much the plan would increase government spending or how the government would raise this additional money.

(f) STREAMLINING OF THE DELIVERY AND PAYMENT SYSTEMS

Each proposal, at least to some degree, would streamline the current health care system and increase coordination of services and payments. Each is also designed to increase efficiency and the appropriate use of services.

In the Pepper Commission's public plan covering medical care (which the Commission estimates would expand coverage to include 24 million additional people), all providers would be paid based on Medicare rules and rates. This plan would replace Medicaid; therefore, more people would be under one regulatory and payment system. The Commission also recommended national practice guidelines and standards of care, as well as a uniform data system, and quality assurance and assessment mechanisms. These provisions would all move toward centralizing and standardizing care.

Senator Mitchell's proposal contains similar provisions. The recommended Federal Health Expenditure Board would set quality standards and national expenditure goals, and would help evaluate the efficiency and quality of providers. The Board would also oversee negotiations of payment rates for providers. Even greater centralization is possible because states would have the option of implementing a single-payer public plan for all residents.

Senator Chafee's bill would develop a standardized benefit package that all insurers would have to follow. Standards for managed care plans would also be developed. The recommended demonstration projects, which would allow states a waiver from federal program requirements so they could implement statewide demonstration projects, could foster an even greater centralized benefit and service delivery system in these states.

The Pepper Commission and PNHP would centralize the long-term care delivery system. The Pepper Commission at the federal level and PNHP at the state level would make similar efforts to avoid duplication and unnecessary administrative functions and to centralize the payment system to make it more equitable, appropriate, and efficient. Providing a single point of entry for all beneficiaries would also eliminate much of the existing fragmentation.

The Pepper Commission would coordinate care through the case manager. As with the Commission's medical care proposal, the federal government would set guidelines and standards to assure consistency and quality of care. Provider payment rates for both home- and community-based care and for nursing-home care would be determined at the federal level and administered by the states in accordance with guidelines and standards set by the federal government.

However, there would still be more than one payment mechanism. Medicare and Medicaid would both still exist for long-term care. Medicaid would be available for those who are less severely disabled but who meet financial qualifications. For the severely disabled, social insurance would replace Medicaid. Consumers would be able to purchase private long-term care insurance to cover cost sharing and to protect additional assets and income in the event of an extended nursing-home stay.

In the PNHP proposal, the state Long-Term Care Planning and Payment Board, along with the network of local, public, long-term care agencies and the panel of assessment agents, would coordinate and centralize care. They would serve as the point of entry for all beneficiaries, certify providers, and verify eligibility for specific services. All payments would come from the state's long-term care operating budget and would be allocated to local long-term care agencies, which would dole out funds to approved providers. Actual payments would be centralized at the state level, which would help limit duplication and excess administrative functions. Thus, the PNHP proposal allows for a greater degree of centralization than the Pepper Commission's proposal. By having only public payments, no private insurance supplements, and no cost sharing, the financing and administrative system is extremely streamlined.

Senator Packwood's proposal would increase coordination of services through the case manager, which would cut down on duplication, centralize administration and service delivery, and foster the delivery of more appropriate care. However, case management would not be provided to everyone and, therefore, would leave much of the current fragmentation of the system intact.

§ 9.5 ADDRESSING THE CURRENT SYSTEM

The goal of each of the proposals is to reform the current health care delivery system in order to make it more affordable, efficient, and appropriate. The implementation of any of these recommendations would address these issues, but there are several problem areas that none of the proposals addresses adequately.

(a) PREVENTIVE SERVICES

Each of the proposals would expand payment and/or availability of some preventive services. Senator Chafee's bill would expand the child immunization program and offer a tax credit for selected preventive services. The bill would also expand community health centers and increase the number of providers in underserved areas. Each of these provisions would likely increase the availability of preventive services. PNHP recommended increasing preventive services but did not mention what these services would be. The Pepper Commission's medical care proposal included prenatal care, well-child care, mammograms, pap smears, colorectal and prostate cancer screening, and "other preventive services that evidence shows are effective relative to costs." Funding for preventive health research was also recommended. The Commission's long-term care proposal included recommendations for research on ways to prevent mortality and morbidity among the severely disabled. The increased availability of social supports could, in many cases, prevent or delay the need for institutionalization. Senator Mitchell's proposal for medical care reform included prenatal and well-baby care, mammograms, pap smears, and well-child care. Senator Packwood's bill would not expand preventive care; however, it would cover prescription drugs.

Except for Senator Packwood's bill, each of these proposals would expand coverage for preventive services well beyond the currently available level. However, they still leave considerable gaps. For instance, none included routine physical exams, routine hearing or vision exams, dental care, or prescription drugs (except for Senator Packwood's bill). Thus, services would still be acute-care-oriented and technology-intensive, and would not include some of the basic services that could prevent many conditions from developing or worsening.

(b) INTEGRATION OF ACUTE AND LONG-TERM CARE

As earlier chapters of this book discuss, the integration of acute and long-term care is crucial in providing effective and appropriate care for the elderly. While it is important to expand the role of each separately, services need to be coordinated in order to meet the complex, interrelated needs of the elderly, particularly those 85 and older. Most of the proposals lack this integration. None of the medical care proposals includes language or specific recommendations that would integrate health and long-term care. In fact, the Pepper Commission's recommendations would make integration difficult. The long-term care plan calls for a case manager to serve as the point of entry for services. The manager designs a plan of care and, although this role is to integrate service delivery, it is limited to various long-term care services. The case manager receives an operating budget based on a per-capita amount, depending on level of disability. Then services are prescribed within this budget, based on need. But what happens if acute care services and long-term services are needed simultaneously or for the same condition? If an elderly person breaks a hip, is hospitalized, and then requires extended home- or community-based care, it is unclear whether acute care and long-term care services would have to be separated for payment. If separated, it is unclear whether the same caregiver could perform services under different funding entities. Would the case manager be able to manage the acute care or at least the transition from acute to long-term care? This clarification is necessary if high-quality care is to be provided.

PNHP did include specific language on the intent to integrate acute and long-term care. At this point, the acute care proposal is not available, and we are hopeful that specific provisions will be included to facilitate this integration.

Senator Packwood's bill would provide some integration by requiring the case manager to consult with the primary care medical provider when outlining and coordinating a long-term care plan. However, the bill would allow Medicaid to cover the first 45 days of care for the functionally and cognitively impaired, after which Title XXI would provide coverage. It is unclear whether coordination between short- and long-term care payment and delivery systems would be possible, especially because it seems that the case manager would not take over until after 45 days.

(c) QUALIFICATIONS FOR NURSING-HOME STAY

The Pepper Commission's proposal did not address the rigidly polarized definitions that are used for short- and long-term nursing-home stays that often result in inappropriate care for acute and long-term care needs. The Commission's social insurance program would have Medicare cover short-term nursing home stays, up to a total of 3 months of care. However, current definitions require that a short-term nursing-home stay must be related to an acute episode of illness. It is unusual for an elderly person to need 3 months of nursing-home care for an acute care illness. Furthermore, under current laws, short-term nursing-home stays for a chronic condition are not publicly financed. It is unclear whether the Commission intended to loosen the definitions for short-term and long-term nursing-home stays so that more appropriate care could be administered and so that people would not have to be hospitalized for an acute care illness before receiving coverage for short-term nursing-home stays.

It is important to note that the deductibles for 3 months of nursing-home care would cost approximately $12,000, a substantial chunk of many elderly persons' savings. None of this would be protected under the Pepper Commission's proposal, which would only protect assets and income for nursing-home stays that exceed 3 months.

(d) APPLYING COST CONTROLS

Several of the proposals include recommendations for development of standards and guidelines, which should help manage what services are to be provided. However, we hope that these will focus on choosing the most efficient and appropriate services, which in many cases may mean changing the emphasis from technology-intensive procedures and recommending such services as annual physical exams. It is unclear whether these standards would address inappropriate settings for service delivery and cost shifting from one setting or service delivery system to another. Would guidelines address such problems as chronic care provided in acute care settings or would they account for the unique care needs of the elderly?

Senator Chafee's proposal—and, to some degree, Senator Mitchell's bill—would contain costs by encouraging enrollment in managed care plans. However, both lack specifics on what "managed care" would include. Definitions of managed care are not specific in either of these proposals. Attention should be given to developing rigorous definitions so that managed care is applied in its intended form to maximize efficiency and appropriate use of services.

The Pepper Commission and PNHP long-term care proposals addressed cost containment through their point-of-entry mechanisms. PNHP said the overall fixed budget given to local long-term care agencies would give them strong incentives to choose cost-effective services, in particular to support informal providers and community-based services in an effort to avoid or delay more costly institutionalization. For this technique to be effective, standards should be developed to guide service choices. Standards are included in the proposal, but they focus only on quality assurance. It is unclear whether they would address issues of efficiency as well as appropriate use of services and care settings.

Senator Packwood's bill attempts to contain costs by requiring case management as a covered service for insurers (particularly in the public program), by having the Standards and Performance Organization determine whether insurers are "using appropriate managed care techniques," and by capping policy benefits at the cost of 2 years of nursing home care. However, as with Senator Chafee's and Senator Mitchell's bills, managed care techniques are not defined. What would they include and how rigorous would the definitions and controls be? Capping nursing-home payments to 2 years of coverage could make the consumer more frugal; however, capping would also serve to shift the costs from partial public payment to total private payment, primarily made out-of-pocket.

The Pepper Commission's long-term care proposal relies primarily on case management to contain costs. However, this approach will not necessarily be effective and so should not be the main focus for cost containment. According to one review of case management and long-term care:

> [T]he success of case management as a means to control the costs and use of long-term care is questionable based on limited research. Those demonstrations that have examined this issue suggest that case management actually increased the cost and use of services (particularly

home- and community-based services) with little or no impact on nursing home or hospital utilization.[9]

The study pointed out that projects reviewed typically conducted case management within the fee-for-service system, providing few incentives for case managers to serve as gatekeepers. According to the same study, demonstrations did not provide sufficient control over the service delivery system to alter provider practice patterns.[10] The Pepper Commission's plan would have similar characteristics.

We suggest that controlling the costs of care will be most effective if the system includes a wide spectrum of managed care techniques. Recommendations should include adequate and thorough definitions and controls, to ensure that managed care techniques are appropriately used.

The ability to contain costs will also be affected by whether various care delivery systems are integrated. For example, as discussed in Chapter 2, when Medicare implemented its prospective payment system (PPS), inpatient hospital stays and costs went down as intended. However, a portion of this cost was shifted to outpatient care. As a result of a fragmented payment and delivery system, there was motivation to redistribute costs rather than try to find better overall methods of delivering care across care settings. Studies show that outpatient expenditures have increased over the past several years, and evidence indicates that inpatient cost containment programs have played a role in this growth.[11] A system that integrates all care settings would be more likely to focus on reforms that contain costs overall, because the motivation to shift from one setting to another would be eliminated.

(e) OVERALL COST OF REFORM

When examining the costs of the various reform proposals, there is a tendency to balk at the feasibility of implementing them because the cost to the public is perceived as too high. However, it is important to keep in mind that many of these proposals would not actually increase total health care expenditures significantly; rather, they would redistribute costs, achieving a more evenly distributed system of cost sharing among the total population. As the PNHP proposal pointed out, although the total cost of the proposal would be between $70 and $75 billion, $52 billion of this is already being paid through private long-term care insurance and out-of-pocket payments. The overall issue is a philosophical one of whether payment for health and long-term care should be the responsibility of only the sick and their families or whether those costs should be spread across the total population through broad-based private insurance programs or public entitlement programs.

§ 9.6   CURRENT AND FUTURE TRENDS

As of this writing, none of these proposals is close to becoming law, but, as a whole, the proposals reflect certain trends that providers can expect.

(a)   MECHANISMS TO COORDINATE CARE

It seems that there will be an organizational structure to oversee and plan the course of care for the elderly. It is also quite possible that the elderly will no longer be coming in for care on their own. They may be advised or directed by a third party to seek care or even to seek specific services. This third party will most likely have direct and on-going contact with the provider. The third party may be a case manager, an agency, a state board, or some other entity. It may control fees, services reimbursed, and services performed. The provider may be expected to work with other providers more closely as the third party tries to coordinate overall care.

Some of these trends have already begun in several states. For example, in 1983, Hennepin County, Minnesota, began its present preadmission screening program for nursing-home applicants. An initial assessment is conducted in the home by a social worker and a nurse, to assess the applicant's physical, social, and mental health and service needs. Recommendations are then made as to whether nursing-home admittance is needed. If the applicant is admitted to a nursing home, a case mix assessment is performed by a nurse after admittance. Although the initial assessment is mandatory, the recommendations do not have to be followed. The final decision is up to the patient and family.[12] The Hennepin County program is a state-mandated program. However, in the future, there could be a federal policy that mandates similar actions nationwide.

(b)   EXPANDING HOME- AND COMMUNITY-BASED SERVICES

The long-term care proposals discussed above suggest that there may be more demand for community- and home-based services as policies begin to provide incentives and even demands that these services be provided and reimbursed. This trend has begun in part already. As pointed out in Chapter 2, with the implementation of Medicare's Prospective Payment System, patients were discharged earlier from the hospital and care was provided in the home. At the same time, because public financing for home-based care was expanded, there has been an increase in home-based care. This trend will most likely continue, as will the demand for trained professionals in the field.

Providers, provider organizations, and professional training entities should be prepared for this demand. Certain areas of the country with proportionately low utilization of home health care services could be left unprepared for such increased demand. The nation as a whole will need to make preparations for this trend.

The National Association for Home Care looked at experiences in European countries where there is broad financing for long-term care. Based on the findings, the Association estimated that at least 500,000 homemakers and home health aides were needed to provide one aide for each 100 persons 65 and older and one aide for each 1,000 persons under 65. This is almost twice the number of available personnel currently in the work force. If policy changes call for home-based services to expand to meet the actual needs of the community, there will be an increased demand for these providers. As the population continues to age, this demand will increase even more. Based on data from Medicare and the 1984 National Long-Term Care Survey, the National Institute on the Aging estimated a need for 370,000 home health aides to serve older persons by 2020. Other analyses have estimated a need for 5 million home health service personnel by 2020.[13] Providers, provider organizations, and provider training organizations should begin to prepare for an increasing demand for home- and community-based providers, particularly those trained in geriatrics.

(c) PREVENTIVE SERVICES

An additional change that is likely to occur is a greater demand for preventive services, although, as mentioned previously, most of the latest legislative recommendations have centered around specific services such as mammograms and prostate cancer screening. Nonetheless, this increase alone will cause a greater demand for physicians trained to care for the elderly.

The past several years have brought a surge in the number of proposals introduced to reform the health and long-term care system. All of the proposals discussed in this chapter would (1) expand the ability to provide services to greater segments of the elderly population, (2) centralize the payment and service delivery system somewhat, and (3) move service delivery toward a need-based rather than a financially driven system. However, the proposals fall short in their ability to integrate acute and long-term care and to control the high level of fragmentation that exists in our current system. They also lack adequate managed care strategies that could contain costs and lead to the provision of more appropriate care. As Chapter 10 discusses, to adequately address the needs of the health and long-term care system for the elderly, we need to develop methods of providing care that are cost-effective and appropriate.

NOTES

[1] The Pepper Commission. *A Call for Action: The Pepper Commission, U.S. Bipartisan Commission on Comprehensive Health Care.* Washington, DC: U.S. Government Printing Office, 1990.

[2] Mitchell, G.S. 1227, HealthAmerica: Affordable Health Care for All Americans. Introduced in the Senate June 5, 1991.

[3] Chafee, J.H.S. 1936, Health Equity and Access Improvement Act of 1991. Introduced in the Senate November 7, 1991.

[4] Packwood, R.S. 1668, Secure Choice. Introduced in the Senate August 2, 1991.

[5] Harrington, C., Cassel, C., Estes, C., Woolhandler, S., and Himmelstein, D. V. "A National Long-Term Care Program for the United States." *Journal of the American Medical Association* (December 1991), *266:* 3023–3029.

[6] Long-Term Care Group, Inc. *Issues in Understanding Activities of Daily Living (ADLs) and Implications for the Design of Long-Term Care Insurance Products.* Unpublished report.

[7] *Ibid.*

[8] *Ibid.*

[9] Polich, C.L., Parker, M., Iversen, L.H., and Korn, K. *Case Management for Long-Term Care: A Review of Experience and Potential* (p. 92). Excelsior, MN: InterStudy, 1989.

[10] *Ibid.* at 21.

[11] Wickizer, T.M., Wheeler, J.R.C., and Feldstein, P.J. "Have Hospital Inpatient Cost-Containment Programs Contributed to the Growth in Outpatient Expenditures?" *Medical Care* (May 1991): 442–450.

[12] Monson, T. Program for Preadmission Screening, Division of Long-Term Care, Department of Health, Hennepin County, Minnesota. Personal communication, May 8, 1992.

[13] National Institute on the Aging. *Personnel for Health Needs of the Elderly Through the Year 2020* (pp. 106–107). Bethesda, MD: Department of Health and Human Services, 1987.

Ten

Meeting Health Care Needs of the Elderly

§ 10.1 OVERVIEW

Over a decade ago, Dr. Robert Butler asked the question "Why survive being old in America?" in a Pulitzer Prize winning book of the same title. Dr. Butler, one of the nation's preeminent gerontologists, challenged our current system of caring for and meeting the needs of the elderly. Those challenges continue to be pertinent as we evaluate our health care financing and delivery system and plan for future needs. We do not do a particularly stellar job of appropriately and cost effectively caring for older Americans, particularly the very old and the very frail. In spite of herculean efforts by individuals and organizations whose mission it is to do just that, the structure of the system defies them.

This book has been a combination of pessimistic projections as well as idealistic visions of the future, and has described real-life efforts to make sense out of a fragmented and confusing health care system. We have shown the rapid growth predicted for the elderly population in the coming decades, particularly when the baby-boom generation reaches age 65. Alongside that prediction is the fact of the striking

245

increase in the very old, those individuals over the age of 85. This fastest growing segment of the population will likely have the most significant impact on future health care costs and utilization, and the current health care system is least suited to meeting their unique needs.

The aging of the population is one of the least appreciated factors contributing to increasing health care costs and utilization in the United States. The fact is, the elderly are the largest users of health care services—again, particularly the very old. They not only have multiple chronic illnesses that require ongoing care, but are also much more likely than are younger adults to experience acute episodes of illness. The results are more visits to the doctor, more days in the hospital, more medications, and so on. Both the chronic and acute illnesses of the elderly lead to and exacerbate decline in their functional status—their ability to carry out the activities of daily living. This decline leads to increased need for long-term care to support and maintain their lives and their health.

It is easy to see that the pattern is circular. With age comes increased chronic and acute illness, which leads to the use of more health care and to limitations in activities of daily living. This condition then increases the need for support and assistance which, if not provided, leads to further deterioration of health and the need for more health care services. It doesn't require in-depth analysis to understand the interrelatedness of these various aspects of care and support to the elderly.

Yet, there is little or no interrelatedness of the financing systems that fund the care needed by and provided to the elderly. The system for financing health and long-term care for the elderly is very fragmented and extremely confusing, even for the most knowledgeable observer. We know that costs are increasing. Some efforts have been made to contain those costs, with little success. There is no question that health care costs cannot be contained successfully within a system that is so fragmented.

The reason is that no one group or program has sufficient incentive to manage those costs. Medicare covers primarily hospital costs and some physician expenses. Medicaid covers primarily long-term care and a variety of other costs for the portion of the elderly who are impoverished. Medigap insurers fund primarily prescription drugs and some hospital and physician expenses. Retiree health plans cover similar services for different groups of seniors. The elderly themselves pay for a significant portion of health and long-term care expenditures, particularly nursing-home care, prescription drugs, home care, and physician care. In fact, the elderly spend about 18 percent of their annual income on health care—more than they spent *before* Medicare was enacted. The Veterans Administration provides health care services for certain elderly veterans; long-term care insurers provide coverage for custodial care; certain state governments provide funding for home care services and other community-based care. The Older Americans Act and Title XX of the Social Security Act provide funding for social services and home-delivered meals. No one group or program has sufficient control or authority over health and long-term care financing for the elderly. Thus, there is no control.

This is a cost-generating system, one with little or no coordination among the parts; there is virtually no opportunity for synergy among the various players. Wonderful programs and service delivery systems are in place to provide care for the elderly. Each is dedicated to a piece of this complicated pie. Each has its own set of rules, regulations, approaches, and biases. Each is blind to the other pieces of the pie.

Before condemning the service delivery system and the organizations currently working to meet the needs of seniors, it is important to recognize that they are a product of the financing system within which they work. In this case, form follows funding, not function. The health and long-term care system for the elderly has been built on a foundation of individual funding sources that were designed for specific purposes. They were certainly not designed with the user— the elderly individual—in mind. Rather, they were designed to accommodate the bureaucracy and the providers of care. Unfortunately, that system is no longer able to meet the needs of the elderly appropriately and cost-effectively.

There are three basic requirements for a health and long-term care system for the elderly that will foster cost and utilization management as well as ensure appropriate care: integrated financing, a benefit package that spans both acute and chronic care, and elimination of the institutional bias that exists in the current system.

§ 10.2 INTEGRATED FINANCING

Enough has been said about the problems associated with a fragmented health care financing system for the elderly. The fragmentation leads to confusion, inappropriate care, and the inability to effectively manage costs.

(a) CONFUSION

Research has repeatedly shown the confusion associated with the current health care system for the elderly. Seniors themselves do not totally understand how the system works and, thus, find it very difficult to ensure appropriate coverage and the security that follows. Even today, the majority of elderly individuals believe that Medicare covers considerably more than it actually does. One of the most prevalent myths is that Medicare will cover the costs associated with a long nursing-home stay. When individuals reach the age of 65 and become eligible for Medicare, they must spend a considerable amount of time and effort to determine how to insure their health care needs. This includes trying to understand Medicare and the gaps in its coverage—a challenge even for health care professionals—and seeking out appropriate supplemental care from a myriad of Medigap policies, Medicare HMOs, retiree plans, and the like. This process, unfortunately, differs for each individual, depending on location (some areas have Medicare HMOs and others don't), employment status (Medicare provides primary coverage for the elderly who are retired, but not for the elderly who are employed by organizations with health care coverage), availability of retiree health plans through a former employer, status as a veteran with service-related disabilities, eligibility for Medicaid, and so on.

In many cases, family members will try to help sort out this myriad of choices, but they may not understand the implications of their choices. Similarly, when an elderly individual experiences a catastrophic illness or requires a nursing-home placement or extended home care, it is the family that often wades through the options for care and financing. "Is a nursing home necessary or can we try home care? If we need a nursing home, how can we find the best one to meet our needs? If we need home care, what kind of services are available? What kind of services do we need? How much does this cost? Who will pay for it?" These are all questions that must be answered by families in crisis, at a time when they might be least capable of making informed decisions. The confusion and difficulty stem from a fragmented financing system that, in many ways, defies logic when viewed from the standpoint of the elderly individual and his or her family.

(b) INAPPROPRIATE CARE

In addition to causing confusion, the fragmented funding can lead to inappropriate care. Because care decisions can be extremely complicated, it is not clear that informed and trained individuals are available to direct people to the right type, combination, and setting of care. In Chapters 4, 5, and 6, we described many programs that have developed to intervene in the fragmented financing system to assess need, develop care plans, make arrangements for care with appropriate providers, and provide follow-up and monitoring to ensure that the care selected continues to be appropriate. These programs have grown out of our need to artificially integrate existing financing and provide logic to an illogical system. These programs have proven successful in coordinating care, but they are not widely available.

Even where these programs do exist, many individuals in need are not aware of them and, as a result, do not access them. Case management programs have worked diligently to become more visible in the community and to perform ongoing outreach. Unfortunately, it is human nature not to pay attention to such things until we need them. By then, it may be too late. The result is that the vast majority of elderly in our country do not have access to or knowledge about the programs that are available to help with their problems. A further result is that they are not always assured the proper care, but rather receive the care for which there is financing and availability. Because our financing system is biased toward acute and institutional care, this often means an excessive use of hospital or nursing-home care.

(c) COSTS AND UTILIZATION

Finally, the fragmentation clearly leads to increased costs and an inability to manage them effectively. The only way to truly manage costs is to have the flexibility and authority to manage across a full continuum of care. Without control over the majority of care provided to an individual, managing costs can quickly become cost shifting to another payer. If a single payer has control over hospital costs, it is possible to manage those costs. It may be expedient, however, to manage those costs by using other services for which the payer has no financial responsibility—outpatient services or skilled nursing facility care, for example. Under these circumstances, *total* costs may not be controlled. In the same way, there may not be incentives to provide the patient the most appropriate care; instead, care is shifted to other payers.

This is one of the issues that has stifled Medicare cost management. In fact, Medicare does not manage care or costs; it manages payment. With coverage of hospital services, for example, Medicare has opted to place hospitals at financial risk for the services provided during the patient stay. Medicare has managed payment to the hospital, providing a fixed cost per patient, depending on the patient's diagnosis. Because the hospital is at financial risk, it has the incentive to manage costs. The initial approach taken by hospitals was to move treatment and procedures to other settings. The results were an increase in outpatient surgery and procedures, and the use of home health care and skilled nursing facility care for postacute recovery. This led to hospital length-of-stay reductions, and presumably, reduction in the hospitals' cost for inpatient care for a particular patient with a given diagnosis. The result for *total* costs of an episode of illness is unclear. What is clear, however, is that costs were shifted to areas in which the hospital did not have financial risk. What will be the next step? Medicare will undoubtedly look for ways to place the hospitals, or other organizations, at risk for other care within an episode of illness, in order to manage payment. But there may well be another place to shift costs . . . . And the beat goes on.

What would happen if all financing for all services were pooled, with one entity placed at financial risk for those services? This is essentially the concept of the health maintenance organization (HMO). In fact, HMOs with Medicare risk contracts approach this ideal. Unfortunately, they mirror the Medicare program. To the extent Medicare is inadequate to meet the total care needs of the elderly, Medicare HMOs will also be inadequate. They do, however, join the Medicare and the Medigap supplement (and, in some cases, the Medicaid and retiree health care) portions of the health care financing pie. What are most often missing are long-term care services and coverage for prescription drugs.

Thus, even within the HMO environment, there remains some fragmentation of funding and service delivery for the elderly. Only the Social HMO and the other demonstration projects described in Chapter 6 begin to overcome this barrier to an appropriate and cost-effective system of providing health and long-term care services to the elderly.

§ 10.3 AN ACUTE AND CHRONIC CARE CONTINUUM

When integrated funding is achieved, there is an opportunity to create a continuum of both acute and chronic care, which is essential to ensuring that appropriate and cost-effective care is provided.

The elderly are high users of both acute and chronic care, because they are likely to have chronic conditions *and* acute episodes of illness.

Even more important, the distinction between what is acute and what is chronic among the elderly is often unclear. In many cases, the acute illnesses and chronic conditions interact in ways that confound medical treatment and the delivery of appropriate care.

Because of the overlap between acute and chronic conditions for the elderly, it is important to model a service delivery and financing system to accommodate those unique needs. We have already discussed integration in financing for acute and chronic care, which is essential to the payments equation. Other requirements are: integrating the service delivery system, and ensuring that the providers of care are adequately trained in the diagnosis and treatment of both acute and chronic conditions in the elderly.

(a) INTEGRATING THE SERVICE DELIVERY SYSTEM

The health and long-term care service delivery system is organized along the fragmented funding lines discussed earlier. The result is that there is an acute care delivery system (primarily, hospitals and physicians) and a long-term care delivery system (primarily, nursing homes and home care agencies). The two intersect in an area typically referred to as postacute care (see Figure 10.1). This segment of the service delivery system largely grew out of efforts by hospitals to reduce costs and lengths of stay associated with Medicare patients. These efforts, spurred by Medicare's Prospective Payment System, placed hospitals at financial risk for this care. As discussed earlier, this risk created incentives to discharge patients to other settings and payment sources. The result was the development and tremendous growth of the postacute

Figure 10.1
The Overlap of Care Systems for the Elderly

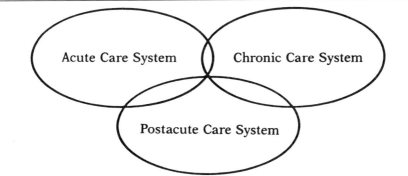

care system, encouraged by the HMO industry and by managed care companies seeking to reduce inpatient hospital costs.

In spite of the incentives created to meld the acute and chronic care systems under such payment mechanisms as Medicare's Prospective Payment System and HMOs, those delivery systems have remained very separate. There are several reasons for this, but history and professional disciplines play a major role.

Acute care has largely been dominated by hospitals and physicians, with nurses playing a significant role in the care of patients. Financing has historically been plentiful, through such funding sources as Medicare and Medigap supplemental insurance. Medicare, being a social insurance program, has had no stigma attached to participation for either the elderly or providers. Medigap insurance, as a private sector program, similarly has had no stigma attached to its use. The providers within the acute care system have been highly respected. Physicians have been esteemed professionals and community leaders. Particularly in smaller towns, hospitals have been akin to the public school as a centerpiece of the town's identity. Acute care has been "where the action is."

Chronic care or long-term care has been the poor second cousin to acute care. Nursing homes have been viewed as a disreputable part of the health care system—they are where people go to die and where no one wants to go. Social workers and nursing assistants have played key roles in the care provided to the elderly. Although critical to the chronic care delivery system, these occupations have received less respect (and financial remuneration) than their counterparts in the acute care system. Even the same professionals (i.e., registered nurses) are paid less and viewed as of less value when they work in a long-term care setting as compared to an acute care setting. Funding sources for long-term care are more likely to be public assistance or welfare programs (e.g., Medicaid), with significant social stigma for participation for both the elderly and providers.

This history and the different professional disciplines involved in acute and long-term care make the integration of the service delivery systems very difficult. The parties, in many cases, do not speak the same language or respect their unique contributions to the health care system for the elderly. Because the acute model dominates the system today, there is fear that, even if we can move to a more integrated service delivery system, it will result in a "medicalization" of the entire continuum. This would not be appropriate from either a cost or quality perspective.

What is needed is an organized delivery system that spans the acute and chronic continuum of care, values the unique expertise and perspectives of the different professional disciplines involved, and can understand the needs of and care for the elderly individual, as a whole.

(b) TRAINING PROVIDERS APPROPRIATELY

The health and long-term care delivery system, however, is not an autonomous entity. It is a compilation of many providers of care, who often work independently to care for individuals. The notion of an organized system of health care for the elderly again conjures up the image of an HMO as the most prevalent existing model of this approach. The HMO is not the only model that can achieve this goal. Yet, in order to develop such an approach, the providers of care must work in a much more integrated fashion than has historically been the case. One model for this is the "community health care network" in which a hospital (or hospitals) align with a network of primary care physicians (either salaried or independent) and specialists, nursing homes, home health agencies, and other ancillary care providers to offer a full continuum of care to a population. The ideal would be several networks within a community from which consumers (or payers) could select. Also ideal would be partnerships between the community network and the payers and managers of care so that appropriate incentives for cost-effective care can be included.

For the elderly population, however, this model requires some adaptation. Of greatest importance is the assurance that the providers that are a part of the network understand and are trained in geriatrics and gerontology. In Chapter 1, we discussed the importance of geriatrics-trained providers. It is clear that the current shortage of such providers

Figure 10.2
Model of a Health Care Partnership

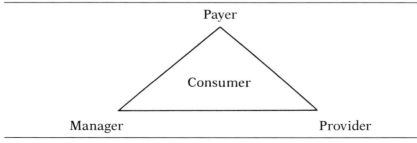

will only worsen as the population ages. In order to meet the needs of this population, we must require geriatrics courses in medical and nursing schools, encourage physicians and nurses to specialize in geriatrics, educate clinical providers in the social aspects of aging so that they can appreciate the interrelationship between the medical and social concerns of the elderly, ensure that the managers of care are thoroughly grounded in the issues associated with aging and the relationship to health care needs, and sensitize the institutional providers of care (primarily hospitals and nursing homes) to the unique needs and requirements of their elderly patients. There is little question that inappropriate and costly care is provided to the elderly because many providers do not understand the dynamics of health, long-term care, and social needs among the elderly, and are in some cases biased against the aged.

If our society is going to be capable of providing necessary care for the elderly in the future, better understanding, communication, and education among the parts of the delivery system are required.

§ 10.4 INSTITUTIONAL BIAS

In addition to a bias toward acute care in our existing financing and delivery system, there is also a bias toward institutional care. Within the acute care system, there has been a bias toward provision of care within the hospital setting. Only recently have there been concerted efforts to move some of that care to outpatient or postacute settings. In postacute and long-term care, there has been a bias toward provision of care within the nursing home. Only recently has there been an effort to use more community-based and home health care.

The funding rules have kept this bias firmly in place, but the institutional bias of the system is not solely related to financing. As a result, an alteration in financing will not necessarily eliminate the bias. This was certainly seen in the movement to prospective payment for hospitals. This financing change created incentives to reduce hospital care, but the preferred location of alternative care has largely been the skilled nursing facility—another institution. There has also been a movement to increase outpatient care—much of it hospital-based, however.

The institutional bias also stems from the need for control over the patient and the care provided. It is much easier for the physician, for example, to be assured that the treatment prescribed is being administered properly when it is being provided inside an institution, where strict rules and protocols are to be followed and documented.

This bias is even stronger for the elderly, possibly because of our society's paternalistic attitude toward this group. Particularly among the very old, there is a tendency to underestimate the individual's ability to make choices and to execute those choices effectively. We doubt elderly persons' ability to take medications appropriately, or supervise home health providers, or understand when to call the physician or hospital when problems occur. There may be many legitimate reasons for these attitudes. Liability is always cited as a justification for maintaining control over the provision of care. However, in many cases, we have a misguided belief that we, as professionals, must protect the elderly from themselves and their "disabilities."

The fact is, the elderly prefer to stay in their home. They would prefer to receive care at home. They feel comfortable making decisions about the care they do and do not want to receive. We should listen to them. Our system should be customer-focused. Today, it is provider-focused.

We also know that institutions are not healthy places for the elderly, especially the frail elderly. When a frail elderly individual enters a hospital, his or her functional status declines and rarely returns to its former level, even after the acute episode has passed. For the sake of quality of life and quality of care, more care should be provided at the place of residence.

Care provided at home is often, though not always, less costly as well. The biggest concern about the cost effectiveness of home health and community-based care is whether people will "come out of the woodwork" to seek this attractive care option. The myth of the "woodwork" effect, however, is not supported by experience. The demonstration projects cited in Chapters 4 and 6 have shown that informal networks of family and friends continue to be the primary caregivers, that the elderly reject formal services as long as possible, and that it is often difficult to convince them to take as much assistance as might be recommended. If home and community-based services were provided within an organized delivery system with integrated funding, the use and costs of the care could be managed effectively. This would ensure that appropriate and necessary care is being provided in the most cost-effective manner.

§ 10.5 WHERE DO WE GO FROM HERE?

Reinventing the health and long-term care system for the elderly will not be an easy or short-term project for anyone. It will require vision and dedicated work. Many believe that it can only occur through a total overhaul of the financing system, which typically implies national health care reform. This notion, however, is misguided. The fundamental problem with the current system is that it is focused on the health care bureaucracy and providers, not on patients and their needs. A centralized, bureaucratized system will only exacerbate this problem, not solve it.

There is somewhat of a contradiction in this view, however. We have stated that integrated funding is required. It is acknowledged that this integration would be potentially simpler through a national health financing scheme. But we have also shown that integration of funding is very possible through other means, like Social HMOs or On Lok, absent national health care reform.

What makes these programs work in spite of all the barriers the existing system has put in place? Visionary leadership, committed and appropriately trained geriatric providers, a focus on the patient, and organized delivery systems that apply managed care principles. The lessons of these programs *can* be translated into improved health and long-term care for the elderly. What we must avoid is waiting for the big fix rather than attending to all the things that we can do to improve care to the elderly. Systemic reform is needed, but we must work simultaneously to create change that will facilitate efforts to improve health and long-term care for the elderly. In the meantime, we need to break out of the malaise that so often surrounds health care today and work individually and collectively toward a system that can meet the health and long-term care needs of the elderly, effectively and cost-efficiently.

Appendixes

Appendix One

Evaluating and Choosing a Public or Private Case Manager

HOW TO DECIDE WHETHER A FAMILY NEEDS THE SERVICES OF A CASE MANAGER

Families are often able to locate solutions and coordinate services for themselves. For example, if the older person is functioning well, has a good deal of help from family and friends, and is not experiencing difficulty or frustration in locating services, then she or he probably does not need the services of a case manager. On the other hand, if the older person is experiencing difficulty in taking care of daily needs (bathing, housework, toileting, driving, eating, and other basic activities); is isolated from family, neighbors, and friends; is having difficulty knowing where to turn and what services can help, or simply wants to do some preventive planning, then the family may want to consider using the services of a case manager. NOT EVERYONE NEEDS A CASE MANAGER!

The following questionnaire* will help with a decision on whether a family member or friend needs a case manager.

Questions for the Individual to Ask Himself or Herself

Are you having problems with walking, bathing, keeping yourself clean, eating, getting out and about, meeting friends?

Have you just gotten out of the hospital and need help, but don't know where to go?

*Expanded from a list devised by Monika White, Ph.D., of Senior Care Network, Huntington Memorial Hospital, Pasadena, CA.

Do you feel you can't get a complete picture of your needs and can't really understand what your problem is?

Have you tried to find information about a problem but can't?

Are you seeking a social or medical service for the first time?

Do you feel that you don't really understand what a particular social service agency is supposed to do for you?

Are you separated from family and friends who could help you?

Do you have people who can help you but who are overwhelmed, ill, unavailable, or living far away?

Do you feel you have no one to talk to or count on for help?

Do you need more than one service and need help coordinating your care?

Are you receiving services from several agencies but still experiencing problems in daily living?

Have you been refused a service or a claim from Medicare, Medicaid, or a similar agency?

Are you considering going into a nursing home? Do you feel as though you need help to seek other solutions—other alternatives?

If you need a nursing home, do you need help locating a good facility to meet your particular needs?

Questions for Families

Do you or other people see the older person's behavior as unmanageable or intolerable?

Have you begun to think about guardianship or conservatorship procedures?

Is the older person having increasing trouble taking care of himself or herself? Does he or she feel lonely and scared and visit the hospital emergency room because he or she feels there is nowhere else to go?

Is the older person having trouble making decisions that used to be routine for him or her?

Is he or she having trouble filling out financial forms and seeking financial help?

HOW TO EVALUATE A CASE MANAGER BEFORE HIRING ONE

Ask for *specific* information about the following:

- Education;
- Experience working with older people and familiarity with community services;

- Professional licenses;
- Fees;
- Special arrangements (if any) he or she has with the agencies to which referrals are made. (Does the case manager get money or other benefits for referrals to a particular home health care agency or nursing home?)

Clients may prefer to hire a case manager who is not linked with a particular service provider; he or she can then make a referral to any agency that best suits the client's needs. There may be less chance of a conflict of interest. On the other hand, some clients may prefer a case manager who owns or controls a home health care agency and who can hire, monitor, and dismiss home health aides.

When working with a case manager, especially one in private practice, *it is important to find out whether he or she has any kind of arrangement with a particular service agency or nursing home.* For example, does the case manager own a nursing home or a home health care agency, or does he or she receive fees from an agency for making referrals to it? Does the case manager refer only to service providers with whom contracts or agreements have been made, or are several options presented to clients for their choice? Ask specifically what services the case manager refers to, provides, and coordinates.

There may be a conflict of interest when the case manager is both *planning* the services and *providing* the services. However, if clients are exhausted and under a lot of stress, it might be simpler to have a trustworthy case manager help with all of the steps.

Developing a Comfortable Relationship with a Case Manager

Hiring a case manager, whether for a short period of time or for many years, is an important decision. In a community with more than one case manager, clients should interview case managers until one is found with whom all family members can trust and feel comfortable.

It is a good idea to find someone who will listen to client needs and customize services to the client's particular situation. This means that clients *must* be open in discussing their situation, even if it requires talking about painful or embarrassing subjects most choose not to disclose to anyone else— mental, emotional, or physical disability, and financial matters, for example. This is the *only* way the case manager will be able to help the family. Before discussing private matters with a case manager, be sure to ask about how confidentiality will be protected, especially if the client and the case manager develop a care plan that involves other family members, friends, or agencies in the community. Families may want to require that the case manager get permission in writing before contacting others.

Generally speaking, families will be most comfortable if they find a case manager who respects their value system, needs, wishes, and ethnic and cultural background. This will become quickly apparent as they talk with the prospective case manager. Are their ideas being listened to or ignored? Are they treated respectfully or talked down to? Are their cultural and ethnic preferences being taken into account?

The Case Manager's Experience with Elderly Persons and Their Families

Because the job of case management involves pulling together a variety of services to meet a family's needs, case managers must be knowledgeable about the services available in the community. Ask the case manager to discuss his or her experience in working with various aspects of community services as well as with families and volunteers. Make certain that the person the family is thinking of hiring has had several years of experience working specifically with older people and their families. Any person hired should have at least some experience working with older people.

What Qualifications and Credentials Do Case Managers Have?

Case managers may have educational degrees in a variety of fields, such as social work, nursing, psychology, gerontology, medicine, and law. In addition, they may have wide experience working with families and older persons in many settings—hospitals, nursing homes, adult day care, protective services, counseling, and private practice. They may also have been caregivers for their own family members and are therefore aware of and sensitive to the family's needs.

The concept and practice of case management is not new, but *private* case management is a more recent phenomenon. Especially when hiring a private case manager who is not a member of a larger agency, check all credentials carefully. Ask for complete educational background and qualifications for doing case management. Ask to be provided with a list of the degrees earned and the active levels of licensing and accreditation. For help, consult the list of case management credentials at the end of this appendix. Many of these degrees represent different levels of education in the field. If there are any doubts about a person's credentials, contact the colleges, universities, or credentialing organizations named, and confirm that the degrees were awarded.

It is important to check a case manager's references. The relationship that the family will build with a case manager over time needs to be one of trust and integrity. Therefore, before hiring a case manager, ask to speak with several other clients with whom he or she has worked. In addition, call a few local agencies such as social services, area agencies on aging, public health nurses, local hospitals, or nursing homes to check the reputation of the case manager. Have they worked with this case manager? Do they make referrals to this particular case manager and, if so, have they been satisfied with the quality of his or her work? Can they refer the family to anyone who has used his or her services? (In most cases, they will have to ask the person's permission before giving out his or her name.)

It is always advisable to compare services and prices of at least two or three case managers, if the family lives in a community where a choice is possible. This will give the family a better sense of which one to hire. When hiring a case manager for a family member who is very frail and incapacitated, and if it is necessary to apply for conservatorship or guardianship status (where one person assumes the legal and financial responsibility for another person), then it is especially important to check the references of the case manager. Conservatorship and guardianship are serious legal and financial steps requiring that those involved have the very highest possible ethical standards. The best interests of the demented or incapacitated person must be protected.

Screening and Hiring the People Who Will Enter the Home

Some case managers actually provide direct care themselves, but most of them prefer instead to plan services and hire home health aides and others to come into the home. Find out what process is used to screen and hire these people. Will the case manager, for example, locate and screen live-in help? How thoroughly does the case manager check the background and references of live-in help? To whom are the workers accountable? How is it determined whether live-ins and home aides are trained? Make sure to get all information needed to feel comfortable before agreeing to let new people come into the home.

Who is the Client?

Determining who the client is can be a problem, when a case manager is working with someone in the family who is mentally incapacitated, such as someone who is very disoriented because of Alzheimer's disease. The case manager must decide whether the client is the older person for whom the plans are being made, the family member who is making the arrangements, or the trust officer or attorney who is paying the bill for case management services. This becomes an important question when the older person is physically, mentally, or emotionally handicapped, or when there is a conflict between what he or she wants and what the family wants—in other words, whenever there is more than one person involved.

Some case managers believe that *the older person is always the client.* Other case managers believe that *the family as a whole is the client.* Still other case managers believe that *whoever is paying the bill* for the services rendered is the client. In any case, it is very important that the case manager listen to and be sensitive to the needs and wishes of the older person. It is always preferable, where possible, to keep the older person for whom plans are being made (even if that person is disoriented) as an important team member in deciding what services will be used and how services are to be monitored.

How Much Will it Cost?

There is considerable variation in the cost of case management services. A public case manager (a government employee who works in a public agency) may charge any amount from zero to whatever the family can afford to pay, based on income. Families can expect to pay nothing for the services if they are eligible under certain income guidelines or if the case manager is being paid by a government program, such as Medicare or Medicaid, to provide services. A private case manager is a privately employed person who charges a fee for his or her services, just as a private physician or attorney would. The private case manager may have a sliding fee scale and may charge little or nothing or as much as $100 or more per hour. The *average* fee nationwide for a private case manager is approximately $80 to $100 per hour.

DECIDING WHETHER TO CHOOSE A PUBLIC OR PRIVATE CASE MANAGER

Only the older person or the family can decide whether to hire a public case manager (a government employee who works in a public agency and whose services are often paid for by Medicare, Medicaid, or some other public program) or a private case manager (a privately employed individual whose services are not usually paid for by public programs and who charges the consumer a fee for his or her services).

Table A.1 lists a few of the advantages of using each, and may help in making a decision.

Both a public and a private case manager can help older persons and their families in filling out Medicaid and Medicare forms. A public case manager is generally more restricted to use of existing community resources in creating a care plan. He or she usually cannot customize services to the degree that a private case manager can.

HOW MUCH SHOULD ONE EXPECT TO PAY A PRIVATE CASE MANAGER?

Private case managers set fees in several different ways:

- An hourly rate fee;
- A sliding fee scale;
- A set rate per service;
- A set rate per session;
- A set rate for a package of services.

Hourly fees set by private case managers range from $60 to $150, with an average of $75 to $100+ per hour. Some private case managers have sliding fees ranging from a low charge to $100+ an hour, depending on the client's income. Most private case managers charge a set fee for the initial assessment (which includes the in-depth evaluation of the client's physical, social,

Table A.1
Advantages of Using Public and Private Case Managers

Public Case Manager	Private Case Manager
1. Services may be free of charge or provided on a sliding fee scale, depending on the client's financial situation.	1. A private case manager may be available nights, weekends, and holidays.
2. In a public agency, the case manager may have established links with a large number of providers.	2. Because private case managers tend to serve fewer clients, they tend to offer more personalized, customized service and attention.
3. A case manager in a public agency is usually subject to more supervision and monitoring than an independent private case manager might be.	3. A private case manager may have more flexibility in developing a creative and innovative plan because he or she is not involved in a bureaucracy.
4. A public case manager may have a better grasp of the eligibility requirements and paperwork necessary to get the services needed.	4. Not everyone may be eligible for public case management services (a client may be financially or geographically ineligible for a public program).
	5. A private case manager may be more responsive and more quickly available, because he or she can avoid long forms and lengthy "intake" procedures.

functional, psychological, and financial situation); this fee may vary from $75 to $400+. Some private case managers charge by the service instead: they receive a set fee for travel expenses, phone consultation, monitoring, psychological assessment, and other services they provide. Others offer a package rate that includes a set amount of time for assessment, establishing a care plan, meetings and consultations, referral services, and monitoring. The "package" rates may vary between $100 to $400 or more.

As wise consumers of case management services, clients need to understand the fees, fee structure, and billing process. Price is not the only factor to look at, but it is definitely important. Get *in writing* a full and complete description of the billing and fee structure, in order to understand what services will be delivered, when, how frequently, where, by whom, for how long a period, and what all the charges will be. For example, will there be added charges if the case manager makes long-distance phone calls, writes up the care plan, contacts the physician, drives to and from the client's home, or writes and mails letters on behalf of the client? Arrange for a detailed monthly accounting of exactly what was done and what the charges are for.

Be certain to determine ahead of time whether the case manager will be paid for hourly services or for a complete job. Find out whether the case manager accepts (and is eligible to receive) private insurance, Medicare, Medicaid, or other forms of payment and whether he or she will do the necessary paperwork. *In most cases, private case management services are not covered by Medicare, health insurance, Medicaid, or private insurance. For that reason, the client and family will probably be required to pay for these services privately, out-of-pocket.*

Availability

One reason to choose to use a private case manager instead of the public system is because private case managers are often available to help with crises in the middle of the night, over holidays, or on weekends. Ask whether there are extra charges for this level of service. What are the hours of operation? When will a case manager be available? Will it always be the same person, and, if not, can the family meet the other persons who may also work with them? What exactly is the family paying for, over what period of time? What services will they be getting, and how available will the case manager be if there are problems? What happens if there are problems with the services that a particular agency is providing? Will the case manager straighten it out and advocate for the client and family?

What if the client has difficulty qualifying for a program? Will the case manager help fill out forms for Medicare, Medicaid, insurance, and other programs, if help is needed? These are questions that families may want to have answered fully, ahead of time, before deciding to hire someone.

LIST OF CASE MANAGEMENT CREDENTIALS

This partial list of degrees, licenses, and certifications is provided to aid in understanding and evaluating the credentials of prospective case managers.

ACSW	Academy of Certified Social Workers
ANP	Adult Nurse Practitioner
ARNP	Advanced Registered Nurse Practitioner
BA	Bachelor of Arts
BHS	Bachelor of Human Services
BS	Bachelor of Science
BSN	Bachelor of Science in Nursing
BSW	Bachelor of Science in Social Work
CFLE	Certified Family Life Educator
CISW	Certified Independent Social Worker
CSA	Community Services Adviser
CSW	Clinical Social Worker/Certified Social Worker
DSW	Doctor of Social Welfare
EdD	Doctor of Education
EdM	Master of Education

LCSW, LICSW, LISW	Licensed Social Worker
LNHA	Licensed Nursing Home Administrator
MA	Master of Arts
MC	Master's Certificate
MD	Medical Doctor
MEd	Master of Education
MFCC	Master in Family and Child Counseling
MM	Master of Management
MPH	Master of Public Health
MPS	Master of Public Service
MS	Master of Science
MSG	Master of Science in Gerontology
MSS	Master of Social Service
MSW	Master of Social Work
NCC	Nursing Clerical Coordinator
PhD	Doctor of Philosophy
RN	Registered Nurse
RPT	Registered Physical Therapist

Appendix Two

Working with the Case Manager

GOALS AND CONTRACTS WITH CASE MANAGERS

Before meeting with a case manager, it is important that the family have some idea of what they want and expect. This may be difficult, because family members may not be familiar with all of the services that are available in the community. AARP's free "Checklist for Concerns/Resources for Caregivers" is recommended. This booklet will help determine what the need is, what solutions are possible, and what resources are available for help. It is important that the family and the case manager together *set goals for the care plan* and *establish a way to evaluate whether the goals have been reached.* Again, a detailed plan of care should be agreed on *in writing.*

Once the family and other care partners have fully evaluated the situation with the help of the case manager, then a plan of care is set up. This is a written plan that clearly tells everyone—the case manager, other health care providers, family, friends, volunteers, and the client—what they have agreed to be responsible for. The care plan may change over time, as the situation changes.

It is also important to reevaluate periodically whether the care plan is being followed and the goals are being accomplished. If they are not, should the goals be changed, should caregivers be doing something differently, or is it necessary to change case managers? In reexamining the performance of the case manager, it is important to assess whether caregivers are fulfilling *their* part of the care plan as well.

WHAT A CASE MANAGER CANNOT DO FOR THE CLIENT/FAMILY

Some people who hire a case manager want to shift all the difficult decisions to him or her. Some families want to avoid discussing painful subjects and making difficult decisions. The case manager can help a family work through and consider all the options. The decisions being considered may not always be comfortable or easy. However, families cannot avoid making decisions and should not expect the case manager to take the responsibility of making decisions. He or she is there to assist in the decision making process.

In addition, many families are dealing with very complex situations that change frequently. Families should not expect the case manager to have "quick fixes" that will resolve these complex and possibly long-standing problems immediately or permanently. As the family situation changes, another evaluation may be needed and new and different solutions found. There are many options and choices for the family (or friends, neighbors, and significant others) to consider; the problems are dynamic and need to be worked through over time. As the situation keeps changing, the solutions must also change.

WORKING WITH A CASE MANAGER: HOW TO GET EXACTLY WHAT A FAMILY NEEDS

If a family decides to hire a case manager, especially a private case manager, they will want to be thorough and well-prepared in interviewing candidates. There are many questions to ask a case manager before allowing him or her to work with the family. A personal meeting is preferable, to allow the family and the case manager the chance to decide whether they can work together effectively. Keep these ideas in mind when interviewing a case manager:

- Ask questions about anything that is not clear.
- The family is purchasing the *education, time,* and *expertise* of a case manager.
- The family has the right to ask and to get answers to questions.
- Don't hesitate to ask a question because someone might think it sounds "stupid" or too simple. *Any* question that any family member has is a legitimate concern.

Write down questions ahead of time. Consider keeping notes on information that is presented during meetings, and refer to them later. Consider developing a written contract with the case manager so that everyone knows what the care plan goals are and how the goals are to be achieved and measured. Review any contracts carefully before signing.

WHERE CAN A CASE MANAGER BE FOUND?

There are many places to find case managers. They work in both public and private agencies, but they are not necessarily easy to find. Don't get discouraged! It may be difficult to find the specific services needed. The system is complicated and, even for those who are very knowledgeable, hard to understand. Case managers can help!

Private case managers—those paid for by clients and families out-of-pocket—can most easily be located by contacting the National Association of Private Geriatric Case Managers (NAPGCM). The address is:

NAPGCM
655 N. Alvernon
Suite 108
Tucson, AZ 85711
(602) 881-8008

The NAPGCM lists are probably the best that are currently available, but many private case managers are not included. One reason is that private case managers are private entrepreneurs and may be difficult to locate. Some social workers, nurses, and others who do this kind of work do not necessarily think of themselves as "private case managers" and do not identify themselves to NAPGCM.

There are, however, many *public* agencies that also provide case management services. Some places to look for case managers are:

Area Agencies on Aging (call the National Association of Area Agencies on Aging at (202) 296-8130 to locate the nearest AAA offices);

County social service agencies;

State or county preadmission screening programs (through preadmission screening, older persons are assessed of their need for nursing-home care; call the state or county health department to see whether a preadmission screening program is available);

The Yellow Pages, under "Social Services" and "Social Workers";

Visiting Nurse Association;

Public health nursing agencies;

Community charitable agencies such as Jewish Family Services or Catholic Charities;

Hospital discharge planners and hospital social workers;

Geriatricians (physicians who specialize in caring for older patients and who may be aware of resources serving the elderly throughout the community);

National Association of Social Workers, (202) 408-8600.

To locate these agencies, try the Yellow Pages of the phone book or call the state, county, or local health department. For help in locating a case manager, call the state or local nursing association, a local university's medical school, or local hospitals.

HOW TO DISMISS A CASE MANAGER: REASONS FOR MAKING A CHANGE

The older person and his or her family are consumers who are paying for a service that may have an important impact on their quality of life. If the family doesn't get answers to questions, if realistic goals are not being met, or if the family has tried unsuccessfully to get things straightened out with the case manager, they may need to dismiss the case manager and seek another. Make sure this option is in the contract that the family draws up and signs with the case manager.

Successful attainment of goals might be another reason why the older person or the family would *curtail* or *terminate* a relationship with a case manager. If, after consultation with the family, care partner, and case manager, the older person decides he or she no longer needs the case manager's assistance, he or she may wish to discontinue the relationship. Most case managers keep their files and records so that, if the situation changes again and the older person wants to get more help, he or she can feel free to call the case manager. Some case managers call former clients every 3 to 6 months to see how they are doing, even though they are no longer paying for the services of the case manager. This ongoing information is also kept in the file; if the older person should decide to contact the case manager again, the data are current.

Appendix Three

Regulations Applicable to Case Managers

The kinds of regulations that apply to case managers depend on at least two factors: (1) the type of education and licensing the case manager has had, and (2) the type of setting in which he or she is practicing.

Most case managers are trained in such professions as social work, nursing, psychology, psychiatry, medicine, or law. If they are licensed to practice a particular profession, they must adhere to that profession's code of ethics. If they violate their professional code of ethics and the violation is reported to their professional regulatory organization, strong sanctions can be brought against them (for example, their license to practice could be revoked or they could be fined or even jailed). Even though a person is licensed in a profession such as social work or nursing, he or she is not necessarily a good or ethical case manager. Private case managers tend to operate with fewer controls and less monitoring than case managers in the public system. Therefore, in choosing to hire and use a private case manager, families must be even more careful about checking credentials.

Case managers who practice in an agency or an institution (a hospital, a nursing home, an area agency on aging, a social services agency, or a mental health center) are usually carefully monitored. Case managers who work alone in private practice are not as closely monitored and, at this time, are not regulated in most states—all the more reason to be a wise consumer. Even though no state yet regulates this profession, organizations such as the National Association of Private Geriatric Care Managers are working to develop standards so that private case managers will regulate themselves.

Appendix Four

Resources for Older Persons and Their Families

PUBLICATIONS AND VIDEOS

Caregiving for the Elderly: Recognizing Your Strengths and Resources, by Gary T. Deimling, David M. Bass, Cheryl Jenson, Linda Morley Bass, and Michael B. Ayers. 1986. The Margaret Blenkner Research Center of The Benjamin Rose Institute, 500 Hanna Building, 1422 Euclid Avenue, Cleveland, OH 44115-1989 (216) 621-7201. This booklet is designed to assist family caregivers in identifying the strengths and resources that may enable them to avoid the stress often associated with caring for an ill or disabled relative.

Caring for Your Parents: A Source Book of Options and Solutions for Both Generations, by H. MacLean. 1987. Lake Worth, FL: Dolphin Books.

Daughters of the Elderly: Building Partnerships in Caregiving, edited by Jane Norris. The Indiana University Press, Tenth & Morton Streets, Bloomington, IN 47405 (812) 335-5429; clothbound and paperback.

Elder Care, by J. Kenny and S. Spicer. 1989. Buffalo, NY: Prometheus Books.

Help! I'm Parenting My Parents, by J. J. Jacobsen. 1988. Tuckahoe, NY: Benchmark Press.

How to Care for Your Parents: A Handbook for Adult Children, by Nora Jean Levin. 1987. Washington, DC: Storm King Press.

How to Survive Your Aging Parents, by B.H. Shulman and R. Berman. 1988. Chicago, IL: Surrey Books.

"In Care of: Families and Their Elders," hosted by Hugh Downs. Videotape: 55 minutes. The Brookdale Center on Aging of Hunter College, 425 E. 25th Street, Room 814, New York, NY 10010 (212) 481-7550. An excellent source; rentable.

My Parents Never Had Sex: Myths and Facts of Sexual Aging, by D.B. Hammond. 1987. Buffalo, NY: Prometheus Books.

On Aging Parents: A Practical Guide to Eldercare, edited by C. Browne and R. Onzuka-Anderson. 1985. Honolulu, HI: University of Hawaii Press.

Parentcare: A Commonsense Guide for Adult Children, by L. Jarvik and G. Small. 1988. Glendale, CA: Crown Publishers, Inc.

Talking with Your Aging Parents, by M.A. Edinberg. 1987. Boston, MA: Shambala Publications, Inc.

The Unfinished Business of Living: Helping Aging Parents Help Themselves, by E.N. Chapman. 1988. Los Altos, CA: Crisp Publications.

Unsung Heroes? A National Analysis and Intensive Local Study of Males and the Elder Caregiving Experience, by L.W. Kaye and J. Applegate; published by The Graduate School of Social Work and Social Research, and by Bryn Mawr (300 Airdale Road, Bryn Mawr, PA 19010). This book is accompanied by *A Practical Guidebook: Involving Men in Caregiver Support Groups.* Also, Kaye and Applegate have just published another book, *Men as Caregivers to the Elderly.* Lexington, MA: Lexington Books.

What Do I Do? How to Care for, Comfort, and Commune with Your Nursing Home Elder, by K. Karr and J. Karr. 1985. Binghamton, NY: The Haworth Press.

When Your Parents Grow Old, by Florence D. Shelley. 1988. San Francisco: Harper & Row.

Women Take Care: The Consequences of Caregiving in Today's Society, by T. Sommers and L. Shields. 1987. Gainesville, FL: Triad Publishing Co.

The following booklets will help you learn more about the issues and services discussed in this book. Many of these resources are available free of charge. Copies may be obtained from: AARP Fulfillment Section, 601 E. Street N.W., Washington, DC 20049; (202) 434-2277.

A Checklist of Concerns/Resources for Caregivers (helps caregivers identify their needs and resources), Stock #D12895.

A Handbook About Care in the Home (describes home care services), Stock #D955.

Before You Buy: A Guide to Long-Term Care Insurance (helps consumers assess long-term care insurance policies), Stock #D12893.

Coping and Caring (for families with Alzheimer's patients), Stock #D12441.

Hand-in-Hand Annotated Bibliography (useful reading materials for caregivers), Stock #D12276.

Home is Where the Care Is (an audiocassette program covering information to help caregivers with daily tasks).

Making Wise Decisions About Long-Term Care (a brochure on long-term care services, providers, and financing), Stock #D12435.

Miles Away and Still Caring (for persons concerned about relatives living at a distance), Stock #D12748.

The Right Place at the Right Time (describes the various types of long-term care services), Stock #D12381.

DIRECTORY

ACTION
1100 Vermont Avenue NW
Washington, DC 20525
(202) 634-9380

Administration on Aging
330 Independence Avenue SW
Washington, DC 20201
(202) 245-0641

Aging Network Services
4400 East-West Hwy., Suite 907
Bethesda, MD 20814
(301) 657-4329

Alliance for Aging Research
2021 K Street NW, Suite 305
Washington, DC 20006
(202) 293-2856

Alzheimer's Association
70 E Lake Street, Suite 600
Chicago, IL 60601
(312) 853-3060

Alzheimer's Disease Education &
  Referral Center
Federal Building, Rm. 6C12
9000 Rockville Pike
Bethesda, MD 20892
(301) 496-1752

American Academy of Dermatology
1567 Maple Avenue
Evanston, IL 60201
(312) 869-3954

American Academy of Family
  Physicians
8880 Ward Parkway
Kansas City, MO 64114-2797
(816) 333-9700

American Academy of Neurology
2221 University Avenue SE
Minneapolis, MN 55414
(612) 623-8115

American Academy of
  Ophthalmology
P. O. Box 7424
San Francisco, CA 94120-7424
(415) 561-8500

American Academy of Orthopaedic
  Surgeons
2222 S Prospect Avenue
Park Ridge, IL 60068
(312) 823-7186

American Academy of
  Otolaryngology-Head &
  Neck Surgery, Inc.
1101 Vermont Avenue NW
Washington, DC 20005
(202) 289-4607

American Academy of Physical
  Medicine and Rehabilitation
122 S. Michigan Avenue
Chicago, IL 60603-6107
(312) 922-9366

American Academy of Physician
  Assistants
950 N Washington Street
Alexandria, VA 22314
(703) 836-2272

American Association of
  Cardiovascular & Pulmonary
  Rehabilitation
7611 Elmwood Avenue
Middleton, WI 53562
(608) 831-6989

American Association for Geriatric
  Psychiatry
P. O. Box 376-A
Greenbelt, MD 20770
(301) 220-0952

American Association of Homes for
  the Aging
1129 - 20th Street NW
Washington, DC 20036-3489
(202) 296-5960

American Association of Retired
  Persons
1909 K Street NW
Washington, DC 20049
(202) 872-4700

American Bar Association
  Commission on the Legal
  Problems of the Elderly
2nd Floor, South Lobby
1800 M Street NW
Washington, DC 20036
(202) 331-2297

American Cancer Society
1599 Clifton Road NE
Atlanta, GA 30329
(404) 320-3333

American Chiropractic Association
1701 Clarendon Boulevard
Arlington, VA 22209
(703) 276-8800

American College of Obstetricians &
  Gynecologists
409 - 12th Street SW
Washington, DC 20024
(202) 638-5577

American College of Physicians
Independence Mall West
6th Street at Race
Philadelphia, PA 19106
(215) 351-2400

American College of Surgeons
55 E Erie Street
Chicago, IL 60611
(312) 664-4050

American Council of the Blind
1010 Vermont Avenue NW
Washington, DC 20005
(202) 393-3666

American Dental Association
211 E Chicago Avenue
Chicago, IL 60611
(312) 440-2860

American Diabetes Association
1660 Duke Street
Alexandria, VA 22314
(703) 549-1500

American Dietetic Association
216 W Jackson Boulevard
Chicago, IL 60606
(312) 899-0040

American Federation for Aging
  Research
725 Park Avenue
New York, NY 10021
(212) 570-2090

American Foundation for the Blind
15 W 16th Street
New York, NY 10011
(212) 620-2147

American Geriatrics Society
770 Lexington Avenue
New York, NY 10021
(212) 308-1414

American Health Care Association
1201 L Street NW
Washington, DC 20005
(202) 842-4444

American Health Foundation
320 E 43rd Street
New York, NY 10017
(212) 953-1900

American Heart Association
7320 Greenville Avenue
Dallas, TX 75231
(214) 750-5397

American Hospital Association
840 N Lake Shore Drive
Chicago, IL 60611
(312) 280-6000

American Lung Association
1740 Broadway
New York, NY 10019-4374
(212) 315-8700

American Medical Association
535 N Dearborn Street
Chicago, IL 60610
(312) 645-5000

American Mental Health Fund
2735 Hartland Road
Falls Church, VA 22043
(703) 573-2200

American Nurses Association
2420 Pershing Road
Kansas City, MO 64108
(816) 474-5720

American Occupational Therapy
  Assoc.
P. O. Box 1725
1383 Piccard Drive
Rockville, MD 20850-4375
(301) 948-9626

American Optometric Association
243 N Lindbergh Boulevard
St. Louis, MO 63141
(314) 991-4100

American Osteopathic Association
142 E Ontario Street
Chicago, IL 60611
(312) 280-5857

American Parkinson's Disease Assoc.
116 John Street
New York, NY 10038
(212) 732-9550

American Pharmaceutical Assoc.
2215 Constitution Avenue NW
Washington, DC 20077-6718
(202) 628-4410

American Physical Therapy Assoc.
1111 N Fairfax Street
Alexandria, VA 22314
(703) 684-2782

American Podiatric Medical Assoc.
9312 Old Georgetown Road
Bethesda, MD 20814
(301) 571-9200

American Psychiatric Association
1400 K Street NW
Washington, DC 20005
(202) 682-6239

American Psychological Association
1200 - 17th Street NW
Washington, DC 20036
(202) 955-7600

American Red Cross
18th & D Streets NW
Washington, DC 20006
(202) 737-8300

American Society on Aging
833 Market Street, Suite 512
San Francisco, CA 94103
(415) 543-2617

American Society for Geriatric
  Dentistry
211 E Chicago Avenue, Suite 1616
Chicago, IL 60611
(312) 440-2660

American Society for Internal
  Medicine
1101 Vermont Avenue NW, Suite 500
Washington, DC 20005
(202) 289-1700

American Society of Plastic and
  Reconstructive Surgeons
444 E Algonquin Road
Arlington Heights, IL 60005
(312) 228-9900

American Speech-Language-Hearing
  Association
10801 Rockville Pike
Rockville, MD 20852
(301) 897-5700

American Tinnitus Association
P. O. Box 5
Portland, OR 97207
(503) 248-9985

Arthritis Foundation
1314 Spring Street NW
Atlanta, GA 30309
(404) 872-7100

Association for Brain Tumor
  Research
2910 W Montrose Avenue
Chicago, IL 60618
(312) 286-5571

Assoc. for Gerontology in Higher
  Education
West Wing 204
600 Maryland Avenue SW
Washington, DC 20024
(202) 484-7505

Assoc. of Sleep Disorders Centers
604 Second Street SW
Rochester, MN 55902
(507) 287-6006

Better Vision Institute
1800 N Kent Street, Suite 1310
Rosslyn, VA 22209
(703) 243-1528

Beverly Foundation
70 S Lake Avenue, Suite 750
Pasadena, CA 91101
(818) 792-2292

B'nai B'rith International
1640 Rhode Island Avenue NW
Washington, DC 20036
(202) 857-6600

Brookdale Center on Aging
425 E 25th Street
New York, NY 10010
(212) 481-4426

Catholic Charities
1319 F Street NW
Washington, DC 20004
(202) 639-8400

Catholic Golden Age
400 Lackawanna Avenue
Scranton, PA 18503
(717) 342-3294

Center for Social Gerontology
117 N First Street, Suite 204
Ann Arbor, MI 48104
(313) 665-1126

Center for the Study of Aging
706 Madison Avenue
Albany, NY 12208
(518) 465-6927

Children of Aging Parents
2761 Trenton Road
Levittown, PA 19056
(215) 945-6900

Concerned Relatives of Nursing
  Home Patients
3130 Mayfield Road
Cleveland Heights, OH 44118
(216) 321-0403

Consumer Information Center
P. O. Box 100
Pueblo, CO 81009

Consumer Product Safety
  Commission
Office of Information & Public
  Affairs
5401 Westbard Avenue
Bethesda, MD 20207
(301) 492-6580

Council of Better Business Bureaus
4200 Wilson Boulevard
Arlington, VA 22209
(703) 276-0133

Delta Society
P. O. Box 1080
Renton, WA 98057-1080
(206) 226-7357

Department of Labor
Consumer Affairs, Rm. S1032
200 Constitution Avenue NW
Washington, DC 20210
(202) 523-6060

DES Action
Long Island Jewish Medical Center
New Hyde Park, NY 11040
(516) 775-3450

Disabled American Veterans
P. O. Box 14301
Cincinnati, OH 45250
(606) 441-7300

Displaced Homemaker Network
1411 K Street NW, Suite 930
Washington, DC 20005
(202) 628-6767

Dizziness & Balance Disorders Assoc.
Resource Center, Rm. 300
1015 Northwest 22nd Avenue
Portland, OR 97210
(503) 229-7348

Elder Craftsmen
135 E 65th Street
New York, NY 10021
(212) 861-5260

Elderhostel
80 Boylston Street, Suite 400
Boston, MA 02116
(617) 426-8056

Elvirita Lewis Foundation
P. O. Box 1539
La Quinta, CA 92253
(619) 397-4552

Environmental Protection Agency
Public Information Center
401 M Street SW
Washington, DC 20460
(202) 382-2080

Episcopal Society for Ministry on
  Aging
317 Wyandotte Street
Bethlehem, PA 18015
(215) 868-5400

Equal Employment Opportunity
  Commission
1801 L Street NW
Washington, DC 20507
(202) 634-6036

Federal Council on Aging
Room 4280 HHS-N
330 Independence Avenue SW
Washington, DC 20201
(202) 245-2451

Federal Trade Commission
Office of Public Affairs, Rm. 421
6th Street & Pennsylvania Avenue NW
Washington, DC 20580
(202) 326-2180

Food and Drug Administration
5600 Fishers Lane
Rockville, MD 20857
(301) 443-3170

Food and Nutrition Information
  Center
National Agricultural Library
  Building
Beltsville, MD 20705
(301) 344-3719

Foundation for Hospice and Home
  Care
519 C Street NE
Washington, DC 20002
(202) 547-7424

Gerontological Society of America
1275 K Street NW, Suite 350
Washington, DC 20005-4006
(202) 842-1275

Gray Panthers
311 S Juniper Street, Suite 601
Philadelphia, PA 19107
(215) 545-6555

Health Care Financing
  Administration
200 Independence Avenue SW
Washington, DC 20201
(202) 245-6145

Health Insurance Association of
  America
1025 Connecticut Avenue NW,
  Suite 1200
Washington, DC 20036
(202) 223-7780

Help for Incontinent People
P. O. Box 544
Union, SC 29379
(803) 579-7900

Hill-Burton Program
Health Resources & Services
  Administration
5600 Fishers Lane
Rockville, MD 20857
(301) 443-5656

Huntington's Disease Society of
  America
140 W 22nd Street, 6th Floor
New York, NY 10011
(212) 242-1968

Hysterectomy Educational Resources
  & Services Foundation
422 Bryn Mawr Avenue
Bala Cynwyd, PA 19004
(215) 667-7757

Japanese-American Citizens League
1765 Sutter Street
San Francisco, CA 94115
(415) 921-5225

John Douglas French Foundation for
  Alzheimer's Disease
11620 Wilshire Boulevard
Los Angeles, CA 90025
(213) 470-5462

Legal Services for the Elderly
132 W 43rd Street, 3rd Floor
New York, NY 10036
(212) 391-0120

Leukemia Society of America
733 Third Avenue
New York, NY 10017
(212) 573-8484

Lupus Foundation of America
1717 Massachusetts Avenue NW
Washington, DC 20036
(202) 328-4550

Make Today Count
101-1/2 S Union Street
Alexandria, VA 22314-3323
(703) 548-9674

Medic Alert Foundation
P. O. Box 1009
Turlock, CA 95381-1009
(209) 668-3333

National Action Forum for Midlife &
  Older Women
c/o Dr. Jane Porcino
P. O. Box 816
Stony Brook, NY 11790-0609

National AIDS Information
Clearinghouse
P. O. Box 6003
Rockville, MD 20850
(301) 762-5111

National Alliance of Senior Citizens
2525 Wilson Boulevard
Arlington, VA 22201
(703) 528-4380

National Arthritis & Musculoskeletal
& Skin Diseases Information
Clearinghouse
P. O. Box AMS
Bethesda, MD 20892
(301) 468-3235

National Association of Area
Agencies on Aging
600 Maryland Avenue SW,
Suite 208W
Washington, DC 20024
(202) 484-7520

National Assoc. of Community
Health Centers
1330 New Hampshire Avenue NW,
Suite 122
Washington, DC 20036
(202) 659-8008

National Association for the Deaf
814 Thayer Avenue
Silver Spring, MD 20910
(301) 587-1788

National Assoc. for Hispanic Elderly
2727 W Sixth Street, Suite 270
Los Angeles, CA 90057

National Assoc. for Home Care
519 C Street NE
Washington, DC 20002
(202) 547-7424

National Assoc. for Human
Development
1424 - 16th Street NW
Washington, DC 20036
(202) 328-2191

National Assoc. of Meal Programs
204 E Street NE
Washington, DC 20002
(202) 547-6340

National Assoc. for Practical Nurse
Education & Services
1400 Spring Street, Suite 310
Silver Spring, MD 20910
(301) 588-2491

National Assoc. of Private Geriatric
Case Managers
655 N. Alvernon, Suite 108
Tucson, AZ 85711
(602) 881-8008

National Assoc. of Social Workers
7981 Eastern Avenue
Silver Spring, MD 20910
(301) 565-0333

National Assoc. of State Units on
Aging
2033 K Street NW, Suite 304
Washington, DC 20006
(202) 785-0707

National Cancer Institute
Office of Cancer Communications
Building 31, Rm. 10A24
9000 Rockville Pike
Bethesda, MD 20892
(301) 496-5583

National Caucus & Center on Black
Aged
1424 K Street NW, Suite 500
Washington, DC 20005
(202) 637-8400

National Center for Health Services
  Research & Health Care Technology
  Assessment
Parklawn Building, Rm. 18-12
5600 Fishers Lane
Rockville, MD 20857
(301) 443-4100

National Center for Health Statistics
3700 East-West Highway
Hyattsville, MD 20782
(301) 436-8500

National Cholesterol Education
  Program
4733 Bethesda Avenue
Bethesda, MD 20814
(301) 951-3260

National Citizens Coalition for
  Nursing Home Reform
1424 - 16th Street NW, Suite L2
Washington, DC 20036
(202) 797-0657

National Clearinghouse for Primary
  Care Information
8201 Greensboro Drive, Suite 600
McLean, VA 22102
(703) 821-8955

National Commission on Working
  Women
1325 G Street NW, Lower Level
Washington, DC 20005
(202) 737-5764

National Committee on the
  Treatment of Intractable Pain
P. O. Box 9553, Friendship Station
Washington, DC 20016
(202) 965-6717

National Consumers League
815 - 15th Street NW, Suite 516
Washington, DC 20005
(202) 639-8140

National Council on the Aging
West Wing 100
600 Maryland Avenue SW
Washington, DC 20024
(202) 479-1200

National Council on Alcoholism
12 W 21st Street, 8th Floor
New York, NY 10010
(212) 206-6770

National Council on Patient
  Information & Education
666 - 11th Street NW, Suite 810
Washington, DC 20001
(202) 347-6711

National Council of Senior Citizens
925 - 15th Street NW
Washington, DC 20005
(202) 347-8800

National Diabetes Information
  Clearinghouse
Box NDIC
Bethesda, MD 20892
(301) 468-2162

National Digestive Diseases
  Information Clearinghouse
Box NDDIC
Bethesda, MD 20892
(301) 468-6344

National Eye Institute
Information Office
Building 31, Room 6A29
Bethesda, MD 20892
(301) 496-5248

National Foundation for Long-Term
  Health Care
1200 - 15th Street NW, Suite 402
Washington, DC 20005
(202) 659-3148

National Geriatrics Society
212 W Wisconsin Avenue
Milwaukee, WI 53203

National Hearing Aid Society
20361 Middlebelt Street
Livonia, MI 48152
(313) 478-2610

National Heart, Lung, & Blood
  Institute
Information Office
Building 31, Room 4A21
9000 Rockville Pike
Bethesda, MD 20892
(301) 496-4236

National High Blood Pressure
  Information Center
4733 Bethesda Avenue
Bethesda, MD 20814
(301) 951-3260

National Hispanic Council on Aging
2713 Ontario Road NW
Washington, DC 20009
(202) 265-1288

National Hospice Organization
1901 N Moore Street, Suite 901
Arlington, VA 22209
(703) 243-5900

National Indian Council on Aging
P. O. Box 2088
Albuquerque, NM 87103
(505) 242-9505

National Information Center on
  Deafness
Gallaudet University
800 Florida Avenue NE
Washington, DC 20002
(202) 651-5051

National Institute on Aging
Public Information Office
Federal Building, Room 6C12
9000 Rockville Pike
Bethesda, MD 20892
(301) 496-1752

National Institute on Alcohol Abuse
  and Alcoholism
5600 Fishers Lane, Room 16-95
Rockville, MD 20857
(301) 443-1677

National Institute of Allergy &
  Infectious Diseases
Office of Communications
Building 31, Room 7A32
9000 Rockville Pike
Bethesda, MD 20892
(301) 496-5717

National Institute of Arthritis &
  Musculoskeletal & Skin Diseases
Information Office
Building 31, Room B2B15
9000 Rockville Pike
Bethesda, MD 20892
(301) 496-8188

National Institute on Deafness &
  Other Communication Disorders
Information Office
9000 Rockville Pike
Bethesda, MD 20892
(301) 496-5751

National Institute of Dental
  Research
Information Office
Building 31, Room 2C35
9000 Rockville Pike
Bethesda, MD 20892
(301) 496-4261

National Institute of Diabetes &
  Digestive & Kidney Diseases
Information Office
Building 31, Room 9A06
9000 Rockville Pike
Bethesda, MD 20892
(301) 496-3583

National Institute on Drug Abuse
Information Office, Room 10A46
5600 Fishers Lane
Rockville, MD 20857
(301) 443-6500

National Institute of General
Medical Sciences
Office of Research Reports
Building 31, Room 4A52
9000 Rockville Pike
Bethesda, MD 20892
(301) 496-7301

National Institute of Mental Health
Public Inquiries Office, Rm. 15C-05
5600 Fishers Lane
Rockville, MD 20857
(301) 443-4513

National Institute of Neurological
Disorders & Stroke
Information Office
Building 31, Room 8A06
9000 Rockville Pike
Bethesda, MD 20892
(301) 496-5751

National Interfaith Coalition on Aging
P. O. Box 1924
Athens, GA 30603
(404) 353-1331

National Kidney Foundation
30 E 33rd Street
New York, NY 10016
(212) 889-2210

National Kidney & Urologic Diseases
Information Clearinghouse
Box NKUDIC
Bethesda, MD 20892
(301) 468-6345

National League for Nursing
10 Columbus Circle
New York, NY 10019-1350
(212) 582-1022

National Library of Medicine
8600 Rockville Pike
Bethesda, MD 20894
(301) 496-5501

National Multiple Sclerosis Society
205 E 42nd Street
New York, NY 10017
(212) 986-3240

National Organization for Rare
Disorders
P. O. Box 8923
New Fairfield, CT 06812
(203) 746-6518

National Organization for Victim
Assistance
717 D Street NW
Washington, DC 20004
(202) 393-6682

National Osteoporosis Foundation
1625 Eye Street NW, Suite 822
Washington, DC 20006
(202) 223-2226

National Pacific/Asian Resource
Center on Aging
2033 Sixth Avenue, Suite 410
Seattle, WA 98121-2524
(206) 448-0313

National Rehabilitation Association
633 S Washington Street
Alexandria, VA 22314
(703) 836-0850

National Rehabilitation Information
Center
8455 Colesville Road, Suite 935
Silver Spring, MD 20910-3319
(301) 588-9284

National Rural Health Care Assoc.
301 E Armour Boulevard, Suite 420
Kansas City, MO 64111
(816) 756-3140

National Safety Council
444 N Michigan Avenue
Chicago, IL 60611-3991
(312) 527-4800

National Self-Help Clearinghouse
33 W 42nd Street
New York, NY 10036
(212) 642-2944

National Senior Citizens Law Center
2025 M Street NW, Suite 400
Washington, DC 20036
(202) 887-5280

National Senior Sports Association
10560 Main Street, Suite 205
Fairfax, VA 22030
(703) 385-7540

National Shut-In Society
P. O. Box 986
Village Station, NY 10014-1986
(212) 222-7699

National Society to Prevent Blindness
500 E Remington Road
Schaumburg, IL 60173
(312) 843-2020

National Stroke Association
300 E Hampden Avenue, Suite 240
Englewood, CO 80110
(303) 762-9922

National Technical Information
  Service
5285 Port Royal Road
Springfield, VA 22161
(703) 487-4600

National Urban League
500 E 62nd Street
New York, NY 10021
(212) 310-9000

National Women's Health Network
1325 G Street NW
Washington, DC 20005
(202) 347-1140

Office of Disease Prevention &
  Health Promotion
Mary Switzer Building, Rm. 2132
330 C Street SW
Washington, DC 20201
(202) 472-5660

Office on Smoking and Health
Park Building, Room 1-10
5600 Fishers Lane
Rockville, MD 20857
(301) 443-1575

Older Women's League
730 - 11th Street NW, Suite 300
Washington, DC 20001
(202) 783-6686

Opticians Association of America
10341 Democracy Lane
P. O. Box 10110
Fairfax, VA 22030
(703) 691-8355

Organization of Chinese Americans
2025 Eye Street NW, Suite 926
Washington, DC 20006
(202) 223-5500

President's Council on Physical
  Fitness & Sports
450 Fifth Street NW, Suite 7103
Washington, DC 20001
(202) 272-3430

Pride Long-Term Home Health Care
  Institute
153 W 11th Street
New York, NY 10011
(212) 790-8864

Public Affairs Committee
381 Park Avenue S
New York, NY 10016

Retirement Research Foundation
1300 W Higgins Road, Suite 214
Park Ridge, IL 60068
(312) 823-4133

The Robert Wood Johnson
  Foundation
P. O. Box 2316
Princeton, NJ 08543-2316
(609) 452-8701

Self-Help for Hard of Hearing People
7800 Wisconsin Avenue
Bethesda, MD 20814
(301) 657-2248

Simon Foundation
Box 835
Wilmette, IL 60091
(312) 864-3913

Skin Cancer Foundation
245 Fifth Avenue, Suite 2402
New York, NY 10016
(212) 725-5176

Social Security Administration
Office of Public Inquiries
6401 Security Boulevard
Baltimore, MD 21235
(301) 594-1234

United Ostomy Association
36 Executive Park, Suite 120
Irvine, CA 92714
(714) 660-8624

United Parkinson Foundation
360 W Superior Street
Chicago, IL 60610
(312) 664-2344

United Seniors Health Cooperative
1334 G Street NW, Suite 500
Washington, DC 20005
(202) 393-6222

U.S. Pharmacopeial Convention
12601 Twinbrook Parkway
Rockville, MD 20852
(301) 881-0666

United Way of America
701 N Fairfax Street
Alexandria, VA 22314-2045
(703) 836-7100

Veterans Administration
Office of Public Affairs
810 Vermont Avenue NW
Washington, DC 20420
(202) 233-2843

Volunteers of America
3813 N Causeway Boulevard
Metairie, LA 70002
(504) 837-2652

Women's Equity Action League
1250 Eye Street NW, Suite 305
Washington, DC 20005
(202) 898-1588

Young Men's Christian Association
101 N Wacker Drive
Chicago, IL 60606
(312) 977-0031

Young Women's Christian Association
726 Broadway
New York, NY 10003
(212) 614-2700

Appendix Five

Pledge of Ethics—The National Association of Private Geriatric Care Managers

I will provide service to you only after I have assessed your needs and you, or a person acting for you, understand and agree to a plan of service, the results that may be expected, and the cost.

I will base my plan of service on goals you, or a person acting for you, have defined, and which enhance the decisions you have made concerning your life.

My first duty is loyalty to you. I will always provide service based on your best interest, even if this conflicts with my interests or the interests of others. However, I reserve the right to terminate my services to you if my reasonable fees are not paid.

I will not end service to you without giving you reasonable notice and alternatives for you to continue to receive the services you need.

I will not substitute my judgment for yours unless I am acting in the role of your guardian, appointed by a Court of Law, or with your approval, or the approval of someone acting for you.

I will hold in trust any confidence you give me, disclosing information to others only with your permission, or if I am compelled to do so by a belief that you will be seriously harmed by my silence, or if the laws of this State require me to do so.

I will refer you only to services and organizations I believe to be appropriate and of good quality. I will fully explain to you any business relationship I have with any service I propose, and give you information on alternatives, if at all possible, so that you, or a person acting for you, can make an informed decision to accept or reject the services I recommend to you.

I will work to assure cooperation between all of the individuals involved in providing service and care to you.

Used with permission of NAPGCM.

I am fully qualified in my profession to provide the services I undertake. I continue to improve my skills and knowledge by participating in professional development programs and maintaining certification and licensing in my profession.

If you, or a person acting for you, believe that I have not behaved in a way that is consistent with this Pledge of Ethics, please discuss your concerns with me. If, after that, you are not satisfied, you can call or write for information about filing a grievance against me:

National Association of Private Geriatric Care Managers
655 North Alvernon Way, Suite 108
Tucson, Arizona 85711
(602) 881-8008

Appendix Six

NAPGCM Standards and Practice Guidelines for Private Geriatric Care Managers

PREAMBLE

These standards have been developed because Private Geriatric Care Management (PGCM) is a human service specialty provided by professionals from diverse backgrounds and academic preparations to a vulnerable and often frail population. No one profession can claim exclusive domain over the knowledge and skills required to provide PGCM services. Thus, private geriatric care managers may be members of formal professions, such as social work, nursing or psychology, or may hold advanced degrees in gerontology, counseling, public health administration, or other fields of human service specialization.

In addition, these Standards have been developed because certain issues of particular concern to private geriatric care managers have not always been included in the standards developed by other organizations. Thus, the purpose of these Standards is to supplement already existing standards of other professions and organizations and to provide guidance to the members of the National Association of Private Geriatric Care Managers in the many complex situations presented by their practices.

Members of NAPGCM are expected to abide by the standards of their respective professions, as well as to these Standards developed specifically for their practices in private geriatric care management.

STANDARD 1

Standard

While the "primary client" usually is the older person whose care needs have instigated the referral to a private geriatric care manager, all others affected by her/his care needs should be considered part of the "client system."

Rationale

In the area of private geriatric care management, the care needs of the older person often have significant consequences for others. The private geriatric care manager's goal is to assist the individual members of the client system to understand fully the issues under consideration and arrive at a solution which allows maximum decision making autonomy for the person receiving care and for the other persons involved with or affected by these care needs.

Guidelines

1) The "primary client" may not be the person who makes the initial contact or the person responsible for payment for services rendered.

2) Members of the "client system" may include:

   —the older person

   —a family member within or outside of the older person's household

   —a paid caregiver

   —friends, neighbors or community agencies

   —a third party with fiduciary responsibilities

   —other professionals, such as a physician, a nurse from a home health care agency, an attorney, etc.

   —the private geriatric care manager (See Standard 6)

3) In the event of conflicting needs within the client system, the goal of professional intervention should be to strive for resolution through a process of review and discussion among the parties, facilitated by the private geriatric care manager.

4) The private geriatric care manager should request assistance of appropriate peers, as needed, to help the client system find an acceptable solution to the conflicts it faces.

STANDARD 2

Standard

To the greatest extent possible, the private geriatric care manager should foster self-determination on the part of the older person.

Rationale

All too often, the older person's goals, values and voiced opinions are overlooked by health care professionals and family members who feel that they have the older person's "best interests at heart." Private geriatric care managers have a responsibility to respect the older person's right to make decisions regarding her/his care.

Guidelines

1) The private geriatric care manager must attempt to involve the older person in all decisions which impact her/his life regardless of the determination of competence.

2) As the older person makes decisions on her/his own behalf, the private geriatric care manager (PGCM) should see that the following factors are understood and discussed. In addition, the PGCM should encourage the older person to communicate, verbally or non-verbally, her/his wishes.

a. The specific information needed to make a given decision

b. The consequences of all decisions

c. Whether or not the consequences of these decisions are in accord with her/personal values and goals

3) If the older person has not comprehended the factors involved in the decision making process and therefore cannot make a responsible self-determination, then the private geriatric care manager should see that all decisions concerning the older person are made by the person(s) with the legal authority to do so.

STANDARD 3

Standard

The private geriatric care manager should respect the older person's and, when applicable, the family's right to privacy by protecting all information which is given in confidence and all information of a confidential nature. It should be made clear to the client the limits of confidentiality as appropriate.

Rationale

The private geriatric care manager (PGCM) generally needs to share information with others in order to fulfill her/his responsibilities. The PGCM utilizes knowledge of the older person's physical and mental status, financial and legal affairs, and family and community supports to assist her/him to achieve maximum well-being. Due care must be exercised at all times to protect the privacy of this information.

Guidelines

1) The information contained in case files is considered privileged and confidential.

2) The private geriatric care manager should obtain a release of information that covers all actions taken on the behalf of the client so that pertinent information can be shared for the benefit of the older person.

3) The private geriatric care manager should act judiciously when sharing information within families and with other professionals.

4) The private geriatric care manager should insure that all consultations and interviews are held in locations which allow for the maximum amount of privacy.

STANDARD 4

Standard

The private geriatric care manager should define her/his role clearly to other professionals.

Rationale

Due to the fact that the specialization of private geriatric care management is a relatively new one, other professionals may not have worked with private geriatric care managers before. Thus, uncertainty may exist as to how each can complement the other's role. It is of utmost importance for all professionals involved in the care of the older person to have a clear understanding of each others' areas of expertise and responsibility.

Guidelines

1) Private geriatric care managers should act only in the roles for which they have the appropriate skills, knowledge and training. She/he should not claim knowledge and skills in roles for which they do not have adequate training and should recommend consultations with specialists as needed.

2) With proper consent the private geriatric care manager should share information concerning the needs of the older person or client system with professional colleagues in a forthright, clear and timely manner.

STANDARD 5

Standard

The private geriatric care manager should strive to provide quality care using a flexible care plan developed in conjunction with the older person and other persons involved in her/his care.

Rationale

A plan of care with the stated recommendations, goals and appropriate interventions must be flexible enough to deal with the older person's changing status. The overall goal is to strive to assist the older person to attain the highest level of health and quality of life that is within her/his particular set of circumstances.

Guidelines

The care plan should:

1) Have a systematic and concise format.

2) Be updated as goals and recommendations are met and needs change.

3) Be acceptable to the older person and the client system.

4) Foster self-determination of the older person while balanced with the person's need for safety. (See Standard 2)

STANDARD 6

Standard

The private geriatric care manager should act in a manner that insures her/his own integrity as well as the integrity of the client system.

Rationale

One of the private geriatric care manager's (PGCM) most important roles is to be an advocate for the older person. At the same time, the PGCM's own values and beliefs must be taken into consideration when working with the older person and client system.

Guidelines

1) After careful consideration of both her/his own values and those of the client system, the private geriatric care manager (PGCM) can appropriately refuse to accept a new case or continue in a case in which she/he is already involved if the PGCM believes that the situation would require compromising her/his own values, beliefs or standards. The PGCM can terminate her/his involvement in an ongoing case by providing timely written notice to allow for alternate arrangements to be made. She/he is obligated to make an effort to refer those cases which she/he is unable to accept to an appropriate resource.

2) If the private geriatric care manager finds her/himself in a circumstance in which the integrity and safety of the older person is at risk (e.g., abuse, neglect or self-neglect) she/he must make a report to the appropriate authority in accordance with national and state laws and regulations.

STANDARD 7

Standard

All fees for private geriatric care management services are to be stated in written form and discussed with the person accepting responsibility for payment prior to the initiation of services.

Rationale

The older person and the family often contact the geriatric care manager at a time of great stress. To prevent any misunderstandings regarding fees it is in the best interest of all parties to have information in written form prior to the initiation of services. If time does not allow for this then all information should be verbally presented.

Guidelines

1) Fees should be charged for services rendered and presented in a clearly itemized statement. These fees should not be based on a percentage of a person's assets.

2) At intake, older people or families determined to be unable to pay for care management services can be referred to community, publicly supported agencies that can provide the necessary services. An older person with an established relationship with a private geriatric care manager (PGCM), but who can no longer pay for services, should not be abandoned. The PGCM must make every effort to provide linkage with a community agency suited to her/his needs.

3) Private geriatric care managers are encouraged to provide free services as a professional responsibility. Free services are to be of equal quality as for persons paying for services.

4) In accordance with state laws, private geriatric care managers should not engage in fee-splitting practices nor should they receive commissions from vendors/professionals, who are providing or may provide in the future, services to the older person.

5) Private geriatric care managers should not pay for her/his services through direct access to client accounts without supervision by a third party.

STANDARD 8

Standard

Advertising and marketing of services should be conducted within all guidelines and laws governing the advertising of professional management services as they relate to the provision of private geriatric care management.

Rationale

Families facing the stresses of coping with complications of aging, dementia, chronic illness or death are vulnerable to claims which suggest a rescue or immediate relief of stressful circumstances. Older persons faced with debilitating illnesses, decreased capacity for judgement and limited financial resources are likewise vulnerable to specious claims.

Guidelines

1) The responsibility for truthful and non-deceptive advertising rests on the private geriatric care manager. All attempts should be made not to use advertising which is deceptive, fraudulent, insincere or falsely disparaging of competitors. Specific caution is urged in the area of misrepresentation by omission or obfuscation of material fact.

STANDARD 9

Standard

The private geriatric care manager who accepts a fiduciary responsibility should act only within her/his knowledge and capabilities and should avoid any activities which might comprise a conflict of interest.

Rationale

When, due to physical frailties or cognitive losses, an older person is not able to handle certain financial transactions, e.g., balancing a checkbook or paying bills and there is no family member or other party to accept these responsibilities the private geriatric care manager acts as a "pay agent." The older person may also need a conservator, guardian or power of attorney.

Guidelines

1) When undertaking pay agent responsibilities the private geriatric care manager should obtain written consent from the older person or a responsible third party with power of attorney.

2) The private geriatric care manager, in her/his role of "pay agent," should not act in the role of financial adviser regarding client's assets or investments, unless qualified to do so. (See Standard 7)

3) The private geriatric care manager (PGCM) should avoid, where possible, self payment or the undertaking of power of attorney, guardianship or conservatorship. If the PGCM has no alternative than to pay for her/his services through direct access to client accounts then this should be done with oversight by a third party. (See Standard 7)

4) When asked to take responsibility for a purchase (of goods or services) not commonly within the "pay agent" agreement, the care manager should conduct appropriate comparative pricing and make the purchase only with the agreement of the older person or a responsible third party.

5) Records of all transactions should be kept current in a format recognized by standard accounting practices, and should be open to inspection by appropriate parties.

STANDARD 10

Standard

The private geriatric care manager should be familiar with laws relating to employment practices and should not knowingly participate in practices that are inconsistent with these laws.

Rationale

Private geriatric care managers (PGCM) are often concerned with private duty caregivers, either in screening and recommending them to clients for hire, or in coordinating and/or supervising their work. In addition, PGCM may employ other professionals or service providers. In either case, they need to be aware of applicable employment and tax laws.

Guidelines

1) Private geriatric care managers should not knowingly participate in employment practices that are not legal, i.e., recommending or employing persons not legally permitted to work, condoning non-payment of wage taxes, or wages that do not meet minimum wage requirements.

2) Private geriatric care managers should use, and recommend that clients use, the appropriate legal and accounting professionals to ensure that applicable laws are followed.

3) Private geriatric care managers may also want to be familiar with the appropriate State and Federal agencies which handle employment practices.

STANDARD 11

Standard

The private geriatric care manager should provide full disclosure regarding business, professional or personal relationships she/he has with each recommended business, agency or institution.

Rationale

When developing a plan of care, the private geriatric care manager (PGCM) often will need to make referrals to businesses, agencies or institutions that can provide needed services. It is important for the older person and his/her family to be informed if the PGCM has a relationship other than objective third party with that agency, e.g., Board of Trustees, ownership, investor, family member.

Guidelines

1) When a referral is made the private geriatric care manager should clarify to the client any special relationship that exists with the recommended business, agency or institution.

2) When the private geriatric care manager has a business, professional or personal relationship with a recommended business, agency or institution, she/he should provide to the client information regarding alternative choices.

STANDARD 12

Standard

The private geriatric care manager should participate in continuing education programs and be a member of her/his respective professional organization in order to enhance professional growth and to provide the highest quality care management.

Rationale

To remain up to date with scientific, cultural, political, legal and social changes in the area of gerontology it is incumbent upon the private geriatric care manager (PGCM) to continually take part in educational programs that will enable her/him to provide the highest quality care management. In addition, both the PGCM and those persons to whom she/he provides services will benefit from the PGCM's participation in her/his respective professional organization. The PGCM thus will practice in accord with that organization's standards, in addition to those specific to private geriatric care management.

Guidelines

Private geriatric care managers should:

1) be certified, if applicable, and/or licensed, as required, in her/his area of expertise.

2) seek peer supervision, as needed.

3) seek consultation with other professions, as needed.

These Standards were adopted by the National Association of Private Geriatric Care Managers on October 20, 1990 at the 6th Annual Meeting held in Washington, D.C., and revised June, 1991.

Appendix Seven

Category "A" Private Geriatric Care Managers

NOTE: Category "A" Membership is offered to a person who is a principal of a business primarily engaged in the practice of client-centered care management services to the elderly and their families, and who holds a degree or substantial equivalent in the field of human services delivery, who is certified or licensed at the independent practice level of such person's state or profession (where applicable), and who has two (2) years' supervised experience in the field of gerontology following such person's advanced degree.

INDEX OF CATEGORY "A" MEMBERS, BY STATE*

Arizona

Nancy Alexander
Complete Care Management
1005 N. Caribe
Tucson, AZ 85710
(602) 886-7602
(800) 669-3949

Paula L. Hurn
Elder Links
2032 East Monterey Way
Phoenix, AZ 85016
(602) 957-4883

Gordon Sloan James
Elder Care Resources Unlimited
Lincoln Centre-Lakeview Suites
11221 North 28th Drive, E. 104
Phoenix, AZ 85029
(602) 548-9348

Arizona (Continued)

Sylvia A. Stevens
Stevens & Associates
612 N. Signal Butte
Apache Jct., AZ 85220
(602) 986-4210

California

Lynn Allen
Senior Care & Family Specialist
5218 Lawton Avenue
Oakland, CA 94618
(510) 655-1551

Anita K. Anderson
P.O. Box 0
El Cerrito, CA 94530
(415) 237-5970

*Used with permission of NAPGCM.

297

California *(Continued)*

Loraine P. Auerbach
American Medical Systems, Inc.
1250 Long Beach Ave.
Suite 328
Los Angeles, CA 90021
(213) 624-2225
(213) 624-2229 FAX

Steven Michael Barlam
Senior Care Management
256 South Robertson Blvd.,
  Suite 709
Beverly Hills, CA 90211
(213) 288-0059
(213) 288-0301 FAX

Julie Barton
E.L.C. Associates
P.O. Box 160249
Cupertino, CA 95016
(415) 968-8028

Toby Bernstein
Elder Assist
140 Woodbine Drive
Mill Valley, CA 94941
(415) 388-5972

Karen Bowman
5150 N Sixth Street
Suite 149
Fresno, CA 93710
(209) 445-3924

Marilyn Carlander
Lifenet, Inc.
1819 State St.
Suite B
Santa Barbara, CA 93101
(805) 687-8766

Jeannine Caryl
Senior Citizen Consultants/
Case Management
7451 Warner Avenue #H
Huntington Beach, CA 92647
(714) 841-8008

California *(Continued)*

Cathy Jo Cress
Cresscare, Case Management
Agency for Elders
230 Fountain Ave., Suite 6
Pacific Grove, CA 93950
(408) 372-0802

Virginia Daugherty
ELC Associates
P.O. Box 160249
Cupertino, CA 95016
(415) 968-8028

Jay A. Deike
Elder Options
1805 Proctor Dr.
Santa Rosa, CA 95404
(707) 579-1485

Maria Estrada
Seniors Support Service
161 Fashion Lane, Suite 107
Tustin, CA 92680
(714) 838-0598

Linda Fodrini-Johnson
Elder Care Placement Services
1844 San Miguel Dr., #101
Walnut Creek, CA 94596
(510) 937-2018

Rita Ghatak
PARD
167 Hamilton Ave.
Palo Alto, CA 94301
(415) 321-6413

Alan Goldberg
Top-Of-The-Line Professional Health
  Care, Inc.
1642 Veteran Avenue
Los Angeles, CA 90024
(213) 479-2832

Harriette R. Grooh
Harriette Grooh & Associates
1112 Sir Francis Drake Boulevard
Kentfield, CA 94904
(415) 924-8311

California *(Continued)*

Evelyne E. Hutkin
Senior Care Services
5333 Mission Center Road
Suite 340
San Diego, CA 92108
(619) 291-4403

Sherry A. Johanson
HealthCare Consultant
12 Barn Road
Mill Valley, CA 94941
(415) 389-1434

Rose Kleiner
Older Adults Care Management
167 Hamilton Avenue
Palo Alto, CA 94301
(415) 329-1411

Jeanne W. Klems
Jeanne W. Klems LCSW
1870 San Lorenzo Ave.
Berkeley, CA 94707
(415) 525-2226

Kyle Laitiner
Lifenet, Inc.
1819 State St., Suite B
Santa Barbara, CA 93101
(805) 687-8766

Mary G. LaNier
Gerontology Consultants
721 Ashland Drive
Huntington Beach, CA 92648
(714) 536-8103

Barbara Larsen
Elder-Connection
P.O. BOX 1061
Grass Valley, CA 95945
(916) 265-4049

Jan E. Lees
1226 Veteran Avenue
Los Angeles, CA 90024
(213) 820-1602

California *(Continued)*

Joyce Marvan-Hyam
Adult Care Services
800 South Broadway
Suite 309
Walnut Creek, CA 94596
(415) 944-5800

Suzanne Fritts McNeely
Senior Planning Services
735 State Street, Suite 106
Santa Barbara, CA 93101
(805) 966-3312

Vida Francis Negrete
1507 Indiana Avenue
South Pasadena, CA 91030
(213) 259-8710

Deborah D. Newquist
Elder Care Resources
2900 Bristol, Suite 206J
Costa Mesa, CA 92626
(714) 854-2990

Mary M. Norcross
Nursing Home/Residential Placement
13623 Valerio St., Unit B
Van Nuys, CA 91405
(818) 376-1411

Carolyn E. Paul
1849 Santa Rosa Court
Claremont, CA 91711
(714) 625-3085

Risha Paz'Soldan
Aging Care Options
12439 Magnolia Blvd., #207
North Hollywood, CA 91607
(818) 700-0209

Becky Peters
Lifespan: Care Management Agency
820 Bay Avenue, Suite 124
Captiola, CA 95010
(408) 475-7211

California (Continued)

Elana Peters
Care Options - Elder Care Mgmt.
2102 Business Center Dr., Suite 130
Irvine, CA 92715
(714) 253-4140
(714) 955-0679 FAX

Myrna Rudman
MLR Associates
P.O. Box 161624
Sacramento, CA 95816
(916) 927-1895

Gabriel Russo
400 Brian Court
Merced, CA 95348
(209) 722-4273

Beverly J. Shannon
Extended Family Associates
820 Walnut St.
San Luis Obispo, CA 93401
(805) 543-3389

Ann Sorgen
P.O. Box 1381
Ross, CA 94957
(415) 461-2356

B.J. Curry Spitler
Age Concerns Inc.
2546 4th Avenue
San Diego, CA 92103
(619) 544-1622
(619) 239-3251 FAX

Emily S. Stuhlbarg
Schapp-Miller-Stuhlbarg
25550 Hawthorne Blvd., #212
Torrance, CA 90505
(213) 375-1968

Jenny P. Thayer
Geriatric Counseling
22318 San Joaquin Drive West
Canyon Lake, CA 92587
(714) 244-6680

California (Continued)

Judith S. Tobenkin
Gerontology Consultants
353 S. Palm Drive
Beverly Hills, CA 90212
(310) 273-3548

Roberta Weissglass
Personal and Financial Services
P.O. Box 31015
Santa Barbara, CA 93130
(805) 563-2436

Nancy Wexler
Gerontology Associates
19225 Rosita Street
Tarzana, CA 91356
(818) 342-3136
(818) 708-8538

Mark Winterman
Alternatives - Senior Care
  Consultant
8009 Lemon Avenue
La Mesa, CA 91941
(619) 464-6560

Colorado

Mary Ann Brown
Elderlink Companion Care
P.O. Box 27154
Lakewood, CO 80227
(303) 972-6782

Louise Brunk
Aging Services
969 S. Pearl St., Suite 207
Denver, CO 80209
(303) 777-3029

Pamela A. Erickson
Professional Respite Care, Inc.
3900 E. Mexico St., Suite 825
Denver, CO 80210
(303) 757-4808

Colorado (Continued)

DeeAnn Groves
Seniors Are Special
1802 16th Street, Suite 2
Greeley, CO 80631
(303) 350-2406

Milton Hanson
Institute for Creative Aging
P.O. Box 3725
Littleton, CO 80161
(303) 795-9682

John H. Reid
Ft. Collins Psychotherapy Group
2362 E. Prospect
Fort Collins, CO 80525
(303) 484-9220

Gordon P. Wolfe
Human Network Systems, Inc.
1410 Grant Street, Suite B-304
Denver, CO 80203
(303) 831-1996
(303) 861-8782 FAX

Connecticut

Louise O. Bernstein
Elder Family Service of Connecticut
37 Columbus Place, Suite 1
Stamford, CT 06907
(203) 329-2750

Mary Fresiello
Gerontological Care Services
135 Trap Falls Extension
Huntington, CT 06484
(203) 926-9643

Alan J. Guire
Extended Care Planning Service
P.O. Box 1632
Middletown, CT 06457
(203) 537-6093

Connecticut (Continued)

Claire Jacobs
Geriatric Counseling Associates
441 Orange Street
New Haven, CT 06511
(203) 785-1496

Eleanor Johnson
Paine-Johnson Agency Inc.
P.O. Box 489
Thomaston, CT 06787
(203) 271-0206

Roberta Litvinoff
Geriatric Counseling Associates
441 Orange Street
New Haven, CT 06511
(203) 785-1496

Irene H. Ross
Ctr. for Interpersonal Relations, Inc.
346 Pomfret Street
Putnam, CT 06260
(203) 928-5967

Delaware

Thomas Posatko
Supportive Care Services, Inc.
507 West Ninth Street
Wilmington, DE 19801
(302) 655-5518

Florida

JoAnn Alderman
Alderman's Inc., Consulting Services
4031 NE 15th Avenue
Fort Lauderdale, FL 33334
(305) 564-4651

Rona S. Bartelstone
Bartelstone Associates
2699 Stirling Road, Suite C304
Fort Lauderdale, FL 33312
(305) 948-8999
(305) 967-6593 FAX

Florida *(Continued)*

Carol F. Bernstein
The Family Connection
2060 South East 17th Street
Pompano Beach, FL 33062
(305) 785-5706

Marian Bruin
Star Systems Consultation &
    Training
206 South Clark Avenue
Tampa, FL 33609
(813) 286-9542

Helen Cogen
Geriatric Counseling & Care
    Management
9 Island Avenue, Suite 707
Miami Beach, FL 33139
(305) 538-3384

Eva J. Corbett
Elder Touch Services, Inc.
7846 Pine Trace Drive
Sarasota, FL 34243
(813) 922-9301

Doris Davis
2920 Clark Road
Suite 202
Sarasota, FL 34231
(813) 922-9301

Joanne Gerard
Long Term Care Consulting Service
11331 South West One Court
Plantation, FL 33325
(305) 472-5556

Irma L. Hausdorff
Adult Management Services
900 N. Federal Highway
Suite 160-8
Boca Raton, FL 33432
(407) 392-1116

Florida *(Continued)*

Maryann Higgins
Connections
540 The Rialto
Venice, FL 34285
(813) 485-7567

Elizabeth E. James
ElderCare of Pinellas, Inc.
4895 112th Street North
P.O. Box 4166
Seminole, FL 34642
(813) 397-0003

O.E. Matos
5330-1 George Street
New Port Richey, FL 34652
(813) 849-2005

Shirley K. Miller
Private Geriatric Care Manager
2017 NE 21st Court
Ft. Lauderdale, FL 33305
(305) 565-1344

Pamela Lenges Overton
Pamela Overton & Associates
Elder Care Management
1871 Cottonwood Trail
Sarasota, FL 34232
(813) 377-4761

Claire Goldberg Plewinski
Senior Care Consultant
1433 Collins Avenue
Miami, FL 33139
(305) 935-1283

Brenda H. Schimmel
Family Partner, Inc.
P.O. Box 12311
Sarasota, FL 34278
(813) 351-1516

Geri Smith
Life Care Continuum, Inc.
1320 S. Federal Highway, Suite 108
Stuart, FL 34994
(407) 288-2273

Florida (Continued)

G. Nadine Smith
Sharing Care
4512 Park Lake Terrace N
Bradenton, FL 34209
(813) 794-1631

Mary Thorman
TLC for Seniors, Inc.
13896 Dominica Drive
Seminole, FL 34646
(813) 595-2000
(800) 729-8907

Barbara R. Whitley
Private Case Management
2078 Minton Road
W. Melbourne, FL 32904
(407) 768-0092

Rina Winckler
Alpha Care Management, Inc.
1020 N.E. 98th St.
Miami, FL 33138
(305) 751-1020

Georgia

Catherine Dwyer
Within Reach
1323 Weatherstone Way
Atlanta, GA 30324
(404) 634-0675

Jane Hamil
Bridging Generations
659 Peachtree Street
Suite 407
Atlanta, GA 30308-1928
(404) 872-7520

Marilyn Peskin-Kaufman
Answers for the Elderly
455 Greenlaurel Drive
Atlanta, GA 30342
(404) 303-0805

Georgia (Continued)

Lucy B. Whelchel
Whelchel & Associates
5315 Woodland Circle
Gainesville, GA 30504
(404) 534-3360

Illinois

Marla Levie Bee
Focus on Aging
4171 Dundee Road, Suite 132
Northbrook, IL 60062
(708) 480-0617

Elizabeth A. Bodie
Elder Link Inc.
2000 North Racine Street,
  Suite 2182
Chicago, IL 60614
(312) 929-4514

Andra J. Ebert
Care Pak Options
P.O. Box 6101
Taylorville, IL 62568
(217) 287-2320

Steven C. Fox
Wellspring Services
179 W. Washington St., Suite 360
Chicago, IL 60602
(312) 201-9696
(312) 201-1374 FAX

Gail Gill
Senior Care Consultants
606 Central
Wilmette, IL 60091
(708) 251-2144

Erica Karp
Northshore Eldercare Management
1019 South Boulevard
Evanston, IL 60202
(708) 866-7466

Illinois *(Continued)*

Sheila McMackin
Wellspring Services
179 W. Washington St.,
  Suite 360
Chicago, IL 60602
(312) 201-9696
(312) 201-1374 FAX

Sara Shevitz Mesirow
Geriatric Resource Consultants
160 Cary Avenue
Highland Park, IL 60035
(708) 432-3490

June C. Ninnemann
CarePlan, Inc.
10520 West Bernice Drive
Palos Park, IL 60464
(708) 524-2070

Curt Paddock
Paddock Health Services, Inc.
4239 War Memorial Dr.
Suite 304
Peoria, IL 61614
(309) 682-7291

Storm Rogers
Aging/Options!
171 Franklin Road
Glencoe, IL 60022
(708) 835-3183

Barbara Sanders
Sanders & Associates
1140 Shady Lane
Wheaton, IL 60187
(708) 260-0012

Mona Thornton
Senior Care Consultants
5048 N. Drake Avenue
Chicago, IL 60625
(312) 588-8670

Indiana

Jane Chapin Frankenstein
Life Care Networks, Inc.
4221 Rurode Lane
Fort Wayne, IN 46809
(219) 747-5016
(219) 422-9077

Hannah F. Zacher
Geriatric Consultants
3637 Rosewood Drive
Fort Wayne, IN 46804
(219) 432-2150

Iowa

Carol Will
Will's Consulting
RR#2, Box 428
Keokuk, IA 52632
(319) 524-7656

Kansas

Cheryl A. Smith
Kansas City Home & Health Care
  Services, Inc.
7922 State Line Rd., Suite 1
Prairie Village, KS 66208
(913) 642-2074

Kentucky

Merrily Orsini
Elder Care Solutions
1220 Bardstown Road
Louisville, KY 40204
(502) 452-9644
(502) 451-3769 FAX

Louisiana

Betty Bartels Landreaux
Care Management Solutions, Inc.
2955 Ridgelake Drive, Suite 112
Metairie, LA 70002
(504) 837-5801

Maine

Jane G. Morrison
Elder Help
46 Lake Street
Auburn, ME 04210
(207) 783-7862

Joan Sud Soreff
25 Highland Street
Portland, ME 04103
(207) 775-2181

Maryland

Mary E. Cress
CressCare Consultants
4313 Elm Street
Chevy Chase, MD 20815
(301) 654-5366

Grace Lebow
Aging Network Services, Inc.
4400 East West Highway, Suite 907
Bethesda, MD 20814
(301) 951-8589

Debra G. Levy
212 Thistle Court
Silver Spring, MD 20901
(301) 593-5285

Gussie Lovelle
The Golden Years Services Inc.
511 North Schroeder Street
Baltimore, MD 21223
(301) 523-1173

Sue McConnell
Adult Care Services, Inc.
1213 Potomac Avenue
Hagerstown, MD 21740
(301) 797-1115

Gail Vander Horst Procter
6 Penny Lane
Baltimore, MD 21209
(301) 653-0821

Maryland (Continued)

Arlene Saks
Social Work Associates, Inc.
101 West Read Street, Suite 622
Baltimore, MD 21201
(301) 727-1717
(301) 938-2429 Pager

Massachusetts

Lucille Alan
960 Trapelo Road
Waltham, MA 02154-4846
(617) 894-8405

Frank E. Baskin
Frank E. Baskin
18 East Meadow Lane
Lowell, MA 01854
(508) 458-1512

Peter S. Belson
Family Logistics
One Kendall Square, Suite 2200
Cambridge, MA 02139
(617) 577-1390
(617) 577-1209 FAX

Jeanne M. Dionne
Generations
104 Nottingham Drive
Centerville, MA 02632
(508) 420-5259

Fran O'Connell
O'Connell Professional Nurse
  Service
397 Appleton Street
Holyoke, MA 01040
(413) 533-1030

Marjorie Osheroff
Long Term Planning Associates, Inc.
5 Sweetwater Street
Saugus, MA 01906
(617) 231-2616

Massachusetts *(Continued)*

Meredith Beit Patterson
109 Seymour Street
Concord, MA 01742
(508) 369-7402

Ann Peck
Geriatric Resource Centre Inc.
20 Morton Road
Newton Centre, MA 02159
(617) 332-7610

Nancy C. Peters
75 Washington Avenue
Cambridge, MA 02140
(617) 354-4899

Anne Smith Sweeney
22 Dartmouth Road
Melrose, MA 02176
(617) 665-4343

Victoria Sears Thaler
Golden Years Counseling Services
P.O. Box 24
Chestnut Hill, MA 02167
(617) 739-1609

Joan Tobin
Elder Network
24 Sevinor Road
Marblehead, MA 01945
(617) 593-1040

Susan Townshend
Long Term Planning Associates, Inc.
5 Sweetwater Street
Saugus, MA 01906
(617) 231-2616

Carol Westheimer
Independent Living, Inc.
1425 Beacon Street
Newton, MA 02168
(617) 332-1710

Michigan

Penny Conn
Farmington Hills Counseling
  Services
32905 W. Twelve Mile Rd., Suite 250
Farmington Hills, MI 48334
(313) 553-8116

Janet L. Howes
Care Planning Associates
4515 West Saginaw
Lansing, MI 48917
(517) 323-8410

Connie D. Knapper
Access Home Care, Inc.
5103 Eastman Place, Suite 229B
Midland, MI 48640
(517) 832-0222

Alan McBroom
Ask Health Care Services, Inc.
24681 Northwestern Hwy.,
  Suite 106
Southfield, MI 48075
(313) 355-1980

Phyllis A. Norman
North Oakland Counseling and
  Geriatric Consultation Center
6401 Citation Drive
Clarkston, MI 48346
(313) 620-1019

Minnesota

Patricia Hanson
Care Management Plus
4460 Oak Chase Way
Eagan, MN 55123
(612) 454-4670

Fran P. Kaschak
Geriatric Family Services
5100 Eden Avenue
Edina, MN 55436
(612) 929-1772

Minnesota (Continued)

Fay Ojile
Care Management PLUS, Inc.
4460 Oak Chase Way
Eagan, MN 55123
(612) 789-2558

Missouri

Cheryl C. Bluestein
Aging Services Network, Inc.
1211 S. Glenstone, Suite 500
Springfield, MO 65804
(417) 865-0300

Ruth Christman Cohen
Creative Care Consultants
14 West 61st Terrace
Kansas City, MO 64113
(816) 444-2231

Constance A. DesChamps
ElderAssist
52 Maryland Plaza
St. Louis, MO 63108
(314) 367-7858
(800) 747-7005

Rebecca Rengo
Aging Consult
P.O. Box 2372
St. Louis, MO 63032
(314) 838-1392

Nebraska

Ruth Muchemore
Parentcare
643 N. 98th St., Suite 253
Omaha, NE 68114
(402) 390-9323

New Hampshire

Terry Ann Black
Long Term Planning Association
P.O. Box 654
Atkinson, NH 03811
(603) 362-5838

New Jersey

Wendy H. Biermann
ElderCare Connections
685 Bloomfield Avenue, Suite 202
Verona, NJ 07044
(201) 239-7599

Patricia C. De Ganahl
Senior Care Services
20 Avenue at the Common, Suite 104
Shrewsbury, NJ 07702-4531
(908) 747-7517

Vicki Doueck
Generations
121 Cedar Lane - 3rd Floor
Teaneck, NJ 07666
(201) 836-5323

Dianne Flanigan
Elder Care Options, Inc.
RD 2 Box 398 Quakertown Road
Pittstown, NJ 08867
(908) 730-6388

Diane Garcia
Diane Garcia, PhD
478 Manchester Ave.
Brick, NJ 08723-5525
(908) 920-8110

Vivian E. Greenberg
Vivian E. Greenberg, A.C.S.W.
106 W. Franklin Avenue, Suite F-122
Pennington, NJ 08534
(609) 737-6365

Lori Lazaroff
Counseling Related to Geriatrics
1500 Kings Highway North,
   Suite 109
Cherry Hill, NJ 08034
(609) 427-0089

Bonnie Malajian
Generations
121 Cedar Lane, 3rd Floor
Teaneck, NJ 07666
(201) 836-5323

New Jersey (Continued)

Janice McCurdy
Bristow-McCurdy
P.O. Box 81
Pennington, NJ 08534
(609) 737-8398

Mary Moser
Mary Moser Associates
58 Hobart Avenue
Summit, NJ 07901
(908) 277-4089

Judith S. Parnes
Elder Life Management, Inc.
P.O. Box 394
Deal, NJ 07723
(908) 776-9104

Connie Rosenberg
Services & Resources for Seniors
930 Mt. Kemble Avenue
Morristown, NJ 07960
(201) 984-3707

Eleanor Rubin
Older Adult Resources & Services,
    Inc.
59 Second Street
South Orange, NJ 07079
(201) 763-8018

Maura C. Ryan
ElderOptions
39 High Point
Cedar Grove, NJ 07009
(201) 857-8856

Kathryn L. Volino
C.O.P.E.
82 Ferndale Avenue
Glen Rock, NJ 07452
(201) 652-3322

Leah Weiss
Older Adult Resources &
    Services, Inc.
59 Second Street
South Orange, NJ 07079
(201) 763-8018

New York

Nancy Ashery
Senior Care Consultants
1 Barstow Road
Great Neck, NY 11021
(516) 466-8864

Susan M. Bagnini
100 Oakland Avenue
Port Washington, NY 11050
(516) 944-8457

Edith W. Bayme
3720 Independence Ave.
Bronx, NY 10463
(212) 884-5749

Dr. Babette Becker
Creative Resources
49 West 12th St., Suite 1 B
New York, NY 10011
(212) 989-8508

Robert C. Bergen
Holiday Plaza
400 Post Avenue, Suite 403
Westbury, NY 11590
(516) 338-5700

Miriam Berman
H.E.L.P. for Elders, Inc.
812 Bromton Drive
Westbury, NY 11590
(516) 334-1131

Maria Bontez
Colly-Bon Associates, Inc.
10 Fiske Place
P.O. Box 2155
Mt. Vernon, NY 10550
(914) 667-2155

Adele R. Brink-Spitzer
Comprehensive Care Management
201 East 17th Street, Apt 4A
New York, NY 10003
(516) 829-7726

New York *(Continued)*

Marie A. Brown
NYCHA
801 Neill Avenue, Suite 23K
Bronx, NY 10462
(212) 409-5926

Gail Busillo
Geriatric Social Work Services
245-27 Walden Avenue
Great Neck, NY 11020
(516) 487-0973

Jerie Charnow
Charnow Associates
240 Mineola Boulevard, Suite 3
Mineola, NY 11501
(516) 747-0034
(516) 747-1415 FAX

Maureen A. Clancy
Maureen Clancy Services
12 East 86 Street, Suite 504
New York, NY 10028
(212) 737-4262

Jane R. Condliffe
Consultants in Care
4726 Independence Avenue
Riverdale, NY 10471
(212) 543-3341

Nancy C. Crawford
Elderly & Family Counseling
  Services
200 MacArthur Drive
Buffalo, NY 14221
(716) 634-0906

Nancy R. Day
Community Medical Counseling
Stone Springs Bldg.
P.O. Box 220
Somers, NY 10589
(914) 276-3864

New York *(Continued)*

Lenise Dolen
Dolen Consulting Systems
290 Quaker Road
Chappaqua, NY 10514
(914) 238-3261
(914) 238-5503 FAX

Robin Eannace-Ullman
2428 Chenango Road
Utica, NY 13502
(315) 793-0090

Jacquelyn A. Efram
House Calls for the Elderly
18 Barnard Avenue
Poughkeepsie, NY 12601
(914) 471-0075

Adele Elkind
343 Old Cedar Road
Hartsdale, NY 10530
(914) 948-9421

Esther Feigenbaum
73-58 189 Street
Flushing, NY 11366
(718) 740-1509

Alice Feldman
One Walworth Terrace
White Plains, NY 10606
(914) 681-1340

Claudia Fine
Claudia Fine Associates
101 Central Park West
New York, NY 10023
(212) 873-4374

Emily H. Fisher
Manhattan Resources, Inc.
140 Riverside Drive
New York, NY 10024
(212) 580-3801

Illese Forgang
405 E. 56th Street
New York, NY 10022
(212) 888-4252

New York *(Continued)*

Joan F. Garofalo
Route 81, Box 83
Oak Hill, NY 12460
(518) 239-4772

Marc Guthartz
Comprehensive Home Care
One East Post Road
P.O. Box 5036
White Plains, NY 10602
(914) 682-3988

Norma B. Heisler
2373 East 7th Street
Brooklyn, NY 11223
(718) 615-5247
(718) 934-9125 Home

Marjorie Hornik
Marjorie Hornik, ACSW
839 West End Ave., Suite 4-C
P.O. Box 1094
New York, NY 10025
(212) 222-8990

Steven Kleitzel
281 Garth Road, Suite C1J
Scarsdale, NY 10583-4039

John Koppenaal, C.S.W.
Shiloh Counseling Center
P.O. Box 436
Germantown, NY 12526
(518) 537-5262

Anne D. Lester
Manhattan Resources, Inc.
140 Riverside Drive
New York, NY 10024
(212) 580-3801

Julie Lomoe-Smith
ElderSource, Inc.
Time Square Professional Park
652 Route 299, Suite 204A
Highland, NY 12528
(914) 883-7824

New York *(Continued)*

Roslyn Robinson Mann
Elder Resources Network
RD 2, Box 259C
Patterson, NY 12563
(914) 878-6707

Leonie Nowitz
Center for Lifelong Growth
400 Central Park West, Suite 3A
New York, NY 10025
(212) 864-5905
(212) 678-5441 FAX

Jane Perlow
Concerned Seniorcare
130 Horace Harding Boulevard
Great Neck, NY 11020
(516) 466-6387
(516) 335-4041

Ellen Lurie Polivy
Lurie Family Assistance Network
326 West 83rd Street
New York, NY 10024
(212) 362-2076

Marsha A. Raines
Marsha A. Raines, C.S.W.
1742 Ridge Road East
Rochester, NY 14622
(716) 266-7444

Eric Ratinetz
Family Care Management, Inc.
7 West Fourteenth Street
New York, NY 10011
(212) 463-9121

Susan Ratner
Professional Care Consultants
35 E 85th Street
New York, NY 10028

Joncie Rowland
Shepard Services
229 E. 67th St.
New York, NY 10028
(212) 737-5510

New York *(Continued)*

Margaret E. Sayers
Laping, Sayers and Associates
1109 Delaware Avenue
Buffalo, NY 14209
(716) 884-3277

Gloria Scherma
Multi-Comprehensive Counseling
1618 West Third Street
Brooklyn, NY 11223
(718) 921-8572

Miriam Scholl
19 Minkel Road
Ossining, NY 10562
(914) 762-7438

Rita Seiden
Elder Family Services
464 Ninth Street
Brooklyn, NY 11215
(718) 788-2461

Jeanne Sharp
Sally Winsby & Company
37 West 57th Street, 14th Floor
New York, NY 10019
(212) 371-4727
(212) 750-7683 FAX

Bernice Shepard
Shepard Services Inc.
229 East 67th Street
New York, NY 10021
(212) 737-5510

Diane K. Sherwood
Sherwood Associates
228 West 260th Street
Riverdale, NY 10471
(212) 548-0609

Mary Ellen Siegel
Mary Ellen Siegel, MSW
75-68 195th Street
Flushing Meadows, NY 11366
(718) 465-1908

New York *(Continued)*

Naomi Solomon
Senior Care Consultants
1 Barstow Rd.
Great Neck, NY 11021
(516) 466-8864

Sandra Steinman
401 E. 80 St., Suite 19B
New York, NY 10021
(212) 517-3103

Andrea Weiler
Private Geriatric Care Manager
7462 Armstrong Road
Manlius, NY 13104
(315) 637-5388

Elaine S. Yatzkan
Elaine S. Yatzkan, CSW, PhD
262 Central Park West
New York, NY 10024
(212) 724-6330

Miriam Zucker
Directions In Aging
1-B Quaker Ridge Road
New Rochelle, NY 10804
(914) 636-7347

North Carolina

Edna Hammer
Greensboro Geriatric Consultants
1101 North Elm Street, Apt. 602
Greensboro, NC 27401
(919) 275-3908

Kimberly Hanchette
Kimberly Hanchette - Geriatric
Case Manager
4104 Converse Drive
Raleigh, NC 27609
(919) 781-5186

North Carolina *(Continued)*

Karen Knutson
OpenCare
2237 Park Road
Charlotte, NC 28203
(704) 377-2273

Ohio

Carolyn Constiner-Lieberman
Health Care Choices, Inc.
479 Terrell Court
Cleveland, OH 44143
(216) 481-2122

Beatrice Feldman
Beatrice Feldman & Associates
23213 Fairmount Blvd.
Beachwood, OH 44122
(216) 292-5530

Robert Lauretig
Alternative Counseling Associates
3789 South Green Road
Cleveland, OH 44122
(216) 292-4409
(216) 382-0991 FAX

Lois J. Mahar
Elder Care Coordinators, Inc.
10219 Edgewater Drive
Cleveland, OH 44102
(216) 574-2446

Phyllis G. Wolk
Caring Connections
2620 Fenick Road
Cleveland, OH 44118
(216) 397-9347

Oklahoma

Lynn Sageser
Sageser & Associates
2 Coventry Court
Edmond, OK 73034
(405) 341-5390

Oregon

Susan Goldsmith
Health Access, Inc.
135 S. W. Ash Street, Suite 530
Portland, OR 97219
(503) 228-3333
(800) 333-8568
(503) 273-8138 FAX

Kathleen C. Milne
Resource Connectors, Ltd.
5520 SW Macadam Ave.,
   Suite 270
Portland, OR 97201
(503) 228-7023

Patricia Percival
Northwest Professional Group
Montgomery Park, Suite 424
2701 NW Vaughn
Portland, OR 97210
(503) 222-4244
(800) 767-3072 referrals

Pennsylvania

Patricia Kern Banzhoff
Patricia Kern Banzhoff, MS, NHA
350 North 25th Street
Camp Hill, PA 17011
(717) 737-2166

Diane M. Bastone
Dignified Aging
138 Sunset Drive
Pittsburgh, PA 15237
(412) 486-8339

Sheila R. Bergman
Comprehensive Health & Human
   Services Inc./Eldercare
8329 High School Road
Elkins Park, PA 19117
(215) 635-6849

Pennsylvania (Continued)

Janice L. Brown
Star Systems Consultation &
  Training
One Winding Drive, Suite 220
Philadelphia, PA 19131
(215) 477-2211

JoAnn M. Burke
12 W Willow Grove Ave., Suite 118
Philadelphia, PA 19118
(215) 836-1280

Margaret Cohn
Family Ties
765 West Hamilton Avenue
State College, PA 16801
(814) 237-1549

Elaine A. Dively
4069 Hill Street
Library, PA 15129
(412) 833-3076

Patricia M. Dwyer
Patricia Dwyer
8200 Flourtown Avenue, Apt. 5B
Wyndmoor, PA 19118
(215) 836-1747

Barbara R. Feinstein
Comprehensive Health & Human
  Services Inc./Eldercare
435 East Lancaster Avenue,
  Suite 211
St. Davids, PA 19087
(215) 688-5579

Jean Hope
Family Options, Inc.
RR 2094
Dushore, PA 18614
(717) 928-9202

Mary M. Korcz
Elder-Service, Inc.
310 Davisville Rd.
Philadelphia, PA 18974
(215) 322-4010

Pennsylvania (Continued)

Anneta Kraus
Geriatric Planning Services
Main Line Bank Fed. Bldg. Suite 201
Two South Orange
Media, PA 19063
(215) 566-6686
(215) 565-5492 FAX

Sybil E. Montgomery
Alternatives in Living LTD
1637 Oakwood Drive
Penn Valley, PA 19072
(215) 667-3154

Roberta Rosenberg
AgeWise Family Services
1250 Glenburnie
Dresher, PA 19025
(215) 659-2111

Carol A. Saez-Henry
Vintage, Inc.
401 North Highland Avenue
Pittsburgh, PA 15206
(412) 361-5003

Sheila L. Saunders
Senior Solutions
44 South Fulton St.
Allentown, PA 18102
(215) 435-6677

Andrea Seewald
Senior Care Consultants
5645 Marlborough Road
Pittsburgh, PA 15217
(412) 421-9171

Thomas Skoloda
P.O. Box 455
Lyndell, PA 19354
(215) 942-2232

Marsha York Solmssen
Intervention Associates
P.O. Box 572
Wayne, PA 19087
(215) 254-9001

Pennsylvania *(Continued)*

Helena A. Stewart
Retirement & Transition Inc.
P.O. Box 451
Bryn Mawr, PA 19010
(215) 527-4578

Catherine C. Thompson
Sterling Care Counseling, Inc.
962 Washington Road
Pittsburgh, PA 15228
(412) 344-5011

Marion Thompson
Intervention Associates, Inc.
P.O. Box 572
Wayne, PA 19087
(215) 254-9001

Jean M. Walsh
Wise Generation Resources Inc.
100 Denniston Avenue
Pittsburgh, PA 15206
(412) 441-4342

Braden L. Walter
Secour Care Management
121 North Highland Avenue
Pittsburgh, PA 15206
(412) 661-6730

Susan P. Weiss
AgeWise Family Services
1250 Glenburnie Lane
Dresher, PA 19025
(215) 659-2111

Rhode Island

Harriet Estrin
Eldercare Options, Inc.
P.O. Box 1527
Kingston, RI 02881
(401) 783-8773

Tennessee

Peg Beehan
2313 Hillsboro Road
Nashville, TN 37212
(615) 386-3333

Darlene Gamble
Total Family Care
3939 Whitebrook Dr.,
Suite 100 Bldg. H
Memphis, TN 38118
(901) 367-0551

Texas

Charlotte Clarke
The Holt House Inc.
709 South Bois d' Arc
Tyler, TX 75701
(903) 592-5553

Leah R. Cohen
Aging Family Services, Inc.
4005 Spicewood Springs Rd.,
   #400-B
Austin, TX 78759
(512) 345-5943

Beth L. Corcoran
Life Directions
P.O. Box 470833
Fort Worth, TX 76147
(817) 732-3688

Sharon Fitch
Kinship Associates
10211 Bridgegate Lane
Dallas, TX 75243
(214) 480-0716

Constance Kilgore
Texas Geriatric Services
12880 Hillcrest, Suite 104
Dallas, TX 75230
(214) 387-4751

Texas *(Continued)*

Joyce A. Robbins
Geriatric Services Inc.
P.O. Box 18223
San Antonio, TX 78218
(512) 822-9494

Geri Sams
Geri-Options
2611 Crestwood
P.O. Box 24457
Denton, TX 76201-2457
(817) 566-0902

Virginia

Celeste D. Galati
Resources for the Elderly
6120 Brandon Avenue, Suite 117
P.O. Box 5252
Springfield, VA 22150
(703) 886-3122

Norah S.R. Knutsen
Mature Options
1910 Byrd Avenue Suite 8
Richmond, VA 23230
(804) 282-0753

Ann E. O'Neil
Care Options for the Elderly
1304 Seaton Lane
Falls Church, VA 22046
(703) 237-9048

Washington

Mary Liz Chaffee
Second Family (McDonald Resources
  for the Aging, Inc.)
1415 Orange Place, North
Seattle, WA 98109
(206) 285-4589

Washington *(Continued)*

Sara Myers
Elder Care Resources
1800 Boylston, #104
Seattle, WA 98122
(206) 324-5695

Mary Lynn Pannen
Sound Options Inc.
917 Pacific Avenue, Suite 608
Tacoma, WA 98402
(206) 572-7008
(800) 628-7649

Jan D. Pitzer
Social Services
3015 37th Avenue, S.W.
Seattle, WA 98126
(206) 935-3020

Polly Pratt
Geriatric Services
1523 East Madison
Seattle, WA 98122
(206) 329-5316

Janet M. Rhode
Northwest Geriatric Care Managers
2208 NW Market Street, Suite 310
Seattle, WA 98107
(206) 783-1902

Wisconsin

Phyllis Mensh Brostoff
Stowell Associates, Inc.
3575 North Oakland Avenue
Milwaukee, WI 53211
(414) 963-2600
(414) 963-2605 FAX

Marianne Ewig
September Managed Care
  For Later Years
830 N. 109th Street, Suite 27
Milwaukee, WI 53226-3740
(414) 774-5800

Wisconsin *(Continued)*

Janice M. Larson
Extended Family, Inc.
1716 Hycrest Drive
Appleton, WI 54914
(414) 749-1117

Barbara Liegel
Regional Services
University of Wisconsin
810 University Bay Drive
Madison, WI 53705
(608) 263-7040

West Virginia

Patricia H. Ahwash
Geriatric Care Management of West
  Virginia
Rt. 7 Box 198
Charleston, WV 25309
(304) 756-9325

DIRECTORY OF FULL-TIME PRACTITIONERS IN GERIATRIC CARE MANAGEMENT

Patricia H. Ahwash, MSW
Geriatric Care Management of West Virginia
Rt. 7 Box 198
Charleston, WV 25309
(304) 756-9325
Years in Full Time Geriatric Care Management: 1
Service Area
Metropolitan Area(s): Charleston
Counties: Kanawha, Putnam, Fayette, Lincoln, Boone
States: WV
Areas of Practice: 1, 2, 3, 5, 6, 7, 8, 9, 10, 11, 12

JoAnn Alderman
Alderman's Inc., Consulting Services
4031 NE 15th Avenue
Fort Lauderdale, FL 33334
(305) 564-4651
Years in Full Time Geriatric Care Management: 2
Service Area
Metropolitan Area(s): South Florida
Counties: Broward, North Dade, Palm Beach
States: FL
Areas of Practice: 1, 2, 3, 5, 7, 8, 9, 10, 11, 12

Data used with permission of NAPGCM.
Key to Areas of Practice:

1. Assessment	5. Counseling	9. Crisis Intervention
2. Placement	6. Advocacy	10. Care Management
3. Education	7. Consultation	11. Entitlements
4. Psychotherapy	8. Info/Referral	12. Home Care

Lynn Allen, MSCC
Senior Care & Family Specialist
5218 Lawton Avenue
Oakland, CA 94618
(510) 655-1551
Years in Full Time Geriatric Care Management: 10
Service Area
Metropolitan Area(s): San Francisco Bay Area
Counties:
States: CA
Areas of Practice: 1, 2, 3, 4, 5, 6, 7, 8, 9, 10, 11, 12

Nancy Ashery, MSW, ASCW
Senior Care Consultants
1 Barstow Road
Great Neck, NY 11021
(516) 466-8864
Years in Full Time Geriatric Care Management: 2.5
Service Area
Metropolitan Area(s): Area Codes 516 & 718
Counties: Queens, Nassau, Western Suffolk
States: NY
Areas of Practice: 1, 2, 3, 4, 5, 6, 7, 8, 9, 10, 11, 12

Mary Jean Ashton, LCSW, RN-MPH
Elder Options, Inc.
128 West Main Street
Westboro, MA 01581
(617) 753-7140
Years in Full Time Geriatric Care Management: 6
Service Area
Metropolitan Area(s): Worcester
Counties: Worcester
States: MA
Areas of Practice: 1, 2, 3, 4, 5, 6, 7, 8, 9, 10, 11, 12

Loraine P. Auerbach, MHCA
American Medical Systems, Inc.
1250 Long Beach Avenue, Suite 328
Los Angeles, CA 90021
(213) 624-2225
(213) 624-2229 FAX
Years in Full Time Geriatric Care Management: 3
Service Area
Metropolitan Area(s): California
Counties:
States: CA
Areas of Practice: 1, 2, 3, 5, 6, 7, 8, 9, 10

Susan M. Bagnini, CSW, ACSW
100 Oakland Avenue
Port Washington, NY 11050
(516) 944-8457
Years in Full Time Geriatric Care Management: 15
Service Area
Metropolitan Area(s): New York
Counties: Nassau, Western Suffolk
States: NY
Areas of Practice: 1, 4, 5, 6, 7, 8, 9, 10, 11

Steven Michael Barlam, MSW, LCSW
Senior Care Management
256 S. Robertson Boulevard, Suite 709
Beverly Hills, CA 90211
(213) 288-0059
(213) 288-0301 FAX
Years in Full Time Geriatric Care Management: 2
Service Area
Metropolitan Area(s): Greater Los Angeles Area, San Gabriel Valley, San
    Fernando Valley, Santa Monica, Beverly Hills
Counties: Los Angeles
States: CA
Areas of Practice: 1, 2, 3, 4, 5, 6, 7, 8, 9, 10, 11

Rona S. Bartelstone, LCSW, BCD
Rona Bartelstone Associates, Inc.
2699 Stirling Road, Suite C304
Fort Lauderdale, FL 33312
(305) 948-8999
Years in Full Time Geriatric Care Management: 10
Service Area
Metropolitan Area(s): Miami, Miami Beach, N. Miami, Hollywood, Ft.
    Lauderdale, Sunrise, Tamarac, Margate, Palm Beach, Boca Raton, Del Ray
    Beach, Boynton Beach
Counties: Dade, Broward, Palm Beach
States: FL
Areas of Practice: 1, 2, 3, 4, 5, 6, 7, 8, 9, 10, 11, 12

Julie Barton, MA
E.L.C. Associates
P.O. Box 160249
Cupertino, CA 95016
(415) 968-8028
Years in Full Time Geriatric Care Management: 5
Service Area
Metropolitan Area(s): Area Codes 408, 415, 510
Counties: Santa Clara, San Mateo, Santa Cruz, Alameda
States: CA
Areas of Practice: 1, 3, 5, 6, 7, 8, 9, 10

Diane M. Bastone, MSW
Dignified Aging
138 Sunset Drive
Pittsburgh, PA 15237
(412) 486-8339

Years in Full Time Geriatric Care Management: 1

Service Area
Metropolitan Area(s): Pittsburgh
Counties: Northern Allegheny County
States: PA
Areas of Practice: 1, 2, 3, 4, 5, 6, 7, 8, 9, 10

Babette Becker, PhD, CSW, NCPP
Creative Resources

58 West 15th Street, 8th Floor   RT #1, Box 34A, North Mountain Road
New York, NY 10011   Copake Falls, NY 12517
(212) 989-8508   (518) 325-5746

Years in Full Time Geriatric Care Management: 10

Service Area
Metropolitan Area(s): Manhattan, Brooklyn, Queens, Bronx
Counties:
States: NY
Areas of Practice: 1, 2, 3, 4, 5, 6, 7, 8, 9, 10, 11, 12

Marla Levie Bee
Focus on Aging
4171 Dundee Road, Suite 132
Northbrook, IL 60062
(708) 480-0617

Years in Full Time Geriatric Care Management:

Service Area
Metropolitan Area(s): Metro Chicago, North & Northwest Suburbs
Counties: Cook, Lake
States: IL
Areas of Practice: 1, 2, 3, 5, 6, 7, 8, 9, 10, 11, 12

Peg Beehan, MSSW, LCSW
2313 Hillsboro Road
Nashville, TN 37212
(615) 386-3333

Years in Full Time Geriatric Care Management:

Service Area
Metropolitan Area(s): Nashville
Counties: Davidson, Williamson
States: TN
Areas of Practice: 1, 2, 3, 4, 5, 7, 8, 9, 10

Peter S. Belson
Family Logistics
One Kendall Square, Suite 2200
Cambridge, MA 02139
(617) 577-1390
(617) 577-1209 FAX
Years in Full Time Geriatric Care Management: 6
Service Area
Metropolitan Area(s): Boston
Counties:
States: MA
Areas of Practice: 1, 2, 3, 4, 5, 6, 7, 8, 9, 10, 11, 12

Robert C. Bergen, MS, MSW, CSW
Holiday Plaza
400 Post Avenue, Suite 403
Westbury, NY 11590
(516) 338-5700
(516) 338-0129 FAX
Years in Full Time Geriatric Care Management: 2
Service Area
Metropolitan Area(s): New York
Counties: Queens, Nassau, Suffolk
States: NY
Areas of Practice: 1, 2, 3, 4, 5, 7, 8, 10

Sheila R. Bergman, MSW, LSW, ACSW, BCD
Comprehensive Health & Human Services Inc./Eldercare
8329 High School Road
Elkins Park, PA 19117
(215) 635-6849
Years in Full Time Geriatric Care Management: 11
Service Area
Metropolitan Area(s): Greater Philadelphia, Southern New Jersey (Area
  codes 215, 609)
Counties: In Pennsylvania: Philadelphia, Montgomery, Delaware, Bucks,
  Chester; In New Jersey: Camden
States: PA, NJ
Areas of Practice: 1, 2, 3, 4, 5, 6, 7, 8, 9, 10, 11, 12

Carol F. Bernstein, ARNP
The Family Connection
2060 South East 17th Street
Pompano Beach, FL 33062
(305) 785-5706

Years in Full Time Geriatric Care Management: 7

Service Area

Metropolitan Area(s): South Florida up to Del Ray Beach
Counties:
States: FL
Areas of Practice: 1, 2, 3, 5, 6, 7, 8, 9, 10, 11, 12

Wendy H. Biermann
ElderCare Connections
685 Bloomfield Avenue, Suite 202
Verona, NJ 07044
(201) 239-7599

Years in Full Time Geriatric Care Management: 1

Service Area

Metropolitan Area(s): New Jersey/Manhattan
Counties:
States: NY, NJ
Areas of Practice: 1, 2, 3, 5, 6, 7, 8, 9, 10, 11, 12

Terry Ann Black, RN
Long Term Planning Association
P.O. Box 654
Atkinson, NH 03811
(603) 362-5838

Years in Full Time Geriatric Care Management: 2

Service Area

Metropolitan Area(s):
Counties:
States: NH
Areas of Practice: 1, 2, 3, 6, 7, 8, 10

Cheryl C. Bluestein, MS, MA, RNC, LCSW, NCC, NCGC
Aging Services Network, Inc.
1211 South Glenstone, Suite 500
Springfield, MO 65804
(417) 865-0300 (417) 864-9420 Pager

Years in Full Time Geriatric Care Management: 4

Service Area

Metropolitan Area(s): Southwest Missouri
Counties: Greene, Taney
States: MO, Northwest AR
Areas of Practice: 1, 2, 3, 4, 5, 6, 7, 8, 9, 10, 11, 12

Elizabeth A. Bodie, MBA, RN
Elder Link Inc.
2000 North Racine Street, Suite 2182
Chicago, IL 60614
(312) 929-4514

Years in Full Time Geriatric Care Management: 3
Service Area
Metropolitan Area(s): Chicago
Counties: Cook, Lake, Will, Kane, DuPage
States: IL, IN, WI, MI
Areas of Practice: 1, 3, 5, 7, 8, 11,
Long Term Care Financial Services

Maria Bontez, PhD
Collybonco Inc.
10 Fiske Place, Suite 421
Mount Vernon, NY 10550
(914) 667-2155
Years in Full Time Geriatric Care Management: 30
Service Area
Metropolitan Area(s): New York City
Counties: Westchester & NYC
States: NY
Areas of Practice: 1, 2, 3, 5, 7, 8, 10, 12

Adele Brink-Spitzer, PhD
Comprehensive Care Management
15 Canterbury Road, Suite 8   201 E. 17th Street, Apt. 4A
Great Neck, NY 11021   New York, NY 10003
(516) 829-7726   (212) 995-8762
Years in Full Time Geriatric Care Management: 4
Service Area
Metropolitan Area(s): New York, all boroughs
Counties: New York, Nassau, Kings, Queens, Bronx, Richmond, Westchester
States: NY
Areas of Practice: 1, 2, 3, 4, 5, 6, 7, 8, 9, 10, 11, 12

Phyllis Mensh Brostoff, MSW
Stowell Associates, Inc.
3575 North Oakland Avenue
Milwaukee, WI 53211
(414) 963-2600
Years in Full Time Geriatric Care Management: 8
Service Area
Metropolitan Area(s): Southeast Wisconsin
Counties: Milwaukee, Racine, Kenosha, Ozaukee, Waukesha, Washington
States: WI
Areas of Practice: 1, 2, 3, 4, 5, 6, 7, 8, 9, 10, 11, 12

Janice L. Brown, MSW, LSW, ACSW
Star Systems Consultation & Training, Inc.
One Winding Drive, Suite 220
Philadelphia, PA 19131
(215) 477-2211
Years in Full Time Geriatric Care Management: 10
Service Area
Metropolitan Area(s): Area Code 215
Counties:
States: PA, NJ, NY
Areas of Practice: 1, 2, 3, 5, 6, 7, 8, 9, 10, 11, 12

Marie A. Brown, MSW, CSW
801 Neill Avenue, Suite 23K
Bronx, NY 10462
(212) 409-5926
Years in Full Time Geriatric Care Management:
Service Area
Metropolitan Area(s): Manhattan, Bronx, Southern Westchester
Counties:
States: NY
Areas of Practice: 1, 2, 3, 4, 5, 6, 7, 8, 9, 10, 11, 12

Mary Ann Brown, RN, MS
Elderlink Companion Care
P.O. Box 27154
Lakewood, CO 80227
(303) 972-6782
Years in Full Time Geriatric Care Management: 3
Service Area
Metropolitan Area(s): Denver Metropolitan area
Counties:
States: CO
Areas of Practice: 1, 3, 6, 7, 10, 12

Marian Bruin, MSW, ACSW, BCD
Star Systems Consultation & Training, Inc.
206 South Clark Avenue
Tampa, FL 33609
(813) 286-9542
Years in Full Time Geriatric Care Management: 12
Service Area
Metropolitan Area(s): Florida Gulf Coast
Counties: Hillsborough, Pinellas, Manatee, Sarasota, Polk
States: FL
Areas of Practice: 1, 2, 3, 5, 6, 7, 8, 9, 10, 11

Louise Brunk, MSS, LCSW, BCD
Aging Services
969 South Pearl Street, Suite 207
Denver, CO 80209
(303) 777-3029
Years in Full Time Geriatric Care Management: 4
Service Area
Metropolitan Area(s): Denver Metropolitan, Boulder
Counties: Denver, Jefferson, Arapahoe, Adams, Douglas, Boulder
States: CO
Areas of Practice: 1, 2, 3, 4, 6, 7, 8, 9, 10, 11

JoAnn M. Burke, PhD, ACSW, RN
12 W. Willow Grove Avenue, Suite 118
Philadelphia, PA 19118
(215) 836-1280
Years in Full Time Geriatric Care Management: 2
Service Area
Metropolitan Area(s):
Counties:
States:
Areas of Practice:

Marilyn Carlander, LCSW
Lifenet, Inc.
1819 State Street, Suite B
Santa Barbara, CA 93101
(805) 687-8766
Years in Full Time Geriatric Care Management: 1
Service Area
Metropolitan Area(s): Santa Barbara, Lompoc, Santa Ynez, Santa Maria
Counties: Santa Barbara, Ventura
States: CA
Areas of Practice: 1, 2, 3, 4, 5, 6, 7, 8, 9, 10, 11, 12

Jeannine Caryl, MSW, LCSW
Senior Citizens Consultants/Case Management
7451 Warner Avenue, #H
Huntington Beach, CA 92647
(714) 841-8008
Years in Full Time Geriatric Care Management: 10
Service Area
Metropolitan Area(s): Long Beach, Huntington Beach
Counties: Orange
States: CA
Areas of Practice: 1, 2, 3, 4, 5, 6, 7, 8, 9, 10

Mary Liz Chaffee, RN
Second Family (McDonald Resources for the Aging, Inc.)
1415 Orange Place, North
Seattle, WA 98109
(206) 285-4589
Years in Full Time Geriatric Care Management: 10
Service Area
Metropolitan Area(s): Seattle
Counties: King, Lower Snohomish
States: WA
Areas of Practice: 1, 2, 3, 6, 7, 8, 10

Jerie Charnow, MSW, PC
Charnow Associates
240 Mineola Boulevard, Suite 3
Mineola, NY 11501
(516) 747-0034
Years in Full Time Geriatric Care Management: 17
Service Area
Metropolitan Area(s): Metropolitan New York
Counties: Nassau, Suffolk, Brooklyn, Queens, New York
States: NY
Areas of Practice: 1, 2, 4, 5, 6, 7, 8, 9, 10, 11, 12

Maureen A. Clancy, RN, CANP
Maureen Clancy Services
12 East 86 Street, Suite 504
New York, NY 10028
(212) 737-4262
Years in Full Time Geriatric Care Management: 10
Service Area
Metropolitan Area(s): Manhattan
Counties: Manhattan
States: NY
Areas of Practice: 1, 2, 3, 5, 6, 7, 8, 9, 10, 12

Charlotte Clarke, ACSW, CSW-ACP, PR
The Holt House Inc.
709 South Bois d' Arc
Tyler, TX 75701
(903) 592-5553
Years in Full Time Geriatric Care Management:
Service Area
Metropolitan Area(s): Area Code 903
Counties: Smith
States: TX
Areas of Practice: 1, 2, 3, 5, 6, 7, 8, 9, 10, 11, 12

Helen Cogen
Geriatric Counseling & Care Management
9 Island Avenue, Suite 707
Miami Beach, FL 33139
(305) 538-3384
Years in Full Time Geriatric Care Management: 8
Service Area
Metropolitan Area(s):
Counties: Dade, South Broward
States: FL
Areas of Practice: 1, 2, 4, 5, 6, 7, 8, 9, 10, 11, 12

Leah R. Cohen, ACSW, CSW-ACP
Aging Family Services, Inc.
4005 Spicewood Springs Road, Suite 400-B
Austin, TX 78759
(512) 345-5943
Years in Full Time Geriatric Care Management: 20
Service Area
Metropolitan Area(s): Austin
Counties: Travis
States: TX
Areas of Practice: 1, 2, 3, 4, 5, 6, 7, 8, 9, 10, 11, 12

Ruth C. Cohen, ACSW, LCSW, LSCSW
Creative Care Consultants
14 West 61st Terrace
Kansas City, MO 64113
(816) 444-2231
Years in Full Time Geriatric Care Management: 6
Service Area
Metropolitan Area(s): Kansas City, Area Codes 816, 913
Counties: In Missouri: Clay, Platte, Jackson
In Kansas: Johnson, Wyandotte
States: MO, KS
Areas of Practice: 1, 2, 3, 4, 5, 6, 7, 8, 9, 10

Jane R. Condliffe, MSW, ACSW, BCD
Consultants in Care
4726 Independence Avenue
Riverdale, NY 10471
(212) 543-3341
Years in Full Time Geriatric Care Management: 6
Service Area
Metropolitan Area(s): Manhattan
Counties: Lower Westchester, Riverdale, Bronx
States: NY
Areas of Practice: 1, 2, 3, 4, 5, 6, 7, 8, 10, 12

Penny Conn, CSW, LPC
Farmington Hills Counseling Services
32905 West Twelve Mile Road, Suite 250
Farmington Hills, MI 48334
(313) 553-8116
Years in Full Time Geriatric Care Management: 8
Service Area
Metropolitan Area(s): Detroit, Windsor
Counties: Oakland, Wayne, Macomb
States: MI
Areas of Practice: 1, 2, 3, 5, 7, 8, 9, 10, 12

Carolyn Constiner-Lieberman, MHSA
Health Care Choices, Inc.
479 Terrell Court
Richmond Heights, OH 44143
(216) 481-2122
Years in Full Time Geriatric Care Management: 3
Service Area
Metropolitan Area(s): Northern Ohio
Counties:
States: OH
Areas of Practice: 1, 2, 3, 5, 6, 7, 8, 10, 12

Eva J. Corbett, BS, RN, ENA
Elder Touch Services, Inc.
7846 Pine Trace Drive
Sarasota, FL 34243
(813) 922-9301
Years in Full Time Geriatric Care Management: 3
Service Area
Metropolitan Area(s): Sarasota, Tampa, St. Petersburg
Counties: Sarasota, Manatee, Charlotte
States: FL
Areas of Practice:

Beth L. Corcoran, BSW, CSW
Life Directions
P.O. Box 470833
Fort Worth, TX 76147
(817) 732-3688
Years in Full Time Geriatric Care Management: 4
Service Area
Metropolitan Area(s): Dallas, Ft. Worth
Counties: Tarrant, Dallas; Johnson, Parker as needed
States: TX
Areas of Practice: 1, 2, 3, 5, 6, 7, 8, 9, 10, 11

Cathy Jo Cress, MSW
Cresscare, Case Management Agency for Elders
230 Fountain Avenue, Suite 6
Pacific Grove, CA 93950
(408) 372-0802
Years in Full Time Geriatric Care Management:
Service Area
Metropolitan Area(s): Monterey, Carmel, Pebble Beach, Salinas
Counties: Monterey
States: CA
Areas of Practice: 1, 2, 3, 5, 6, 7, 8, 9, 10, 12

Mary E. Cress, LSW
CressCare Consultants
4313 Elm Street
Chevy Chase, MD 20815
(301) 654-5366
Years in Full Time Geriatric Care Management: 5
Service Area
Metropolitan Area(s): Area Codes 301, 703, 202
Counties: Montgomery, Washington, DC;
In Virginia: Fairfax Cross Country Network
States: MD, VA, DC
Areas of Practice: 1, 2, 3, 5, 6, 7, 8, 10, 11, 12

Virginia Daugherty, RN, MA
E.L.C. Associates
P.O. Box 160249
Cupertino, CA 95016
(415) 968-8028
Years in Full Time Geriatric Care Management: 6
Service Area
Metropolitan Area(s): Area Codes 408, 415, 510
Counties: Santa Clara, San Mateo, Santa Cruz, Alameda
States: CA
Areas of Practice: 1, 3, 5, 6, 7, 8, 9, 10

Nancy R. Day, MSW

Community Medical Counseling
Stone Springs Building, P.O. Box 220
Somer, NY 10589
(914) 276-3864

Center for Behavioral Psychotherapy
23 Old Mamaroneck Road
White Plains, NY 10605
(914) 761-4082 ext. 20

Years in Full Time Geriatric Care Management: 14
Service Area
Metropolitan Area(s): New York City, White Plains, Danbury
Counties: In New York: Westchester, Putnam;
In Connecticut: Fairfield
States: NY, CT, NJ
Areas of Practice: 1, 2, 3, 4, 5, 6, 7, 8, 9, 10, 11, 12

Jay A. Deike, MSSW, ACSW
Elder Options
1805 Proctor Drive
Santa Rosa, CA 95404
(707) 579-1485
Years in Full Time Geriatric Care Management: 4
Service Area
Metropolitan Area(s): Santa Rosa
Counties: Sonoma
States: CA
Areas of Practice: 1, 2, 3, 5, 6, 7, 8, 9, 10, 12

Constance A. DesChamps, MA, LPC
ElderAssist
52 Maryland Plaza
St. Louis, MO 63108
(800) 747-7005 (314) 367-7858
Years in Full Time Geriatric Care Management: 3
Service Area
Metropolitan Area(s): Greater St. Louis & Metropolitan East Illinois
Counties: In Missouri: St. Louis, St. Charles, Jefferson, Franklin; In Illinois:
   St. Clair, Madison
States: IL, MO
Areas of Practice: 1, 2, 3, 4, 5, 6, 7, 8, 9, 10, 11, 12

Lenise Dolen, PhD
Dolen Consulting Systems
290 Quaker Road
Chappaqua, NY 10514
(914) 238-3261
Years in Full Time Geriatric Care Management: 9
Service Area
Metropolitan Area(s): In New York: Riverdale, Westchester;
In Connecticut: Fairfield
Counties: Westchester, Putnam, Rockland
States: NY, CT
Areas of Practice: 1, 2, 3, 4, 5, 6, 7, 8, 9, 10, 11, 12

Vicki Doueck, MSW, ACSW, CSW
Generations
121 Cedar Lane - 3rd Floor
Teaneck, NJ 07666
(201) 836-5323
Years in Full Time Geriatric Care Management: 14
Service Area
Metropolitan Area(s): Northern New Jersey, Manhattan
Counties: Bergen, Passaic, Morris, Hudson, Rockland, & Westchester
States: NJ, NY
Areas of Practice: 1, 2, 3, 4, 5, 6, 7, 8, 9, 10, 11, 12

Catherine Dwyer, LCSW
Within Reach
1323 Weatherstone Way
Atlanta, GA 30324
(404) 634-0675
Years in Full Time Geriatric Care Management: 2
Service Area
Metropolitan Area(s): Metro Atlanta
Counties:
States: GA
Areas of Practice: 1, 2, 3, 4, 5, 6, 7, 8, 9, 10, 11

Patricia M. Dwyer
Patricia Dwyer
8200 Flourtown Avenue, Apartment #5B
Wyndmoor, PA 19118
(215) 836-1747
Years in Full Time Geriatric Care Management:
Service Area
Metropolitan Area(s): Chestnut Hill Area of Philadelphia
Counties: Montgomery (Eastern)
States: PA
Areas of Practice: 1, 4, 5, 7, 9

Robin Eannace-Ullman, MPS
2428 Chenango Road
Utica, NY 13502
(315) 793-0090
Years in Full Time Geriatric Care Management: 6
Service Area
Metropolitan Area(s):
Counties: Oneioa, Madison, Herkimer, Schenectady, Otsego, Lewis
States: NY
Areas of Practice: 1, 2, 3, 5, 7, 8, 9, 10, 11, 12

Andra J. Ebert, RN, LSW
Care Pak Options
P.O. Box 6101
Taylorville, IL 62568
(217) 287-2320
Years in Full Time Geriatric Care Management: 1
Service Area
Metropolitan Area(s):
Counties: Christian, Shelby, Montgomery (40 Mile Radius)
States: IL
Areas of Practice: 1, 2, 3, 6, 7, 8, 9, 10

Jacquelyn A. Efram, CSW, ACSW
House Calls for the Elderly
18 Barnard Avenue
Poughkeepsie, NY 12601
(914) 471-0075
Years in Full Time Geriatric Care Management: 12
Service Area
Metropolitan Area(s): Poughkeepsie
Counties: Dutchess (Mid Hudson River Region 1/2 way between NYC and
  Albany)
States: NY
Areas of Practice: 1, 2, 3, 4, 5, 6, 7, 8, 9, 10, 11

Pam Erickson, RN
Professional Respite Care, Inc.
3900 E. Mexico Street, Suite 825
Denver, CO 80210
(303) 757-4808
Years in Full Time Geriatric Care Management: 8
Service Area
Metropolitan Area(s):
Counties: Adams, Arapahoe, Denver, Jefferson
States: CO
Areas of Practice: 1, 2, 3, 5, 6, 7, 8, 9, 10, 12

Maria Estrada, MSW, LCSW
Seniors Support Service
161 Fashion Lane, Suite 107
Tustin, CA 92680
(714) 838-0598
Years in Full Time Geriatric Care Management: 3
Service Area
Metropolitan Area(s): Orange County (all cities)
Counties: Orange County
States: CA
Areas of Practice: 1, 2, 3, 4, 5, 6, 7, 8, 9, 10, 12

Harriet Estrin, EdD
Eldercare Options, Inc.
P.O. Box 1527
Kingston, RI 02881
(401) 783-8773
Years in Full Time Geriatric Care Management: 5
Service Area
Metropolitan Area(s):
Counties:
States: RI
Areas of Practice: 1, 2, 3, 5, 6, 7, 8, 9, 10, 11, 12

Marianne Ewig, MSW, ACSW
September Managed Care For Later Years
830 N. 109th Street, Suite 27
Milwaukee, WI 53226-3740
(414) 774-5800

Years in Full Time Geriatric Care Management: 3
Service Area
Metropolitan Area(s): Greater Milwaukee, Area Code 414
Counties: Milwaukee, Ozaukee, Waukesha, Washington, Racine, Walworth
States: WI
Areas of Practice: 1, 2, 3, 5, 6, 7, 8, 9, 10, 11

Barbara R. Feinstein, ACSW, MSW, LSW, BCD
Comprehensive Health & Human Services Inc./Eldercare
435 East Lancaster Avenue, Suite 211
St. Davids, PA 19087
(215) 688-5579

Years in Full Time Geriatric Care Management: 11
Service Area
Metropolitan Area(s): Greater Philadelphia (Area Code 215), Southern New
    Jersey (Area Code 609)
Counties: In PA: Philadelphia, Montgomery, Delaware, Bucks, Chester; In NJ:
    Camden
States: PA, NJ
Areas of Practice: 1, 2, 3, 4, 5, 6, 7, 8, 9, 10, 11, 12

Beatrice Feldman, MSW
Beatrice Feldman & Associates
23213 Fairmount Boulevard   25000 Great Northern Corp. Ctr. #300
Beachwood, OH 44122   N. Olmsted, OH 44070
(216) 292-5530   (216) 779-3280

Years in Full Time Geriatric Care Management: 5
Service Area
Metropolitan Area(s): Cleveland
Counties: Cuyahoga, Lake, Geauga
States: OH
Areas of Practice: 1, 2, 3, 4, 5, 6, 7, 8, 9, 10, 11, 12

Claudia Fine, MSW, MPH, CSW
Claudia Fine Associates
101 Central Park West
New York, NY 10023
(212) 873-4374

Years in Full Time Geriatric Care Management: 4
Service Area
Metropolitan Area(s): Manhattan, Bronx—Will see clients from other areas
    in our office.
Counties:
States: NY
Areas of Practice: 1, 2, 3, 4, 5, 6, 7, 8, 9, 10, 11, 12

Emily H. Fisher, MS, EdM
Manhattan Resources, Inc.
140 Riverside Drive
New York, NY 10024
(212) 580-3801
Years in Full Time Geriatric Care Management: 7
Service Area
Metropolitan Area(s): New York City Metropolitan Area
Area Codes 201, 203, 212, 516, 718
Counties:
States: NY
Areas of Practice: 1, 2, 3, 7, 8, 10, 12

Sharon Fitch, ACSW, ACP
Kinship Associates
10211 Bridgegate Lane
Dallas, TX 75243
(214) 480-0716
Years in Full Time Geriatric Care Management:
Service Area
Metropolitan Area(s): Dallas, Ft. Worth
Counties:
States: TX
Areas of Practice: 1, 2, 3, 4, 5, 6, 7, 8, 9, 10, Bereavement

Dianne Flanigan, MSW
Elder Care Options, Inc.
RD 2 Box 398 Quakertown Road
Pittstown, NJ 08867
(908) 730-6388
Years in Full Time Geriatric Care Management: 2
Service Area
Metropolitan Area(s):
Counties: Hunterdon, Sussex, Warren
States: NJ
Areas of Practice: 1, 2, 5, 6, 7, 8, 9, 10

Linda Fodrini-Johnson, MA, MFCC
Elder Care Placement Services
1844 San Miguel Drive, Suite 101
Walnut Creek, CA 94596
(510) 937-2018
Years in Full Time Geriatric Care Management: 7
Service Area
Metropolitan Area(s):
Counties: Contra Costa, Alameda
States: CA
Areas of Practice: 1, 2, 3, 4, 5, 6, 7, 8, 9, 10, 11

Illese Forgang
405 E. 56th Street
New York, NY 10022
(212) 888-4252
Years in Full Time Geriatric Care Management: 2
Service Area
Metropolitan Area(s): New York City
Counties: New York
States: NY
Areas of Practice: 1, 2, 4, 5, 6, 7, 8, 9, 10, 11, 12

Steven C. Fox, DO, MS
Wellspring Services
179 W. Washington Street, Suite 360
Chicago, IL 60602
(312) 201-9696
Years in Full Time Geriatric Care Management: 7
Service Area
Metropolitan Area(s): Chicago
Counties: Cook, Will, Dupage, Lake, McHenry
States: IL, IN
Areas of Practice: 1, 2, 3, 4, 6, 7, 8, 9, 10

Celeste D. Galati, ACSW, LSW
Resources for the Elderly
P.O. Box 5252
6120 Brandon Avenue, Suite 117
Springfield, VA 22150
(703) 886-3122
Years in Full Time Geriatric Care Management: 5
Service Area
Metropolitan Area(s): Washington, D.C.
Counties:
States:
Areas of Practice: 1, 2, 3, 6, 7, 8, 9, 10

Darlene Gamble, MS
Total Family Care
3939 Whitebrook Drive, Suite 100 Building H
Memphis, TN 38118
(901) 367-0551
Years in Full Time Geriatric Care Management:
Service Area
Metropolitan Area(s): Memphis (Area Code 901)
Counties: Shelby
States: TN
Areas of Practice: 1, 2, 5, 7, 8, 9, 10, 12

Diane Garcia, MSW, PhD
Diane Garcia, Ph.D.
478 Manchester Avenue
Bricktown, NJ 08723-5225
(908) 920-8110
Years in Full Time Geriatric Care Management: 2
Service Area
Metropolitan Area(s): Jersey Shore Area
Counties: South Monmouth, Ocean
States: NJ
Areas of Practice: 1, 2, 3, 4, 5, 6, 7, 8, 9, 10, 11, 12

Joan F. Garofalo, MSW, QCSW-R
Route 81, Box 83
Oak Hill, NY 12460
(518) 239-4772
Years in Full Time Geriatric Care Management: 5
Service Area
Metropolitan Area(s): Capital Region
Counties:
States: NY
Areas of Practice: 1, 2, 3, 4, 5, 6, 7, 8, 9, 10, 11, 12

Joanne Gerard, MSW
Long Term Care Consulting Service
11331 South West One Court
Plantation, FL 33325
(305) 472-5556
Years in Full Time Geriatric Care Management: 9
Service Area
Metropolitan Area(s): Greater Ft. Lauderdale
Counties: Broward, South Palm Beach
States: FL
Areas of Practice: 1, 2, 3, 5, 6, 7, 8, 9, 10, 11

Rita Ghatak, LCSW, PhD
PARD
167 Hamilton Avenue
Palo Alto, CA 94301
(415) 321-6413
Years in Full Time Geriatric Care Management: 9
Service Area
Metropolitan Area(s):
Counties:
States: CA
Areas of Practice: 3, 7, 8

Gail Gill, LCSW
Senior Care Consultants
606 Central
Wilmette, IL 60091
(708) 251-2144
Years in Full Time Geriatric Care Management: 2
Service Area
Metropolitan Area(s): Metro Chicago Area
Counties:
States: IL
Areas of Practice: 1, 2, 3, 4, 5, 6, 7, 8, 9, 10, 11, 12

Alan Goldberg, MS, MSW, MSG, LCSW
Top-Of-The-Line Professional Health Care, Inc.
1642 Veteran Avenue
Los Angeles, CA 90024
(213) 479-2832
Years in Full Time Geriatric Care Management: 7
Service Area
Metropolitan Area(s): Beverly Hills, Santa Monica, Los Angeles
Counties:
States: CA
Areas of Practice: 1, 2, 3, 4, 5, 6, 7, 8, 9, 10, 11, 12

Susan Goldsmith, MSW, LCSW, BCD
Health Access, Inc.
135 SW Ash Street, Suite 530
Portland, OR 97219
(503) 228-3333   (800) 333-8568
Years in Full Time Geriatric Care Management: 12
Service Area
Metropolitan Area(s): Portland, Vancouver, Washington
Counties: In Oregon: All counties;
In Washington: Clark
States: OR, Southwest WA
Areas of Practice: 1, 2, 3, 4, 5, 6, 7, 8, 9, 10, 11, 12

Harriette R. Grooh, MFCC
Harriette R. Grooh & Associates
1112 Sir Francis Drake Blvd.   1730 Divisadero Street
Kentfield, CA 94904   San Francisco, CA 94115
(415) 924-8311   (415) 924-8311
Years in Full Time Geriatric Care Management: 14
Service Area
Metropolitan Area(s): San Francisco, San Jose, Oakland, Sacramento
Counties: San Francisco, San Mateo, Marin, Santa Clara, Contra Costa,
   Sonoma, Napa, Alameda
States: CA, National referrals
Areas of Practice: 1, 2, 3, 5, 6, 7, 8, 9, 10, 11, 12,
Serve trust depts from CA, OR, WA

DeeAnn Groves, MA
Seniors Are Special
1802 16th Street #2
Greeley, CO 80631
(303) 350-2406

Years in Full Time Geriatric Care Management: 3

Service Area
Metropolitan Area(s): Greeley, Northern Colorado
Counties: Greeley, Weld, Larimer, Ft. Morgan
States: CO
Areas of Practice: 1, 2, 3, 5, 6, 7, 8, 9, 10, 11

Marc Guthartz, MSW
Comprehensive Home Care
One East Post Road
White Plains, NY 10601
(914) 682-3988

Years in Full Time Geriatric Care Management: 10

Service Area
Metropolitan Area(s):
Counties: Westchester County
States: NY
Areas of Practice: 1, 5, 9, 10, 12

Jane Hamil, MSW, CFP
Bridging Generations
659 Peachtree Street, Suite 407
Atlanta, GA 30308-1928
(404) 872-7520

Years in Full Time Geriatric Care Management: 1

Service Area
Metropolitan Area(s): Metropolitan Atlanta
Counties: Cobb, N. Fulton, Givinnett
States: GA
Areas of Practice: 1, 2, 3, 5, 6, 7, 8, 9, 10

Kimberly Hanchette
Kimberly Hanchette - Geriatric Case Manager
4104 Converse Drive
Raleigh, NC 27609
(919) 781-5186

Years in Full Time Geriatric Care Management: 1

Service Area
Metropolitan Area(s): Raleigh, Durham, Chapel Hill
Counties: Orange, Durham, Wake
States: NC
Areas of Practice: 1, 2, 3, 5, 6, 7, 8, 9, 10, 12

Milton Hanson, LCSW
Institute for Creative Aging
P.O. Box 3725
Littleton, CO 80161
(303) 795-9682
Years in Full Time Geriatric Care Management:
Service Area
Metropolitan Area(s): Metropolitan Denver
Counties: Statewide
States: All States
Areas of Practice: 1, 2, 3, 5, 7, 8, 11

Patricia Hanson, RN
Care Management Plus
4460 Oak Chase Way
Eagan, MN 55123
(612) 454-4670
Years in Full Time Geriatric Care Management: 4
Service Area
Metropolitan Area(s): Minneapolis - St. Paul
Counties: 7 Metro Counties
States: MN
Areas of Practice: 1, 2, 3, 5, 6, 7, 8, 9, 10, 11, 12

Irma L. Hausdorff, PhD
Adult Management Services
900 N. Federal Highway, Suite 160-8
Boca Raton, FL 33432
(407) 392-1116
Years in Full Time Geriatric Care Management: 10
Service Area
Metropolitan Area(s): Boca Raton, Deerfield Beach, West Palm Beach
Counties: Palm Beach, N. Broward
States: FL
Areas of Practice: 1, 2, 3, 7, 8, 9, 10,
health claim filing

Maryann Higgins, BSW, MA
Connections
540 The Rialto
Venice, FL 34285
(813) 485-7567
Years in Full Time Geriatric Care Management: 11
Service Area
Metropolitan Area(s): Tampa, Sarasota, Venice, Englewood, North Port, Port
  Charlotte
Counties: Sarasota, Charlotte, Hillsborough, Pasco
States: FL
Areas of Practice: 1, 2, 3, 4, 5, 6, 7, 8, 9, 10, 12

Marjorie Hornik, MSW, ACSW
839 West End Avenue, Suite 4-C
P.O. Box 1094
New York, NY 10025
(212) 222-8990
Years in Full Time Geriatric Care Management: 1
Service Area
Metropolitan Area(s): Manhattan
Counties:
States: NY
Areas of Practice: 1, 2, 5, 6, 7, 8, 9, 10, 11

Janet L. Howes, MSW
Care Planning Associates
4515 West Saginaw
Lansing, MI 48917
(517) 323-8410
Years in Full Time Geriatric Care Management: 1
Service Area
Metropolitan Area(s): Lansing
Counties: Eaton, Ingham, Clinton
States: MI
Areas of Practice: 1, 2, 3, 4, 5, 6, 7, 8, 9, 10, 11

Paula L. Hurn, ACSW, CSW, MSW
Elder Links
2032 East Monterey Way
Phoenix, AZ 85016
(602) 957-4883
Years in Full Time Geriatric Care Management: 5
Service Area
Metropolitan Area(s): Phoenix, Scottsdale, Glendale, Sun City, Sun City West
Counties: Western Maricopa
States: AZ
Areas of Practice: 1, 2, 3, 4, 5, 6, 7, 8, 9, 10, 11, 12

Evelyne E. Hutkin, MSSW, LCSW, BCD
Senior Care Services
5333 Mission Center Road, Suite 340
San Diego, CA 92108
(619) 291-4403
Years in Full Time Geriatric Care Management: 8
Service Area
Metropolitan Area(s): San Diego
Counties: San Diego
States: CA
Areas of Practice: 1, 2, 3, 4, 5, 6, 7, 8, 9, 10, 11, 12

Elizabeth E. James, MSN, ARNP
ElderCare of Pinellas, Inc.
4895 112 Street North
St. Petersburg, FL 33708
(813) 397-0003
Years in Full Time Geriatric Care Management: 5
Service Area
Metropolitan Area(s): St. Petersburg, Seminole, Largo, Clearwater, Beaches
Counties: Pinellas, Pasco
States: FL
Areas of Practice: 1, 2, 3, 5, 6, 7, 8, 9, 10

Gordon Sloan James, PhD, ACSW
Elder Care Resources Unlimited
Lincoln Centre-Lakeview Suites
11221 North 28th Drive, E. 104
Phoenix, AZ 85029
(602) 548-9348
Years in Full Time Geriatric Care Management: 1
Service Area
Metropolitan Area(s): Phoenix
Counties: Maricopa
States: AZ
Areas of Practice: 1, 2, 3, 4, 5, 6, 7, 8, 9, 10, 11, 12

Eleanor Johnson
Paine-Johnson Agency, Inc.
P.O. Box 489
Thomaston, CT 06787
(203) 271-0206
Years in Full Time Geriatric Care Management: 3.5
Service Area
Metropolitan Area(s): Bridgeport to Terrington
Counties: Lichfield, New Haven, Fairfield
States: CT
Areas of Practice: 1, 2, 3, 5, 6, 7, 8, 10, 11

Erica Karp, MSW, LCSW
Northshore Eldercare Management
1019 South Boulevard
Evanston, IL 60202
(708) 866-7466
Years in Full Time Geriatric Care Management: 12
Service Area
Metropolitan Area(s): Metropolitan Chicago
Counties: Cook
States: IL
Areas of Practice: 1, 2, 3, 4, 5, 6, 7, 8, 9, 10, 11, 12

Fran P. Kaschak, MSW, LCSW
Geriatric Family Services
5100 Eden Avenue
Edina, MN 55436
(612) 929-1772
Years in Full Time Geriatric Care Management: 6
Service Area
Metropolitan Area(s): Twin Cities, Minneapolis, St. Paul
Counties: 7 county Metropolitan area
States: MN
Areas of Practice: 1, 2, 3, 4, 5, 6, 7, 8, 9, 10, 11, 12,
                   life planning

Constance Kilgore, CSW, ACP
Texas Geriatric Services
12880 Hillcrest, Suite 104
Dallas, TX 75230
(214) 387-4751
Years in Full Time Geriatric Care Management: 5
Service Area
Metropolitan Area(s): Dallas, Ft. Worth, North Texas Area Codes 817, 214, 903
Counties: Dallas, Denton, Collin, Tarrant, Ellis
States: TX
Areas of Practice: 1, 2, 3, 4, 5, 6, 7, 8, 9, 10, 12,
                   Chemical Dependency & Substance Abuse

Rose Kleiner, LCSW
Older Adults Care Management
167 Hamilton Avenue
Palo Alto, CA 94301
(415) 329-1411
Years in Full Time Geriatric Care Management: 9
Service Area
Metropolitan Area(s): San Francisco, San Jose, San Mateo, Santa Clara
Counties:
States: CA
Areas of Practice: 1, 3, 4, 5, 7, 8, 10, 12

Jeanne W. Klems, MA, LCSW
Jeanne W. Klems LCSW
1870 San Lorenzo Ave.
Berkeley, CA 94707
(415) 525-2226
Years in Full Time Geriatric Care Management: 1.5
Service Area
Metropolitan Area(s): Oakland, Berkeley, Richmond
Counties: Alameda, Contra Costa
States: CA
Areas of Practice: 1, 2, 3, 4, 5, 6, 7, 8, 9, 10

Connie D. Knapper, RN, MS
Access Home Care, Inc.
5103 Eastman Place, Suite 229B
Midland, MI 48640
(517) 832-0222
Years in Full Time Geriatric Care Management: 4
Service Area
Metropolitan Area(s): Bay City, Midland, Saginaw
Counties: Saginaw, Midland, Bay, Gratist
States: MI
Areas of Practice: 1, 2, 3, 5, 6, 7, 8, 9, 10, 11, 12

Norah S. R. Knutsen, MSN, RN, CS
Mature Options
1910 Byrd Avenue, Suite 8
Richmond, VA 23230
(804) 282-0753
Years in Full Time Geriatric Care Management: 1
Service Area
Metropolitan Area(s): Richmond and surrounding area
Counties:
States: VA
Areas of Practice: 1, 2, 3, 5, 6, 7, 8, 9, 10, 11, 12

Karen Knutson, MSN, MBA
OpenCare
2237 Park Road
Charlotte, NC 28203
(704) 377-2273
Years in Full Time Geriatric Care Management: 1
Service Area
Metropolitan Area(s): Charlotte
Counties: Mecklenburg, Gaston
States: NC
Areas of Practice: 1, 2, 3, 4, 5, 6, 7, 8, 9, 10, 12

Mary M. Korcz
Elder-Service, Inc.
310 Davisville Road
Warminster, PA 18974
(215) 322-4010
Years in Full Time Geriatric Care Management: 2
Service Area
Metropolitan Area(s):
Counties: Philadelphia, Bucks, Montgomery, Delaware
States: PA, NJ, DE
Areas of Practice: 1, 2, 3, 5, 6, 7, 8, 9, 10, 12

Anneta Kraus, RN
Geriatric Planning Services
Main Line Federal Bldg, Suite 201
Two South Orange
Media, PA 19063
(215) 566-6686
Years in Full Time Geriatric Care Management: 11
Service Area
Metropolitan Area(s): Greater Philadelphia
Counties: Delaware, Chester
States: PA
Areas of Practice: 1, 2, 3, 5, 6, 7, 8, 9, 10, 11

Kyle Laitiner, LCSW
Lifenet, Inc.
1819 State Street, Suite B
Santa Barbara, CA 93101
(805) 687-8766
Years in Full Time Geriatric Care Management:
Service Area
Metropolitan Area(s): Santa Barbara, Ventura, Kern, San Luis Obispo
Counties:
States: CA
Areas of Practice: 1, 2, 3, 5, 6, 7, 8, 9, 10, 11, 12

Betty Bartels Landreaux, BCSW
Care Management Solutions, Inc.
2955 Ridgelake Drive, Suite 112
Metairie, LA 70002
(504) 837-5801
Years in Full Time Geriatric Care Management:
Service Area
Metropolitan Area(s): LA, Southern MS, AL, Northwest FL
Counties:
States: LA, MS, AL, FL
Areas of Practice: 1, 2, 3, 4, 5, 6, 7, 8, 9, 10, 11, 12

Mary G. LaNier, MA
Gerontology Consultants
721 Ashland Drive
Huntington Beach, CA 92648
(714) 536-8103
Years in Full Time Geriatric Care Management: 4
Service Area
Metropolitan Area(s):
Counties: Orange
States: CA
Areas of Practice: 1, 2, 3, 5, 6, 7, 8, 9, 10, 12

Barbara Larsen, MEd
Elder-Connection
P.O. Box 1061
Grass Valley, CA 95945
(916) 265-4049
Years in Full Time Geriatric Care Management: 1
Service Area
Metropolitan Area(s):
Counties: Nevada
States: CA
Areas of Practice: 1, 3, 6, 7, 8, 10

Janice M. Larson, MSN, NP
Extended Family, Inc.
1716 Hycrest Drive
Appleton, WI 54914
(414) 749-1117
Years in Full Time Geriatric Care Management: 1
Service Area
Metropolitan Area(s): Northeast Wisconsin
Counties: Outagomie, Winnebago, Calumet
States: WI
Areas of Practice: 1, 2, 3, 6, 7, 8, 9, 10

Robert Lauretig
Alternative Counseling Associates
3789 South Green Road
Cleveland, OH 44122
(216) 292-4409
Years in Full Time Geriatric Care Management: 25
Service Area
Metropolitan Area(s): Cleveland, Akron, Canton
Counties: Cuyahoga, Summit
States: OH
Areas of Practice: 1, 2, 3, 4, 5, 7, 8, 9, 10, 11, 12

Lori Lazaroff, MSW
Counseling Related to Geriatrics
1500 Kings Highway North, Suite 109
Cherry Hill, NJ 08034
(609) 427-0089
Years in Full Time Geriatric Care Management: 5
Service Area
Metropolitan Area(s): Southern NJ, Philadelphia PA
Counties:
States: NJ, PA
Areas of Practice: 1, 2, 3, 4, 5, 6, 7, 8, 9, 10, 11, 12

Grace Lebow, MSW, LCSW
Aging Network Services, Inc.
4400 East-West Highway, Suite 907
Bethesda, MD 20814
(301) 951-8589
Years in Full Time Geriatric Care Management: 9
Service Area
Metropolitan Area(s): Area Codes 202, 301, 703
Counties: Montgomery, Upper Prince Georges, Metropolitan D.C. & Fairfax
States: MD, DC, Northern VA
Areas of Practice: 1, 2, 3, 4, 5, 6, 7, 8, 9, 10, 12

Jan E. Lees, LCSW, MSW, MSG
1226 Veteran Avenue
Los Angeles, CA 90024
(213) 820-1602
(213) 477-3097 FAX
Years in Full Time Geriatric Care Management:
Service Area
Metropolitan Area(s): Los Angeles
Counties: Los Angeles
States: CA
Areas of Practice: 1, 2, 3, 4, 5, 6, 7, 8, 9, 10

Anne D. Lester, MS
Manhattan Resources, Inc.
140 Riverside Drive
New York, NY 10024
(212) 580-3801
Years in Full Time Geriatric Care Management: 7
Service Area
Metropolitan Area(s): New York City Metropolitan area
Counties: Area Codes 201, 203, 212, 516, 718
States: NY
Areas of Practice: 1, 2, 3, 7, 8, 10, 12

Debra G. Levy, LICSW
212 Thistle Court
Silver Spring, MD 20901
(301) 593-5285
Years in Full Time Geriatric Care Management: 3
Service Area
Metropolitan Area(s): Washington DC & Suburbs
Counties:
States: MD, DC
Areas of Practice: 1, 2, 3, 4, 5, 6, 7, 8, 9, 10, 11, 12

Julie Lomoe-Smith, MA, MFA, ATR
ElderSource, Inc.
Time Square Professional Park
652 Route 299, Suite 204A
Highland, NY 12528
(914) 883-7824
Years in Full Time Geriatric Care Management: 1.5
Service Area
Metropolitan Area(s): Kingston, Newburgh, Poughkeepsie
Counties: Ulster, Dutchess, Orange
States: NY
Areas of Practice: 1, 2, 3, 4, 5, 6, 7, 8, 9, 10, 11, 12

Gussie Lovelle
The Golden Years Services Inc.
511 North Schroeder Street
Baltimore, MD 21223
(301) 523-1173
Years in Full Time Geriatric Care Management:
Service Area
Metropolitan Area(s): Baltimore
Counties: Surrounding counties
States: MD
Areas of Practice: 1, 2, 3, 6, 7, 8, 9, 10, 11, 12

Lois J. Mahar, RN, C
Elder Care Coordinators, Inc.
10219 Edgewater Drive
Cleveland, OH 44102
(216) 574-2446
Years in Full Time Geriatric Care Management: 3
Service Area
Metropolitan Area(s): Cleveland
Counties: Cuyahoga & Surrounding
States: OH
Areas of Practice: 1, 2, 3, 6, 7, 8, 9, 10

Bonnie Malajian, MSW, ACSW
Generations
121 Cedar Lane, 3rd Floor
Teaneck, NJ 07666
(201) 836-5323
Years in Full Time Geriatric Care Management: 14
Service Area
Metropolitan Area(s): Northern New Jersey, Manhattan
Counties: Bergen, Passaic, Morris, Hudson, Rockland, Westchester
States: NJ, NY
Areas of Practice: 1, 2, 3, 4, 5, 6, 7, 8, 9, 10, 11, 12

Joyce Marvan-Hyam, RN, MPA/HSA
Adult Care Services
800 South Broadway, Suite 309
Walnut Creek, CA 94596
(415) 944-5800
Years in Full Time Geriatric Care Management: 14
Service Area
Metropolitan Area(s):
Counties: Alameda, Contra Costa
States: CA
Areas of Practice: 1, 2, 3, 6, 7, 8, 9, 10, 12

O. E. Matos, MDPA
5330-1 George Street
New Port Richey, FL 34652
(813) 849-2005
Years in Full Time Geriatric Care Management: 15
Service Area
Metropolitan Area(s): Hudson, Holiday, Tarpon Springs
Counties: Pasco
States: FL
Areas of Practice: 1, 2, 3, 4, 5, 6, 7, 8, 9, 10

Alan McBroom, MSW
Ask Health Care Services, Inc.
24681 Northwestern Highway, Suite 106
Southfield, MI 48075
(313) 355-1980
Years in Full Time Geriatric Care Management: 5
Service Area
Metropolitan Area(s): Area Codes 313, 517, 616
Counties: Detroit, Tri-County
States: MI
Areas of Practice: 1, 2, 3, 5, 6, 7, 8, 10, 12

Janice McCurdy, MSW
Bristow-McCurdy
P.O. Box 81
Pennington, NJ 08534
(609) 737-8398
Years in Full Time Geriatric Care Management: 15
Service Area
Metropolitan Area(s): Central New Jersey
Counties:
States: NJ
Areas of Practice: 1, 2, 3, 5, 6, 7, 8, 9, 10, 11

Sheila McMackin, MSW, LCSW, ACSW
Wellspring Services
179 West Washington Street, Suite 360
Chicago, IL 60602
(312) 201-9696
Years in Full Time Geriatric Care Management: 5
Service Area
Metropolitan Area(s): Chicago
Counties: Cook, DuPage, Will, Lake, McHenry
States: IL, IN, WI
Areas of Practice: 1, 2, 3, 4, 5, 6, 7, 8, 9, 10, 11, 12

Suzanne Fritts McNeely, MSW
Senior Planning Services
735 State Street, Suite 106
Santa Barbara, CA 93101
(805) 966-3312
Years in Full Time Geriatric Care Management: 2
Service Area
Metropolitan Area(s): Santa Barbara
Counties: Santa Barbara
States: CA
Areas of Practice: 1, 2, 3, 5, 6, 7, 8, 9, 10, 11, 12

Sara Shevitz Mesirow, MA
Geriatric Resource Consultants, Inc.
160 Cary Avenue
Highland Park, IL 60035
(708) 432-3490
Years in Full Time Geriatric Care Management: 8
Service Area
Metropolitan Area(s): Chicago
Counties: Cook, Lake
States: IL
Areas of Practice: 1, 2, 3, 5, 6, 7, 8, 9, 10, 12

Shirley K. Miller, MSW, ACSW
Private Geriatric Care Manager
2017 Northeast 21st Court
Ft. Lauderdale, FL 33305
(305) 565-1344
Years in Full Time Geriatric Care Management: 3.5
Service Area
Metropolitan Area(s): Greater Ft. Lauderdale, Pompano
Counties: Broward, Dade, Palm Beach
States: FL
Areas of Practice: 1, 2, 3, 5, 6, 7, 8, 9, 10, 11, 12

Kathleen C. Milne, RN, BSN
Resource Connectors, Ltd.
5520 SW Macadam Avenue, Suite 270
Portland, OR 97201
(503) 228-7023
Years in Full Time Geriatric Care Management: 6
Service Area
Metropolitan Area(s): Portland, Vancouver
Counties: Multnomah, Washington, Clackamas, Clark
States: OR, WA
Areas of Practice: 1, 2, 3, 4, 5, 6, 7, 8, 9, 10, 11, 12

Sybil E. Montgomery, PhD, LSW
Alternatives in Living LTD
1637 Oakwood Drive
Penn Valley, PA 19072
(215) 667-3154
Years in Full Time Geriatric Care Management: 5
Service Area
Metropolitan Area(s):
Counties: Philadelphia, Montgomery, Delaware
States: PA
Areas of Practice: 1, 2, 3, 4, 5, 6, 7, 8, 9, 10, 11, 12, Medicare approved
  provider for mental health services

Mary Moser, BSN, RN, MA
Mary Moser Associates
58 Hobart Avenue
Summit, NJ 07901
(908) 277-4089
Years in Full Time Geriatric Care Management: 1
Service Area
Metropolitan Area(s): Northern & Central New Jersey
Counties: Essex, Union, Morris
States: NJ
Areas of Practice: 1, 2, 3, 5, 6, 7, 8, 9, 10, 11, 12

Ruth Muchemore, MS, RN
Parentcare
643 North 98th Street, Suite 253
Omaha, NE 68114
(402) 390-9323
Years in Full Time Geriatric Care Management: 16
Service Area
Metropolitan Area(s): Omaha
Counties:
States: NE
Areas of Practice: 1, 2, 3, 4, 5, 6, 7, 8, 9, 10, 11, 12

Vida Francis Negrete, RN, DrPH
1507 Indiana Avenue
South Pasadena, CA 91030
(213) 259-8710
Years in Full Time Geriatric Care Management:
Service Area
Metropolitan Area(s): Los Angeles, San Gabriel Valley
Counties: Los Angeles
States: CA
Areas of Practice: 1, 3, 6, 7, 8, 10

Deborah D. Newquist, MSW, PhD
Elder Care Resources
2900 Bristol, Suite 206J
Costa Mesa, CA 92626
(714) 854-2990
Years in Full Time Geriatric Care Management: 4
Service Area
Metropolitan Area(s): Leisure World, Anaheim, Huntington Beach, Laguna
    Hills, Tustin, Irvine, Santa Ana, Fullerton
Counties: Orange
States: CA
Areas of Practice: 1, 2, 3, 5, 6, 7, 8, 9, 10

June C. Ninnemann, ACSW, LCSW
CarePlan, Inc.
10520 West Bernice Drive   1010 West Lake Street, #204
Palos Park, IL 60464   Oak Park, IL 60301
(708) 524-2070   (708) 524-2070
Years in Full Time Geriatric Care Management: 3
Service Area
Metropolitan Area(s):
Counties: Cook
States: IL
Areas of Practice: 1, 2, 3, 4, 5, 6, 7, 8, 9, 10, 12

Mary M. Norcross, PhD
Nursing Home/Residential Placement
13623 Valerio Street, Unit B
Van Nuys, CA 91405
(818) 376-1411
Years in Full Time Geriatric Care Management: 8
Service Area
Metropolitan Area(s): Van Nuys & Surrounding Area
Counties:
States: Various States By Appointment
Areas of Practice: 1, 2, 3, 5, 6, 7, 8, 9, 10, 12

Leonie Nowitz, MSW, ACSW
Center for Lifelong Growth
400 Central Park West, Suite 3A
New York, NY 10025
(212) 864-5905
Years in Full Time Geriatric Care Management: 2
Service Area
Metropolitan Area(s): Manhattan, consultations in Brooklyn, Bronx, Queens
Counties: New York
States: NY
Areas of Practice: 1, 2, 3, 4, 5, 6, 7, 8, 9, 10, 11, 12,
Housing Options

Fran O'Connell, RN, BSN
O'Connell Professional Nurse Service, Inc.
397 Appleton Street
Holyoke, MA 01040
(413) 533-1030
Years in Full Time Geriatric Care Management:
Service Area
Metropolitan Area(s): Holyoke, Chicopee, Springfield
Counties: Hampden, Hampshire
States: MA
Areas of Practice: 1, 2, 3, 7, 8, 10

Ann E. O'Neil, RN, MSN, CS
Care Options for the Elderly
1304 Seaton Lane
Falls Church, VA 22046
(703) 237-9048
Years in Full Time Geriatric Care Management: 3
Service Area
Metropolitan Area(s): Metropolitan Washington, D.C., Area Codes 202, 301, 703
Counties: Northern Virginia, Washington D.C.
In Maryland: Montgomery
States: VA, MD, DC
Areas of Practice: 1, 2, 3, 5, 6, 7, 8, 9, 10, 11, 12

Fay Ojile, RN
Care Management PLUS, Inc.
4460 Oak Chase Way
Eagan, MN 55123
(612) 789-2558
Years in Full Time Geriatric Care Management: 4
Service Area
Metropolitan Area(s): Minneapolis, St. Paul
Counties:
States: MN
Areas of Practice: 1, 2, 3, 6, 8, 10

Merrily Orsini, MSSW
Elder Care Solutions
1220 Bardstown Road
Louisville, KY 40204
(502) 452-9644
(800) 633-5723

Years in Full Time Geriatric Care Management: 10

Service Area
Metropolitan Area(s): Louisville, Southern Indiana
Counties: In Kentucky: Jefferson
In Indiana: Floyd, Clark
States: KY, IN
Areas of Practice: 1, 2, 3, 5, 7, 8, 9, 10, 11, 12

Marjorie Osheroff, BSN, RN, MSM
Long Term Planning Associates, Inc.
5 Sweetwater St.
Saugus, MA 01906
(617) 231-2616

Years in Full Time Geriatric Care Management: 6

Service Area
Metropolitan Area(s): Area Codes 617, 508, 413
Counties: All MA
States: MA
Areas of Practice: 1, 2, 3, 6, 7, 8, 10, 11

Pamela Lenges Overton, RN
Pamela Overton & Associates
Elder Care Management
1871 Cottonwood Trail
Sarasota, FL 34232
(813) 377-4761

Years in Full Time Geriatric Care Management: 3

Service Area
Metropolitan Area(s): Bradenton & Sarasota
Counties:
States: FL
Areas of Practice: 1, 2, 3, 5, 6, 7, 8, 9, 10, 11

Curt Paddock, MPA
Paddock Health Services, Inc.
4239 War Memorial Drive, Suite 304
Peoria, IL 61614
(309) 682-7291

Years in Full Time Geriatric Care Management: 2

Service Area
Metropolitan Area(s): Peoria, Bloomington-Normal, Springfield
Counties: Peoria, Tazewell, Woodford, McLean, Fulton, Sangamon
States: IL
Areas of Practice: 1, 2, 3, 5, 6, 7, 8, 10, 11, 12

Mary Lynn Pannen, BSN, RN, C
Sound Options Inc.
917 Pacific Avenue, Suite 608
Tacoma, WA 98402
(206) 572-7008   (800) 628-7649
Years in Full Time Geriatric Care Management: 2
Service Area
Metropolitan Area(s): Tacoma, Seattle, Olympia
Counties: King, Pierce, Kitsap
States: WA
Areas of Practice: 1, 2, 3, 6, 7, 8, 10, 12

Judith S. Parnes, MSW, ACSW
Elder Life Management, Inc.
P.O. Box 394
Deal, NJ 07723
(908) 776-9104
Years in Full Time Geriatric Care Management: 4
Service Area
Metropolitan Area(s):
Counties: Middlesex, Monmouth, Ocean
States: NJ
Areas of Practice: 1, 2, 3, 4, 5, 6, 7, 8, 9, 10, 11

Meredith Beit Patterson, MSW, LICSW
109 Seymour St.
Concord, MA 01742
(508) 369-7402
Years in Full Time Geriatric Care Management: 4
Service Area
Metropolitan Area(s): West of Boston within 495 Belt
Counties: Metro West
States: MA
Areas of Practice: 1, 2, 3, 4, 5, 6, 7, 8, 10, 11

Risha Paz'Soldan, LCSW
Aging Care Options
12439 Magnolia Boulevard, #207
North Hollywood, CA 91607
(818) 700-0209
Years in Full Time Geriatric Care Management: 10
Service Area
Metropolitan Area(s):
Counties: Los Angeles County
States: CA
Areas of Practice: 1, 2, 3, 4, 5, 6, 7, 8, 9, 10, 11, 12

Ann Peck, BS
Geriatric Resource Centre Inc.
20 Morton Road
Newton Centre, MA 02159
(617) 332-7610
Years in Full Time Geriatric Care Management: 11
Service Area
Metropolitan Area(s): Boston & Suburbs
Counties:
States: MA
Areas of Practice: 1, 2, 5, 7, 8, 9, 10, 12

Patricia Percival, RCSW
Northwest Professional Group
Montgomery Park, Suite 424
2701 NW Vaughn
Portland, OR 97210
(503) 222-4244   (800) 767-3072 for referrals
Years in Full Time Geriatric Care Management: 10
Service Area
Metropolitan Area(s): Portland
Counties: Multnomah, Washington, Clackamas & Willamette Valley
States: OR, Southwest WA
Areas of Practice: 1, 2, 3, 4, 5, 6, 7, 8, 9, 10, 11, 12

Jane Perlow, MA, LNHA
Concerned Seniorcare
130 Horace Harding Boulevard
Great Neck, NY 11020
(516) 466-6387   (516) 335-4041
Years in Full Time Geriatric Care Management: 2
Service Area
Metropolitan Area(s): Metropolitan New York, All 5 Boroughs
Counties: Nassau, Suffolk, Westchester
States: NY, FL Transfers
Areas of Practice: 2, 6, 7, 8, 11

Marilyn Peskin-Kaufman, MSSA
Answers for the Elderly
455 Greenlaurel Drive
Atlanta, GA 30342
(404) 303-0805
Years in Full Time Geriatric Care Management: 2
Service Area
Metropolitan Area(s): Atlanta
Counties: Cobb, DeKalb, Fulton, Cherokee
States: GA
Areas of Practice: 1, 2, 3, 5, 6, 7, 8, 9, 10, 11, 12

Becky Peters, RN
Lifespan: Care Management Agency
820 Bay Avenue, Suite 124
Capiola, CA 95010
(408) 475-7211
Years in Full Time Geriatric Care Management:
Service Area
Metropolitan Area(s): Santa Cruz
Counties: Santa Cruz
States: CA
Areas of Practice: 1, 2, 3, 5, 6, 7, 8, 9, 10, 11, 12

Elana Peters, MA
Care Options - Elder Care Mgmt.
2102 Business Center Drive, Suite 130
Irvine, CA 92715
(714) 253-4140
Years in Full Time Geriatric Care Management: 5
Service Area
Metropolitan Area(s): Los Angeles, Inland Empire
Counties: Orange, Los Angeles
States: CA
Areas of Practice: 1, 2, 3, 5, 6, 7, 8, 9, 10

Nancy C. Peters
75 Washington Avenue
Cambridge, MA 02140
(617) 354-4899
Years in Full Time Geriatric Care Management: 2
Service Area
Metropolitan Area(s): All of Massachusetts
Counties:
States: MA
Areas of Practice: 1, 2, 3, 5, 6, 7, 8

Jan D. Pitzer
Social Services
3015 37th Avenue SW
Seattle, WA 98126
(206) 935-3020
Years in Full Time Geriatric Care Management: 11.5
Service Area
Metropolitan Area(s): Seattle, Tacoma
Counties: Snohomish, Pierce
States: WA
Areas of Practice: 1, 2, 3, 5, 6, 7, 8, 10, 12

Claire Goldberg Plewinski, MSW
Senior Care Consultant
1433 Collins Avenue
Miami, FL 33139
(305) 935-1283   (305) 538-5743
Years in Full Time Geriatric Care Management: 1
Service Area
Metropolitan Area(s): Miami Beach, North Miami Beach, Hollywood
Counties: Dade, Broward
States: FL
Areas of Practice: 1, 2, 3, 5, 6, 7, 8, 9, 10, 11, 12

Thomas Posatko, MSW
Supportive Care Services, Inc.
507 West Ninth Street
Wilmington, DE 19801
(302) 655-5518
Years in Full Time Geriatric Care Management: 10
Service Area
Metropolitan Area(s):
Counties:
States: DE, Southeast PA
Areas of Practice: 1, 2, 6, 7, 8, 10, 11, 12

Polly Pratt, MSW, CSW
Geriatric Services
1523 East Madison
Seattle, WA 98122
(206) 329-5316
Years in Full Time Geriatric Care Management: 8
Service Area
Metropolitan Area(s): Seattle
Counties: King County, San Juan Islands
States: WA
Areas of Practice: 1, 2, 4, 5, 6, 7, 10

Gail Vander Horst Procter
6 Penny Lane
Baltimore, MD 21209
(301) 653-0821
Years in Full Time Geriatric Care Management:
Service Area
Metropolitan Area(s): Baltimore
Counties: Anne, Arendel, Howard, Baltimore, Harford
States: MD
Areas of Practice: 1, 2, 3, 4, 5, 6, 7, 8, 9, 10, 11

Marsha A. Raines, MSW, CSW
Marsha A. Raines, CSW
1742 Ridge Road East
Rochester, NY 14622
(716) 266-7444
Years in Full Time Geriatric Care Management: 5
Service Area
Metropolitan Area(s): Rochester, New York
Counties: Monroe
States: NY
Areas of Practice: 1, 2, 3, 4, 5, 6, 7, 8, 9, 10, 11

Eric Ratinetz, MSW, ACSW
Family Care Management, Inc.
7 West Fourteenth Street
New York, NY 10011
(212) 463-9121
Years in Full Time Geriatric Care Management: 6
Service Area
Metropolitan Area(s): Metropolitan New York
Counties:
States: NY
Areas of Practice: 1, 2, 3, 4, 5, 6, 7, 8, 9, 10, 11, 12

John H. Reid, MA
Ft. Collins Psychotherapy Group
2362 East Prospect
Fort Collins, CO 80525
(303) 484-9220
Years in Full Time Geriatric Care Management:
Service Area
Metropolitan Area(s): Ft. Collins, Loveland
Counties: Larimer
States: CO
Areas of Practice: 1, 2, 4, 5, 6, 8, 9, 10

Rebecca Rengo
Aging Consult
P.O. Box 2372
St. Louis, MO 63032
(314) 838-1392
Years in Full Time Geriatric Care Management: 2.5
Service Area
Metropolitan Area(s): St. Louis Area Codes 314 & 618
Counties: In MO: St. Louis, Jefferson, St. Charles, Franklin; In IL: Madison,
    St. Clair
States: MO, IL
Areas of Practice: 1, 2, 3, 4, 5, 6, 7, 8, 9, 10, 11

Janet M. Rhode, RN, ARNP, MN
Northwest Geriatric Care Managers
2208 NW Market Street, Suite 310
Seattle, WA 98107
(206) 783-1902
Years in Full Time Geriatric Care Management: 8
Service Area
Metropolitan Area(s): Seattle
Counties: King
States: WA
Areas of Practice: 1, 2, 3, 4, 5, 6, 7, 8, 10, 12

Joyce A. Robbins, MSW, CSW
Geriatric Services Inc.
P.O. Box 18223   8634 Crownhill
San Antonio, TX 78218   San Antonio, TX 78209
(512) 822-9494   (512) 822-9494
Years in Full Time Geriatric Care Management: 6
Service Area
Metropolitan Area(s): San Antonio
Counties: Bexar, Area Code 512
States: TX
Areas of Practice: 1, 2, 3, 4, 5, 6, 7, 8, 9, 10, 11, 12

Storm Rogers
Aging/Options!
171 Franklin Road
Glencoe, IL 60022
(708) 835-3183
Years in Full Time Geriatric Care Management:
Service Area
Metropolitan Area(s): Chicago
Counties: Northern Cook
States: IL
Areas of Practice: 1, 2, 3, 4, 5, 6, 7, 8, 9, 10, 12

Roberta Rosenberg, MSW
AgeWise Family Services
1250 Glenburnie
Dresher, PA 19025
(215) 659-2111
Years in Full Time Geriatric Care Management: 2
Service Area
Metropolitan Area(s): Area Codes 215, 609
Counties: Philadelphia, Montgomery, Bucks, Delaware
States: PA, Southern NJ
Areas of Practice: 1, 2, 3, 4, 5, 6, 7, 8, 9, 10, 11, 12

Irene H. Ross
Ctr. for Interpersonal Relations, Inc.
346 Pomfret Street
Putnam, CT 06260
(203) 928-5967
Years in Full Time Geriatric Care Management: 5
Service Area
Metropolitan Area(s): 10 towns of Northeast Connecticut, adjacent Rhode
    Island, Massachusetts
Counties: Windham, New London
States: Northeastern CT, MA, RI
Areas of Practice: 1, 2, 3, 4, 5, 6, 7, 8, 9, 10, 11, 12

Joncie Rowland
Shepard Services
229 East 67th St.
New York, NY 10028
(212) 737-5510
Years in Full Time Geriatric Care Management: 15
Service Area
Metropolitan Area(s): Area Code 212
Counties: New York, Kings, Bronx
States: NY
Areas of Practice: 1, 2, 4, 5, 6, 7, 8, 9, 10

Eleanor Rubin, MA
Older Adult Resources & Service, Inc.
59 Second Street
South Orange, NJ 07079
(201) 763-8018
Years in Full Time Geriatric Care Management: 6
Service Area
Metropolitan Area(s): Northern & Central New Jersey
Counties: Essex, Union, Somerset, Morris, Passaic
States: NJ
Areas of Practice: 1, 2, 3, 5, 6, 7, 8, 9, 10, 11, 12

Gabriel Russo
400 Brian Court
Merced, CA 95348
(209) 722-4273
Years in Full Time Geriatric Care Management: 7
Service Area
Metropolitan Area(s): Merced, Atwater, Chowchila, Los Banos
Counties: Merced
States: CA
Areas of Practice: 1, 2, 3, 4, 5, 7, 8, 9, 12

Carol A. Saez-Henry
Vintage, Inc.
401 North Highland Avenue
Pittsburgh, PA 15206
(412) 361-5003
Years in Full Time Geriatric Care Management: 18
Service Area
Metropolitan Area(s): Pittsburgh
Counties: Allegheny
States: PA
Areas of Practice: 1, 3, 5, 6, 7, 8, 9, 10, 11

Lynn Sageser, MSW
Sageser & Associates
2 Coventry Court
Edmond, OK 73034
(405) 341-5390
Years in Full Time Geriatric Care Management:
Service Area
Metropolitan Area(s): Metropolitan Oklahoma City
Counties:
States: OK
Areas of Practice: 1, 2, 3, 5, 6, 7, 8, 9, 10, 11, 12

Arlene Saks, MSW, LCSW
Social Work Associates, Inc.
101 West Read Street, Suite 622
Baltimore, MD 21201
(410) 727-1717   (410) 938-2429 Pager
Years in Full Time Geriatric Care Management: 13
Service Area
Metropolitan Area(s): All of state
Counties: All counties in Maryland
States: MD, D.C.
Areas of Practice: 1, 2, 3, 4, 5, 6, 7, 8, 9, 10, 11, 12

Geri Sams, CSW-ACP, ACSW
Geri-Options
2611 Crestwood
P.O. Box 24457
Denton, TX 76204-2457
(817) 566-0902
Years in Full Time Geriatric Care Management:
Service Area
Metropolitan Area(s): Denton County area
Counties: Denton, Wise, Cooke
States: TX
Areas of Practice: 1, 2, 3, 5, 6, 7, 8, 9, 10, 11

Barbara Sanders, MA, LSW
Sanders & Associates
1140 Shady Lane
Wheaton, IL 60187
(708) 260-0012
Years in Full Time Geriatric Care Management: 8
Service Area
Metropolitan Area(s): Chicago Suburbs
Counties: DuPage, East Kane, West Cook
States: IL
Areas of Practice: 1, 2, 3, 4, 5, 6, 7, 8, 9, 10, 11, 12
Durable Power of Attorney & Guardianship

Sheila L. Saunders, MS
Senior Solutions
44 South Fulton Street
Allentown, PA 18102
(215) 435-6677
Years in Full Time Geriatric Care Management: 9
Service Area
Metropolitan Area(s): Allentown, Bethlehem, Easton, Quakertown, Poconos
Counties: Lehigh, Northampton, Bucks, Berks, & Carbon
States: PA
Areas of Practice: 1, 2, 3, 5, 6, 7, 8, 9, 10, 11, 12

Margaret E. Sayers, GNP
Laping, Sayers and Associates
1109 Delaware Avenue
Buffalo, NY 14209
(716) 884-3277
Years in Full Time Geriatric Care Management: 2
Service Area
Metropolitan Area(s): Buffalo, New York
Counties: Erie, Niagara
States: NY
Areas of Practice: 1, 2, 3, 4, 5, 6, 7, 8, 9, 10

Brenda H. Schimmel, MSW
Family Partner, Inc.
P.O. Box 12311
Sarasota, FL 34278
(813) 351-1516
Years in Full Time Geriatric Care Management: 7
Service Area
Metropolitan Area(s): Sarasota, Bradenton, Venice
Counties: Sarasota, Manatee
States: FL
Areas of Practice:

Miriam Scholl, MSW, CSW
19 Minkel Road
Ossining, NY 10562
(914) 762-7438
Years in Full Time Geriatric Care Management: 4
Service Area
Metropolitan Area(s): New York City
Counties: Westchester
States: NY
Areas of Practice: 1, 2, 5, 6, 7, 8, 10, 11, 12

Andrea Seewald, MSW
Senior Care Consultants
5646 Marlborough Road
Pittsburgh, PA 15217
(412) 421-9171
Years in Full Time Geriatric Care Management: 1
Service Area
Metropolitan Area(s): Metropolitan Pittsburgh
Counties: Allegheny, Westmoreland, Beaver, Butler
States: Southwestern PA
Areas of Practice: 1, 2, 3, 5, 6, 7, 8, 9, 10

Rita Seiden, PhD, CSW
Elder Family Services
464 Ninth Street
Brooklyn, NY 11215
(718) 788-2461
Years in Full Time Geriatric Care Management: 8
Service Area
Metropolitan Area(s): Brooklyn, Staten Island, Nassau
Counties: Kings, Nassau, Richmond
States: NY
Areas of Practice: 1, 2, 3, 4, 5, 6, 7, 8, 10, 11, 12

Beverly J. Shannon, MA
Extended Family Associates
820 Walnut Street
San Luis Obispo, CA 93401
(805) 543-3389
Years in Full Time Geriatric Care Management: 3
Service Area
Metropolitan Area(s): Area Code 805
San Luis Obispo
Counties:
States: CA
Areas of Practice: 1, 2, 5, 6, 7, 8, 9, 10, 11, 12

Jeanne Sharp, MPH
Sally Winsby & Company
37 West 57th Street, 14th Floor
New York, NY 10019
(212) 371-4727
Years in Full Time Geriatric Care Management: 7
Service Area
Metropolitan Area(s): Greater New York City
Counties: Manhattan, Queens, Kings, Richmond, Bronx, Nassau
States: NY
Areas of Practice: 1, 2, 3, 5, 6, 7, 8, 9, 10, 11, 12

Bernice Shepard, MSW
Shepard Services Inc.
229 East 67th Street
New York, NY 10021
(212) 737-5510
Years in Full Time Geriatric Care Management: 15
Service Area
Metropolitan Area(s): Area Code 212
Counties: New York, Kings, Bronx
States: NY
Areas of Practice: 1, 2, 4, 5, 6, 7, 8, 9, 10

Diane K. Sherwood, MSW, ACSW
Sherwood Associates
228 West 260th Street
Riverdale, NY 10471
(212) 548-0609
Years in Full Time Geriatric Care Management: 1
Service Area
Metropolitan Area(s): Bronx, Manhattan
Counties: Westchester
States: NY, Long distance caregiving nationally
Areas of Practice: 1, 2, 3, 5, 6, 7, 8, 9, 10, 11, 12

Mary Ellen Siegel, MSW
75-68 195th Street
Fresh Meadows, NY 11366
(718) 465-1908
Years in Full Time Geriatric Care Management: 7
Service Area
Metropolitan Area(s): Queens, Manhattan, Nassau
Counties:
States: New York
Areas of Practice: 1, 2, 3, 4, 5, 6, 7, 8, 9, 10, 11, 12

Thomas Skoloda, PhD
P.O. Box 455
Lyndell, PA 19354
(215) 942-2232
Years in Full Time Geriatric Care Management: 10
Service Area
Metropolitan Area(s):
Counties: Westchester
States: PA
Areas of Practice: 1, 2, 3, 4, 5, 7, 8, 9, 10

Cheryl A. Smith, MA
Kansas City Home & Health Care Service, Inc.
7922 State Line Road, Suite 1
Prairie Village, KS 66208
(913) 642-2074
Years in Full Time Geriatric Care Management: 6
Service Area
Metropolitan Area(s): Kansas City, MO & Kansas City, KS
Counties: In Missouri: Jackson, Clay County
In Kansas: Johnson
States: KS, MO
Areas of Practice: 1, 2, 3, 5, 6, 7, 8, 9, 10, 12

G. Nadine Smith, RN, BSN
Sharing Care
4512 Park Lake Terrace N
Bradenton, FL 34209
(813) 794-1631
Years in Full Time Geriatric Care Management:
Service Area
Metropolitan Area(s): Manatee County
Counties: Manatee
States: FL
Areas of Practice: 1, 2, 3, 6, 7, 8, 9, 10, 11

Geri Smith, MSW, LCSW, BCD
Life Care Continuum, Inc.
1320 South Federal Highway, Suite 108
Stuart, FL 34994
(407) 288-2273
Years in Full Time Geriatric Care Management: 6
Service Area
Metropolitan Area(s): Stuart, Port St. Lucie, Jupiter
Counties: Martin, St. Lucie, North Palm Beach
States: FL
Areas of Practice: 1, 2, 3, 4, 5, 6, 7, 8, 9, 10, 11, 12

Marsha York Solmssen, MSS, ACSW, LSW
Intervention Associates
P.O. Box 572
Wayne, PA 19087
(215) 254-9001
Years in Full Time Geriatric Care Management: 8
Service Area
Metropolitan Area(s): Philadelphia
Counties: Philadelphia, Bucks, Chester, Montgomery, Delaware
States: Southeastern PA
Areas of Practice: 1, 2, 3, 5, 6, 7, 8, 9, 10, 11, 12

Naomi Solomon, MSW, ACSW, BCD
Senior Care Consultants
1 Barstow Road
Great Neck, NY 11021
(516) 466-8864
Years in Full Time Geriatric Care Management: 2.5
Service Area
Metropolitan Area(s): Area Codes (516) & (718)
Counties: Queens, West Suffolk, Nassau
States: NY
Areas of Practice: 1, 2, 3, 4, 5, 6, 7, 8, 9, 10, 11, 12

Joan Sud Soreff
25 Highland Street
Portland, ME 04103
(207) 775-2181
Years in Full Time Geriatric Care Management: 5
Service Area
Metropolitan Area(s): Portland, South Maine
Counties: Rockingham, New Hampshire
States: ME, NH
Areas of Practice: 1, 3, 4, 5, 6, 7, 8, 9, 10, 11

Ann Sorgen, MA, RN
P.O. Box 1381
Ross, CA 94957
(415) 461-2356
Years in Full Time Geriatric Care Management: 7
Service Area
Metropolitan Area(s): San Francisco Bay Area
Counties: Marin, Sonoma, Contra Costa, San Mateo, Santa Clara
States: CA
Areas of Practice: 1, 2, 3, 4, 5, 6, 7, 8, 9, 10

B. J. Curry Spitler, MSW, PhD, LCSW
Age Concerns Inc.
2546 4th Avenue
San Diego, CA 92103
(619) 544-1622
Years in Full Time Geriatric Care Management: 10
Service Area
Metropolitan Area(s): San Diego
Counties:
States: CA
Areas of Practice: 1, 2, 3, 4, 5, 6, 7, 8, 9, 10, 11, 12

Sandra Steinman, MA, CSW, DSW
401 East 80 Street, Suite 19B
New York, NY 10021
(212) 517-3103
Years in Full Time Geriatric Care Management: 12
Service Area
Metropolitan Area(s): Metropolitan New York
Counties:
States: NY, NJ, CT
Areas of Practice: 1, 3, 4, 5, 7, 8, 9

Sylvia A. Stevens, MSW, ACSW
Stevens & Associates
612 North Signal Butte
Apache Jct., AZ 85220
(602) 986-4210
Years in Full Time Geriatric Care Management: 10
Service Area
Metropolitan Area(s): Mesa, East Mesa
Counties:
States: AZ
Areas of Practice: 1, 2, 5, 6, 7, 8, 10, 12

Helena A. Stewart, RN, MSG
Retirement & Transition Inc.
P.O. Box 451
Bryn Mawr, PA 19010
(215) 527-4578
Years in Full Time Geriatric Care Management: 3
Service Area
Metropolitan Area(s): Greater Philadelphia
Counties: Philadelphia, Delaware, Chester, Montgomery, Bucks
States: PA
Areas of Practice: 1, 2, 3, 5, 6, 7, 8, 10, 12

Emily S. Stuhlbarg
Schapp - Miller - Stuhlbarg
25550 Hawthorne Blvd. #212   215 Long Beach Blvd., Suite 414
Torrance, CA 90505   Long Beach, CA 90802
(213) 375-1968   (213) 491-0390
Years in Full Time Geriatric Care Management: 6
Service Area
Metropolitan Area(s): Torrance, Long Beach
Counties: Southeast and Southwest Los Angeles, Orange
States: CA
Areas of Practice: 1, 2, 3, 5, 6, 7, 8, 10, 11, 12, Conservatorship

Victoria Sears Thaler
Golden Years Counseling Services
P.O. Box 24
Chestnut Hill, MA 02167
(617) 739-1609
Years in Full Time Geriatric Care Management: 18
Service Area
Metropolitan Area(s): Metropolitan Boston, Outer Cape Cod
Counties: Norfolk, Suffolk, Middlesex, Barnstable
States: MA
Areas of Practice: 1, 2, 4, 5, 7, 8, 10, Long term monitoring

Jenny P. Thayer
Geriatric Counseling
22318 San Joaquin Drive West
Canyon Lake, CA 92587
(714) 244-6680
Years in Full Time Geriatric Care Management: 7
Service Area
Metropolitan Area(s): Riverside, Corona, Lake Elsinor
Counties: Riverside
States: CA
Areas of Practice: 1, 2, 5, 7, 8, 9, 10, 11, 12

Catherine C. Thompson, PhD, ACSW
Sterling Care Counseling, Inc.
962 Washington Road
Pittsburgh, PA 15228
(412) 344-5011
Years in Full Time Geriatric Care Management: 3
Service Area
Metropolitan Area(s): Greater Pittsburgh
Counties: Allegheny, Butler, Beaver, Washington
States: PA
Areas of Practice: 1, 2, 3, 4, 5, 6, 7, 8, 9, 10, 11

Marion Thompson, MSW, LSW, BCD
Intervention Associates, Inc.
P.O. Box 572
Wayne, PA 19087
(215) 254-9001
Years in Full Time Geriatric Care Management: 8
Service Area
Metropolitan Area(s): Philadelphia
Counties: Philadelphia, Montgomery, Delaware, Bucks, Chester
States: Southeastern PA
Areas of Practice: 1, 2, 3, 4, 5, 6, 7, 8, 9, 10, 11, 12

Mary Thorman
TLC for Seniors, Inc.
13896 Dominica Drive
Seminole, FL 34646
(813) 595-2000   (800) 729-8907
Years in Full Time Geriatric Care Management:
Service Area
Metropolitan Area(s): Clearwater, Dunedin, Clearwater Beach, Largo,
    Seminole, St. Petersburg, Suncoast Beaches, Pinellas Park
Counties: Pinellas
States: FL
Areas of Practice: 1, 2, 3, 5, 6, 7, 8, 9, 10, 11

Mona Thornton, LCSW
Senior Care Consultants
5048 North Drake
Chicago, IL 60625
(312) 588-8670
Years in Full Time Geriatric Care Management: 1
Service Area
Metropolitan Area(s): Metro Chicago
Counties:
States: IL
Areas of Practice: 1, 2, 3, 4, 5, 6, 7, 8, 9, 10, 11, 12

Judith S. Tobenkin, MS, MSG
Gerontology Consultants
353 S. Palm Drive
Beverly Hills, CA 90212
(310) 273-3548
Years in Full Time Geriatric Care Management: 8
Service Area
Metropolitan Area(s): Area Code 213, Greater Los Angeles San Fernando
    Valley, Los Angeles
Counties: Santa Monica, Beverly Hills
States: CA
Areas of Practice: 1, 2, 3, 4, 5, 6, 7, 8, 9, 10, 11, 12

Susan Townshend, RN
Long Term Planning Assoc., Inc.
5 Sweetwater Street
Saugus, MA 01906
(617) 231-2616
Years in Full Time Geriatric Care Management: 6
Service Area
Metropolitan Area(s): Area codes 413, 617, 508
Counties: All MA Counties
States: MA
Areas of Practice: 1, 2, 3, 6, 7, 8, 10, 11

Kathryn L. Volino
C.O.P.E. - Creative Options in
Planning for the Elderly
82 Ferndale Avenue
Glen Rock, NJ 07452
(201) 652-3322
Years in Full Time Geriatric Care Management: 8
Service Area
Metropolitan Area(s): Northern New Jersey
Counties: Bergen, Passaic, Morris & Hudson
States: NJ
Areas of Practice: 1, 2, 3, 5, 6, 7, 8, 9, 10, 11, 12

Jean M. Walsh, RN, MSN
Wise Generation Resources Inc.
100 Denniston Avenue
Pittsburgh, PA 15206
(412) 441-4342
Years in Full Time Geriatric Care Management: 2.5
Service Area
Metropolitan Area(s): Greater Pittsburgh, Area Code 412
Counties: Allegheny, Westmoreland, Butler, Beaver, Washington
States: PA
Areas of Practice: 1, 2, 3, 5, 6, 7, 8, 9, 10, 11, 12

Braden L. Walter, PhD
Secour Care Management
121 North Highland Avenue
Pittsburgh, PA 15206
(412) 661-6730
Years in Full Time Geriatric Care Management:
Service Area
Metropolitan Area(s): Metropolitan Pittsburgh
Counties: Allegheny, Surrounding area
States: PA
Areas of Practice: 1, 2, 3, 4, 5, 6, 7, 8, 9, 10, 11, 12

Leah Weiss, MSW, ACSW
Older Adult Resources & Services, Inc.
59 Second Street
South Orange, NJ 07079
(201) 763-8018
Years in Full Time Geriatric Care Management: 6
Service Area
Metropolitan Area(s): Northern and Central New Jersey
Counties: Essex, Union, Somerset, Morris, Passaic
States: NJ
Areas of Practice: 1, 2, 3, 5, 6, 7, 8, 9, 10, 11, 12

Susan P. Weiss, MA
AgeWise Family Services
1250 Glenburnie Lane
Dresher, PA 19025
(215) 659-2111
Years in Full Time Geriatric Care Management: 20
Service Area
Metropolitan Area(s): Area Codes 215, 609
Counties: Philadelphia, Montgomery, Bucks, Delaware
States: PA, Southern NJ
Areas of Practice: 1, 2, 3, 4, 5, 6, 7, 8, 9, 10, 11, 12

Roberta Weissglass, MEd
Personal and Financial Services
P.O. Box 31015
Santa Barbara, CA 93130-1015
(805) 563-2436
Years in Full Time Geriatric Care Management: 6
Service Area
Metropolitan Area(s): Santa Barbara
Counties: Santa Barbara
States: CA
Areas of Practice: 1, 2, 3, 5, 6, 7, 8, 9, 10, 12

Carol Westheimer
Independent Living, Inc.
1425 Beacon Street
Newton, MA 02168
(617) 332-1710
Years in Full Time Geriatric Care Management: 19
Service Area
Metropolitan Area(s): Greater Boston area to Route 495
Counties:
States: MA
Areas of Practice: 1, 2, 3, 5, 6, 7, 8, 9, 10, 12

Nancy Wexler
Gerontology Associates
19225 Rosita Street
Tarzana, CA 91356
(818) 342-3136(818) 708-8538
Years in Full Time Geriatric Care Management: 10
Service Area
Metropolitan Area(s): Area Codes 310, 213, 818, 805
Counties: Ventura, Los Angeles
States: CA
Areas of Practice: 1, 2, 3, 4, 5, 6, 7, 8, 9, 10, 11, 12

Lucy B. Whelchel, MA
Whelchel & Associates
5315 Woodland Circle
Gainesville, GA 30504
(404) 534-3360
Years in Full Time Geriatric Care Management: 1.5
Service Area
Metropolitan Area(s): Metropolitan Atlanta
Counties: Hall, Fulton, DeKalb, Cobb, Gwinnett
States: GA
Areas of Practice: 1, 2, 3, 6, 7, 8, 9, 10

Barbara R. Whitley, MSW, MEd
Private Case Management
2078 Minton Road
West Melbourne, FL 32904
(407) 768-0092
Years in Full Time Geriatric Care Management: 2
Service Area
Metropolitan Area(s): Melbourne, Cocoa, Palm Bay
Counties: Brevard
States: FL
Areas of Practice: 1, 2, 3, 5, 6, 7, 8, 9, 10, 11

Carol Will, RN, MA
Will's Consulting
RR #2, Box 428
Keokuk, IA 52632
(319) 524-7656
Years in Full Time Geriatric Care Management: 4
Service Area
Metropolitan Area(s): Keokuk
Counties: In Iowa: Lee; In Illinois: Hancock;
In Missouri: Clark
States: IA, IL, MO
Areas of Practice: 1, 2, 3, 6, 7, 8, 9, 10

Rina Winckler
Alpha Care Management, Inc.
1020 NE 98th Street
Miami, FL 33138
(305) 751-1020
Years in Full Time Geriatric Care Management: 10
Service Area
Metropolitan Area(s): Miami, Ft. Lauderdale, Palm Beach, Boca Raton
Counties: Dade, Broward, Palm Beach
States: FL
Areas of Practice: 1, 2, 3, 4, 5, 6, 7, 8, 9, 10, 11, 12

Mark Winterman, MSW, MSG
Alternatives-Senior Care Consultants
8009 Lemon Avenue
La Mesa, CA 91941
(619) 464-6560
Years in Full Time Geriatric Care Management: 1
Service Area
Metropolitan Area(s): San Diego
Counties: San Diego
States: CA
Areas of Practice: 1, 2, 3, 5, 6, 7, 8, 9, 10, 11

Gordon P. Wolfe, SMW, LCSW
Human Network Systems, Inc.
1410 Grant Street, Suite B304
Denver, CO 80203
(303) 831-1996
Years in Full Time Geriatric Care Management: 6
Service Area
Metropolitan Area(s): Denver Metro area and Mtn. area code (303)
Counties:
States: CO
Areas of Practice: 1, 2, 3, 5, 6, 7, 8, 9, 10, 11

Hannah F. Zacher
Geriatric Consultants
3637 Rosewood Drive
Fort Wayne, IN 46804
(219) 432-2150
Years in Full Time Geriatric Care Management: 6
Service Area
Metropolitan Area(s): Indiana
Counties: Allen, DeKalb, Kosciusko
States: IN
Areas of Practice: 1, 2, 3, 4, 5, 6, 7, 8, 10

Miriam Zucker, MSW
Directions in Aging
1-B Quaker Ridge Road
New Rochelle, NY 10804
(914) 699-6963
Years in Full Time Geriatric Care Management: 4
Service Area
Metropolitan Area(s): Greater New York, Lower Connecticut
Counties: Westchester, Fairfield, Upper Bronx
States: NY, CT
Areas of Practice: 1, 2, 3, 5, 6, 7, 8, 9, 10, 11

DIRECTORY OF PART-TIME PRACTITIONERS IN GERIATRIC CARE MANAGEMENT

Lucille Alan
960 Trapelo Road
Waltham, MA 02154-4846
(617) 894-8405
Years in Geriatric Care Management: 13
Service Area
Metropolitan Area(s): Metro West Boston
Counties:
States: MA
Areas of Practice: 1, 3, 4, 5, 7, 8

Nancy Alexander, JD, MSW, ACSW, CISW
Complete Care Management
1005 North Caribe
Tucson, AZ 85710
(602) 886-7602
(800) 669-3949
Years in Geriatric Care Management: 6
Service Area
Metropolitan Area(s): Arizona
Counties:
States: AZ
Areas of Practice: 1, 2, 3, 4, 5, 6, 7, 8, 9, 10, 11, 12, Legal Support Service, Nursing Support Service

Anita K. Anderson, CSW
P.O. Box 0
El Cerrito, CA 94530
(415) 237-5970

Years in Geriatric Care Management:

Service Area
Metropolitan Area(s): San Francisco, East Bay
Counties: Contra Costa, Alameda
States: CA
Areas of Practice: 1, 2, 3, 4, 5, 6, 7, 8, 9, 10, 11

Patricia Kern Banzhoff, MS, NHA
350 North 25th Street
Camp Hill, PA 17011
(717) 737-2166

Years in Geriatric Care Management: 1.5

Service Area
Metropolitan Area(s): Harrisburg and neighboring
Counties: Dauphin, Cumberland, Perry, Northern York, Western Lancaster, Lebanon
States: PA
Areas of Practice: 1, 2, 3, 4, 5, 7, 8, 9, 10

Edith W. Bayme, MSW, CSW
3720 Independence Avenue
Bronx, NY 10463
(212) 884-5749

Years in Geriatric Care Management: 4

Service Area
Metropolitan Area(s): Area Codes: 212, 718, 914
Counties: New York City, Bronx, lower Westchester
States: NY
Areas of Practice: 1, 2, 4, 5, 6, 7, 8, 9, 10, 11, 12

Frank E. Baskin, BCD
18 East Meadow Lane
Lowell, MA 01854
(508) 458-1512

Years in Geriatric Care Management: 8

Service Area
Metropolitan Area(s): Merrimack Valley
Counties: Essex, Middlesex, Suffolk
States: MA
Areas of Practice: 1, 2, 3, 4, 5, 6, 7, 8, 9, 10

Miriam Berman
H.E.L.P. for Elders, Inc.
812 Bromton Drive
Westbury, NY 11590
(516) 334-1131

Years in Geriatric Care Management: 1

Service Area
Metropolitan Area(s): New York City
Counties: Nassau, Western Suffolk
States: NY
Areas of Practice: 1, 2, 5, 6, 7, 8, 9, 10, 11

Louise O. Bernstein, MSW, ACSW, CISW
Elder Family Service of Connecticut
37 Columbus Place, Suite 1
Stamford, CT 06907
(203) 329-2750
(203) 847-3582
Years in Geriatric Care Management: 3
Service Area
Metropolitan Area(s):
Counties: Fairfield
States: CT
Areas of Practice: 1, 2, 3, 5, 6, 7, 8, 9, 10, 11

Toby Bernstein
Elder Assist
140 Woodbine Drive
Mill Valley, CA 94941
(415) 388-5972
[no information provided]

Karen Bowman
5150 North Sixth, Suite 149
Fresno, CA 93710
(209) 445-3924
Years in Geriatric Care Management: 1
Service Area
Metropolitan Area(s):
Counties: Kings, Madera
States: CA
Areas of Practice: 1, 2, 3, 5, 6, 7, 8, 9, 10, 12

Gail Busillo, CSW, BCD
Geriatric Social Work Services
245-27 Walden Avenue
Great Neck, NY 11020
(516) 487-0973
Years in Geriatric Care Management: 4
Service Area
Metropolitan Area(s): Area Codes 516, 718
Counties: Nassau, Queens
States: NY
Areas of Practice: 1, 2, 3, 4, 5, 6, 7, 8, 9, 10

Margaret Cohn, RN, PhD
Family Ties
765 West Hamilton Avenue
State College, PA 16801
(814) 237-1549
Years in Geriatric Care Management: 2
Service Area
Metropolitan Area(s):
Counties: Centre
States: PA
Areas of Practice: 1, 2, 3, 4, 5, 6, 7, 8, 9, 10, 11

Nancy C. Crawford, CSWR, BCD
Elderly & Family Counseling Service
200 MacArthur Drive
Buffalo, NY 14221
(716) 634-0906
Years in Geriatric Care Management: 8
Service Area
Metropolitan Area(s): Greater Buffalo
Counties: Erie
States: NY
Areas of Practice: 1, 2, 3, 4, 5, 6, 7, 8, 9, 10, 11, 12

Doris Davis, ACSW, LCSW
2920 Clark Road, #202
Sarasota, FL 34231
(813) 922-9301
Years in Geriatric Care Management:
Service Area
Metropolitan Area(s): Sarasota, Bradenton, Venice
Counties: Manatee, Sarasota
States: FL
Areas of Practice: 1, 2, 5, 7, 8, 9, 10, 11

Patricia C. de Ganahl, RN
Senior Care Services
20 Avenue at the Common, Suite 104
Shrewsbury, NJ 07702-4531
(908) 747-7517
Years in Geriatric Care Management: 4
Service Area
Metropolitan Area(s): Red Bank Area
Counties: Monmouth
States: NJ
Areas of Practice: 1, 2, 3, 5, 6, 7, 8, 9, 10, 11, 12

Jeanne M. Dionne, LCSW
Generations
104 Nottingham Drive
Centerville, MA 02632
(508) 420-5259
Years in Geriatric Care Management: 5
Service Area
Metropolitan Area(s): Barnstable, Cape Cod & the Islands
Counties:
States: MA
Areas of Practice: 1, 2, 5, 6, 7, 8, 9, 10, 12

Elaine A. Dively, ACSW, LSW
4069 Hill Street
Library, PA 15129
(412) 833-3076
Years in Geriatric Care Management: 1
Service Area
Metropolitan Area(s): Pittsburgh Area
Counties:
States: PA
Areas of Practice: 1, 2, 3, 5, 6, 7, 8, 9, 10, 12

Adele Elkind, CSW
343 Old Cedar Road
Hartsdale, NY 10530
(914) 948-9421
Years in Geriatric Care Management: 20
Service Area
Metropolitan Area(s): All of New York State
Counties:
States: NY
Areas of Practice: 1, 2, 3, 4, 5, 6, 7, 8, 9

Esther Feigenbaum, MSW, CSW
73-58 189 Street
Flushing, NY 11366
(718) 740-1509
Years in Geriatric Care Management: 8
Service Area
Metropolitan Area(s): Queens, Nassau, Brooklyn, Bronx, Westchester,
  Manhattan
Counties:
States: NY
Areas of Practice: 1, 2, 3, 4, 5, 6, 7, 8, 9, 10, 11, 12

Alice Feldman
One Walworth Terrace
White Plains, NY 10606
(914) 681-1340
Years in Geriatric Care Management: 20
Service Area
Metropolitan Area(s): Westchester
Counties:
States: NY
Areas of Practice: 1, 2, 3, 6, 7, 8, 10, 12

Jane Chapin Frankenstein, ACSW
Life Care Networks, Inc.
4221 Rurode Lane
Fort Wayne, IN 46809
(219) 747-5016
(219) 422-9077
Years in Geriatric Care Management: 20
Service Area
Metropolitan Area(s):
Counties:
States: IN
Areas of Practice: 1, 2, 3, 4, 5, 6, 7, 8, 9, 10, 11, 12

Mary Fresiello, RN, BS
Gerontological Care Services
135 Trap Falls Extension
Huntington, CT 06484
(203) 926-9643
Years in Geriatric Care Management: 10
Service Area
Metropolitan Area(s): Huntington
Counties:
States: CT
Areas of Practice: 1, 2, 3, 5, 6, 7, 8, 9, 10, 12

Vivian E. Greenberg, ACSW
106 West Franklin Avenue, Suite F-122
Pennington, NJ 08534
(609) 737-6365
Years in Geriatric Care Management: 16
Service Area
Metropolitan Area(s):
Counties: Mercer
States: NJ
Areas of Practice: 3, 4, 5, 6, 7, 8

Alan J. Guire
Extended Care Planning Service
P.O. Box 1632
Middletown, CT 06457
(203) 537-6093
[no information provided]

Edna Hammer, MSW, ACSW, Diplomat Status
Greensboro Geriatric Consultant
1101 North Elm Street, Apt. 602
Greensboro, NC 27401
(919) 275-3908
Years in Geriatric Care Management: 10
Service Area
Metropolitan Area(s): High Point, Salisbury
Counties:
States: NC
Areas of Practice: 1, 2, 3, 4, 5, 7, 8, 9, 10, 11, 12

Norma B. Heisler, MSW
2373 East 7th Street
Brooklyn, NY 11223
(718) 615-5247
Years in Geriatric Care Management: 3
Service Area
Metropolitan Area(s): Brooklyn
Counties: Kings
States: NY
Areas of Practice: 1, 3, 4, 5, 6, 7, 8, 9, 11

Jean Hope
Family Options, Inc.
RR 2094
Dushore, PA 18614
(717) 928-9202
[no information provided]

Claire Jacobs, BA, BSW
Geriatric Counseling Associates
441 Orange Street
New Haven, CT 06511
(203) 785-1496
Years in Geriatric Care Management: 10
Service Area
Metropolitan Area(s): New Haven, Milford, Hamden
Counties: All of New Haven
States: CT
Areas of Practice: 1, 2, 3, 5, 6, 7, 8, 9, 10, 11, 12

Sherry A. Johanson, BSN, MPA
HealthCare Consultant
12 Barn Road
Mill Valley, CA 94941
(415) 389-1434

Years in Geriatric Care Management: 3

Service Area
Metropolitan Area(s): San Francisco, San Jose, Oakland, Richmond,
  Berkeley, Sacramento
Counties: Marin, Sonoma, San Francisco, Santa Clara, San Mateo, Napa,
  Alemeda, Contra Costa
States: CA
Areas of Practice: 1, 2, 3, 5, 7, 8, 9, 10, 12

Steven Kleitzel
281 Garth Road, #C1J
Scarsdale, NY 10583-4039

[no information provided]

John Koppenaal, CSW
Shiloh Counseling Center
P.O. Box 436
Germantown, NY 12526
(518) 537-5262

Years in Geriatric Care Management:

Service Area
Metropolitan Area(s):
Counties: Dutchess, Columbia, Ulster
States: NY
Areas of Practice: 1, 2, 3, 4, 5, 6, 7, 8, 9, 10, 11, 12

Roberta Litvinoff
Geriatric Counseling Associates
441 Orange Street
New Haven, CT 06511
(203) 785-1496

Years in Geriatric Care Management: 10

Service Area
Metropolitan Area(s): New Haven, Milford, Hamden
Counties: All of New Haven
States: CT
Areas of Practice: 1, 2, 3, 5, 6, 7, 8, 9, 10, 11, 12

Roslyn Robinson Mann
Elder Resource Network
RD 2, Box 259C
Patterson, NY 12563
(914) 878-6707

Years in Geriatric Care Management: 15

Service Area
Metropolitan Area(s):
Counties: N. Westchester, Putnam, Dutchess, Fairfield
States: NY, CT
Areas of Practice: 1, 2, 3, 5, 6, 7, 8, 9, 10, 11, 12

Sue McConnell
Adult Care Services, Inc.
1213 Potomac Avenue
Hagerstown, MD 21740
(301) 797-1115
[no information provided]

Jane G. Morrison, MSW, LSW
Elder Help
46 Lake Street
Auburn, ME 04210
(207) 783-7862
Years in Geriatric Care Management: 12

Service Area
Metropolitan Area(s): Southern & Central Maine
Counties: York, Cumberland, Franklin
States: ME
Areas of Practice: 1, 2, 3, 5, 6, 7, 8, 9, 10, 11, 12

Sara Myers, MA
Elder Care Resources
1800 Boylston, Suite 104
Seattle, WA 98122
(206) 324-5695
Years in Geriatric Care Management:

Service Area
Metropolitan Area(s): Seattle
Counties: King
States: WA
Areas of Practice: 1, 2, 3, 4, 5, 6, 7, 10

Phyllis A. Norman
North Oakland Counseling and Geriatric Consultation Center
6401 Citation Drive
Clarkston, MI 48346
(313) 620-1019
Years in Geriatric Care Management: 9

Service Area
Metropolitan Area(s):
Counties: Oakland, McComb, Genesee
States: MI
Areas of Practice: 1, 2, 3, 4, 5, 6, 7, 8, 9, 10

Carolyn E. Paul
1849 Santa Rosa Court
Claremont, CA 91711
(714) 625-3085
[no information provided]

Ellen Lurie Polivy, CSW, CEAP
Lurie Family Assistance Network
326 West 83rd Street
New York, NY 10024
(212) 362-2076
Years in Geriatric Care Management: 2
Service Area
Metropolitan Area(s): New York Metro Area
Counties:
States: NY
Areas of Practice: 1, 2, 3, 4, 5, 6, 7, 8, 9, 10, 11, 12

Susan Ratner
Professional Care Consultants
35 East 85th Street
New York, NY 10028
[no information provided]

Connie Rosenberg, MPS, RN, C
Services & Resources for Seniors
930 Mt. Kemble Avenue
Morristown, NJ 07960
(201) 984-3707
Years in Geriatric Care Management: 4.5
Service Area
Metropolitan Area(s): Northern New Jersey Area Codes 201, Part of 908
Counties:
States: NJ
Areas of Practice: 1, 2, 3, 5, 6, 7, 8, 9, 10, 11, 12

Myrna Rudman, LCSW
MLR Associates
P.O. Box 161624
Sacramento, CA 95816
(916) 927-1895
Years in Geriatric Care Management: 10
Service Area
Metropolitan Area(s): Sacramento & Surrounding Area
Counties:
States: CA
Areas of Practice: 1, 2, 3, 4, 5, 6, 7, 8, 10

Maura C. Ryan, PhD, RN, C
ElderOptions
39 High Point
Cedar Grove, NJ 07009
(201) 857-8856
Years in Geriatric Care Management: 2.5
Service Area
Metropolitan Area(s): Northern New Jersey
Counties:
States: NJ
Areas of Practice: 1, 2, 3, 5, 6, 7, 8, 9, 10, 12

Gloria Scherma, MPS
Multi-Comprehensive Counseling
1618 West Third Street
Brooklyn, NY 11223
(718) 921-8572
Years in Geriatric Care Management: 10
Service Area
Metropolitan Area(s): Area Codes: 212, 718, 914, 516
Counties:
States: NY
Areas of Practice: 1, 2, 3, 4, 5, 6, 7, 8, 9, 10, 11, 12

Anne Smith Sweeney
22 Dartmouth Road
Melrose, MA 02176
(617) 665-4343
Years in Geriatric Care Management: 6
Service Area
Metropolitan Area(s): Melrose & Surrounding Areas
Counties:
States: MA
Areas of Practice: 1, 2, 3, 5, 6, 7, 8, 9, 10, 11, 12

Joan Tobin
Elder Network
24 Sevinor Road
Marblehead, MA 01945
(617) 593-1040
[no information provided]

Andrea Weiler, MSW, CSW, ACSW
Private Geriatric Care Manager
7462 Armstrong Road
Manlius, NY 13104
(315) 637-5388

Years in Geriatric Care Management: 1

Service Area
Metropolitan Area(s):
Counties: Onondaga
States: NY
Areas of Practice: 1, 2, 3, 5, 6, 7, 8, 9, 10, 11, 12, PRI, Screen

Phyllis G. Wolk
Caring Connections
2620 Fenick Road
Cleveland, OH 44118
(216) 397-9347

Years in Geriatric Care Management: 3.5

Service Area
Metropolitan Area(s): Cleveland, Eastside Suburbs
Counties: Cuyahoga
States: OH
Areas of Practice: 1, 2, 3, 5, 6, 7, 8, 9, 10, 12

Elaine S. Yatzkan, CSW, PhD
262 Central Park West
New York, NY 10024
(212) 724-6330

Years in Geriatric Care Management: 15

Service Area
Metropolitan Area(s): New York, New Jersey
Counties: Lower Westchester
States: NY
Areas of Practice: 1, 2, 3, 4, 5, 7, 8, 9, 10, 11, 12

Glossary

This glossary is designed to explain the health and social services that may be or become available in the community. The glossary should be of use in discussions with the family, physician, case manager, and other service providers. In a community that does not have a needed service, individuals might want to get together with families, service providers, or physicians, to try to establish the service. Scanning this glossary will provide a better understanding of the wide range of services that are available, whether the client lives alone, with family or friends, or in a nursing home. Some people use several of these services together to remain active and healthy.

adult day care.   Social, recreational, and/or limited health care provided in a group setting during daytime hours. Some programs focus on health and personal care; others focus on social or recreational activities. Both types (and combinations) generally provide transportation and a noon meal, in addition to other services. The goal of adult day care is to keep the client as independent as possible and to provide a rest for the care partner. Services may include nursing; counseling; social services; rehabilitative services; medical and health care monitoring; exercise sessions; field trips; recreational activities; physical, occupational, and speech therapy; medication administration; well-balanced meals; and transportation to and from the center.

board and care facilities.   These facilities provide housing, supervision, and care, but do not offer skilled nursing or other medical services. Board and care facilities are not licensed to receive

385

reimbursement under Medicare and Medicaid programs. In some states, financial help may be obtained through a state supplement to Supplemental Security Income (SSI) when the client lives in a board and care facility.

case management. A systematic process of assessment, planning, service coordination and/or referral, monitoring, and reassessment, to help the client find and use the community services (such as health care) that are needed.

chore services. Services that help in the home and yard—putting storm windows up and taking screens down, minor home repairs, snow removal, lawn care, heavy house cleaning, and so on.

client counseling. For the purposes of this glossary, "client counseling" refers to short-term, problem-solving-oriented sessions between the client and the case manager.

companion services. A program to provide the client with regular company and a visitor, usually in the home.

congregate meals. Meal programs that serve healthful, inexpensive meals 1 to 5 days a week at a convenient location, and that provide a chance to visit with friends and join in activities.

counseling. Programs that help client and family to resolve emotional, interpersonal, or stress problems with the help of a trained therapist or social worker.

diagnosis related groups (DRGs). The payment system used by Medicare to reimburse hospital care for Medicare patients. The hospital receives a fixed amount of money (based on one chief diagnosis) to care for each patient.

emergency financial assistance or material aid. Money or goods from government agencies or private charities, provided as help during a time of crisis.

emergency shelter. Housing on a short-term basis, provided if the client needs emergency housing because of fire, theft, physical or mental abuse, or other situations beyond his or her control.

employment assistance. Employment services that help the client find work. If he or she is 55 or older and meets certain income requirements, the client can be trained and referred to job openings with local employers.

escort or transportation services.   Services that help the client get around if he or she can't do so alone. Services are often provided by volunteers. A volunteer might pick the client up at home to take him or her to a doctor's appointment, or spend an afternoon with the client running errands.

estate management.   A service through which the client's money and property are managed by someone else.

financial counseling.   Advice given to the client on basic financial management. The advice can affect the client and his or her property, particularly as it relates to maintaining the client's long-term financial independence and using his or her funds and assets.

foster care (adult).   The client's placement with a family, if living alone is no longer possible but when entering a nursing home is not necessary.

"friendly visitors" or reassurance programs.   Programs, which go by several different names, in which someone either visits or telephones the client regularly if he or she lives alone. A volunteer usually provides the service. Not only does the client have a friendship with the visitor or caller, but he or she can help spot problems the client may be experiencing and notify others who can offer help.

group home.   Residence with others, arranged for a client if he or she cannot live in his or her own home or a foster home, but a nursing home is not necessary. Some group homes offer psychological and social counseling in addition to general supervision, meals, and a home-like environment.

guardianship or conservatorship.   Designation of another person, the guardian or conservator is often an attorney or trust officer in a bank, to manage the client's legal and financial affairs, property, living arrangements, and medical decisions if the client is no longer able to do so.

health services—dental.   Programs that help the client keep teeth, gums, and dentures in good condition.

health services—medical.   Programs that provide the client with medical services, medications, and equipment.

health services—mental.   Programs to help the client improve his or her emotional well-being.

home-delivered meals. Hot, nutritious meals brought to the client's home 1 to 7 days a week if he or she cannot prepare meals alone.

home health aide services. Personal care services provided in-home (help with grooming, toileting, bathing, eating, walking, and so on).

home health care. Nursing, social work, and rehabilitation services given in the client's own home. Usually coordinated by one service provider, case management is often a key part of home care. Home health care is recognized as an increasingly important alternative to hospitalization and nursing-home care if the client does not need professional supervision 24 hours a day. The client may find it possible to remain home for the duration of an illness. Home care allows some people a way to shorten their hospital stay and, in many cases, can prevent or delay readmission to the hospital. A variety of health services are available through home health care programs. All services must be under the direction of a physician.

homemaker services. In-home help consisting of light housekeeping, meal preparation, grocery shopping, laundry, general shopping assistance, and some limited personal grooming and care.

hospice programs. Programs that help the client and significant others if the client is ill and dying. Some services—pain relief, symptom management, and supportive services—are provided in-home. The client is admitted to a hospital if his or her doctor deems it necessary.

housing placement. Help with locating a place to live, often in senior housing or retirement living communities.

ICF-I (Intermediate Care Facility-I). The federal certification level for long-term care beds in a facility for elderly persons who need licensed nursing services, supervision, and supportive services. The level of care in ICF-I is less intense than that required by persons in a skilled nursing facility (SNF), and more intense than care in ICF-II.

ICF-II (Intermediate Care Facility-II). Also called "board and care," "sheltered housing," and "domiciliary care." The federal certification level for long-term care beds in a facility for elderly persons who need room, board, and personal and daily maintenance care.

information and referral (I & R). Information and referral programs operated by many public and private agencies (such as local Area Agencies on Aging) to help the client and his or her family locate services in the community.

legal services.   Services providing advice and representation to the client in legal matters. A licensed attorney or trained paralegal can help the client with questions about health care, income tax, public benefits (social security, Medicare, Medicaid, SSI, food stamps), employment, consumer complaints, nursing-home resident rights, utilities, guardianship/conservatorship, wills, and estates.

Medicaid (Title XIX).   A federal–state program designed to pay for health care for some low-income individuals, including older persons who meet certain income and asset requirements set by the states. Medicaid pays for almost half of all nursing-home costs in the United States.

Medicare (Title XVIII).   The main federal funding source for paying for health care services rendered to people over age 65. *Part A* pays for inpatient hospital coverage. *Part B* pays for physician care and other related care costs.

nursing home placement.   Help with finding and entering a nursing home.

occupational therapy.   Treatment by a trained occupational therapist to help the client be as self-reliant as possible in activities of daily living, such as dressing, eating, grooming, and toileting.

physical therapy.   Treatment by a trained physical therapist, under the direction of a physician, to relieve pain and develop, maintain, or restore a client's ability to function. Treatment may include the use of exercise, heat, water, light, or massage, and is often prescribed for persons who have problems moving and walking.

preadmission screening (PAS).   A complete evaluation and assessment to determine whether the client needs to be in a nursing home or can stay at home with the help of family and friends and community services. More than half of the states in the United States have PAS programs, some of which also provide case management services.

psychotherapy.   Treatment of mental or emotional disorders by psychological means.

residential repair and renovation.   Programs that help the client keep his or her home in good repair and prevent major problems. For example, volunteers might come to the home and patch a leaky roof, repair faulty plumbing, insulate drafty walls, or repaint the house.

respite care.   Temporary care for the family member when a caregiver is taking care of a family member and needs a brief period of rest and relaxation. Respite care can be provided in-home, at the family's home, in a foster home, or in a nursing home, and may last for a few hours, a full day, a weekend, a week, or a month.

retirement planning.   Help in preparing for the financial, social, and personal aspects of retirement.

self-help/mutual aid support groups.   Person-to-person ways of helping a client and family to cope with stresses and illnesses. The client meets with others who are experiencing the same problems and exchanges emotional support and solutions. Common issues dealt with in support groups related to aging include: caregiver stress, coping with death and dying, adjustment to nursing-home placement or retirement, arthritis, cancer, poststroke adjustment, Alzheimer's disease, and many others.

senior center.   A place for the client to meet and socialize with other older persons. Most centers also provide health screening, information and referral services, or other services similar to those found in adult day care settings. Some senior centers serve as meal sites, transportation dispatch centers, information and referral offices, health screening clinics, recreational centers, social service agency branch offices, mental health counseling clinics, employment agencies for older workers, volunteer coordinating centers, and community meeting halls.

shared housing and home matching.   Living arrangement where two or more people share a house or apartment and keep their own private bedroom. In home-matching programs, potential home or apartment sharers are introduced to home or apartment seekers. Shared housing arrangements have three main benefits: (1) the financial advantage of splitting the rent, utilities, and other home expenses; (2) the sharing of homemaking jobs; and (3) the friendship of others. Arrangements for shared housing can be made by individuals or by a public or private agency (such as Lutheran Social Services Share-a-Home).

skilled nursing facility (SNF).   The most medically intensive of the three federal certification levels for long-term care beds (ICF-I, ICF-II, SNF). Generally, it includes rehabilitation, convalescent or rehabilitative services, and/or special treatments by licensed nurses (such as administration of medications and application of dressings).

speech therapy.   Help from a trained speech therapist for clients who have problems with written or spoken language or hearing.

telephone hotline.   Also called "24-hour hotline," "telephone reassurance." Telephone hotline programs offer regular telephone contact with people who ask how the client is doing and help the client overcome loneliness, if needed.

transportation services.   Help for clients in traveling from their homes to community services, health care providers, and other places in the community.

Index

393